Integrated Behaviora

MW01254617

Mary R. Talen • Aimee Burke Valeras
Editors

Integrated Behavioral Health in Primary Care

Evaluating the Evidence, Identifying the Essentials

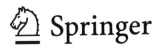 Springer

Editors
Mary R. Talen
Northwestern Family Medicine Residency
Erie Family Health Center
Chicago, IL, USA

Aimee Burke Valeras
NH Dartmouth Family Medicine Residency
Concord Hospital Family Health Center
Concord, NH, USA

ISBN 978-1-4614-6888-2 (hardcover)   ISBN 978-1-4614-6889-9 (eBook)
ISBN 978-1-4939-2909-2 (softcover)
DOI 10.1007/978-1-4614-6889-9
Springer New York Heidelberg Dordrecht London

Library of Congress Control Number: 2013936941

Springer is part of Springer Science+Business Media (www.springer.com)

To our families:
Thomas, Aaron, and Emily
Andy, Ayanna, and Alique

Foreword

The Landscape of Integrated Behavioral Health Care Initiatives

Five decades ago, orthodoxy reigned in the canons of medical science: medical breakthroughs, scientific discoveries, and lifesaving procedures were occurring at an ever-increasing pace, and new specialties and subspecialties were brought into existence to accommodate these new discoveries and incorporate them into clinical care. Medical progress was understood as inexorably linked to deeper and more narrowly focused biological and biochemical inquiry. Biomedicine reigned supreme. The generalist heart of the health care system was being hollowed out, disappearing, supplanted by an explicit priority for specialism and a burgeoning army of specialists and subspecialists.

A few observers noticed that this biomedical hyper-specialization, however conducive to discoveries at the molecular level, was also exacerbating the fragmentation in an already-fragmented health care system. Within such a system, clinicians were unable to make good use of these marvelous discoveries. Diseases were understood, but patients weren't getting healthier. This problem led to three developments: (1) a new, more comprehensive, and integrated model of medical science and health care, the biopsychosocial model; (2) a new appreciation of the shortfalls in health care; and (3) recommendations to redesign the health care system with a foundation of primary care, to better remedy these perceived shortfalls (vide the Millis, Willard, and Folsom Reports).

Family Medicine was born, and took off, together with General Internal Medicine and General Pediatrics, to heal this fragmentation and to lay in a foundation for our health care system that was personal, coordinated, and comprehensive. Behavioral health was baked into Family Medicine from the beginning, principally as a training requirement. But there were many problems with this initial rollout:

- First, there was little agreement on what was meant by integration, behavior, and other basic terms.
- Second, the research support was thin and inconsistent.

- Third, there were unanticipated difficulties with actually incorporating behavioral health care into primary care effectively. Local variations in the primary care settings, and the context in which they existed, made it difficult to arrive at general principles – implementation was maddeningly local.
- Fourth, there were plenty of behavioral clinicians around, but they hadn't worked in primary settings. Transition from one setting, culture, and paradigm was jarring.
- Fifth, there are costs associated with integration that were difficult or even impossible to cover, particularly in a fee-for-service, behavioral carve-out environment.
- Finally, purchasers, payers, and even patients had no experience with this kind of care, didn't realize its advantages, and as a result, weren't particularly motivated to advocate for it.

This is not how the world of integrated behavioral–primary care looks today. In fits and starts, there has been significant progress on many of these fronts. This kind of integrated care turns out to be a very good idea, with solid evidence (that can be found in the pages that follow) behind it. There have been beautiful conceptual formulations of how this kind of care can look, how behavioral and primary care clinicians can be trained to work together, and how clinics, payers, purchasers, and policymakers can respond to this opportunity and succeed.

The notion of integrated primary care has taken hold and looks like it is here to stay. But there are still problems aplenty. The very growth of interest in whole-person primary care itself creates problems. For the first time, it is becoming impossible to keep up with the literature – with the trials, demonstration projects, pilots, and innovations across the nation. We have not yet developed the means to learn from the experience of others. We still suffer from a crippling lack of agreement about our terms, criteria, prerequisites, and principles. We have not yet made a sufficiently compelling case for integration that disrupting the status quo seems worth it to those doing well today. We don't know how to design trials for these incredibly complex, multilevel transformations that will tell us whether we are making progress. So today, even though we can be heartened by the ever-widening support for and adoption of integrated forms of care, there remains resistance, confusion, and challenge in the field of integrated care.

Talen and Valeras, along with their distinguished authors, understand the state of the field, the problems and barriers we are facing, and what must be done next. They have aimed this book squarely at the problems in the field *today*. It is fitting that in a field that avers the primacy of integration and coherence, this book advances this field's coherence. To begin, the reader will find a rigorous and defensible shared lexicon, an early report on a beautiful pre-empirical research effort still under way that clears out one of the most consistent impediments to progress in science. Other authors have reviewed the scattered and inconsistent literature on clinical integration and pulled it into a useful, internally consistent framework – they have organized wildly variable evidence and data into a sensible, consistent matrix that is easy to read and use. Now we can see where we are! Now we can see what to do next, from the simple to the complex. And this is not only true for clinical or operational dimensions of collaboration, but also the policy, macro dimension, as well.

It will take good policy to sustain collaborative care, and this book points the way ahead for policymakers and funders.

Finally, this volume reminds us that collaboration goes beyond those in primary care and those in the behavioral sciences. We must collaborate with the patient, the patient's family, the patient's community, and others. Some of the principles are the same, and yet effective collaboration requires that we approach each of these partners humbly, carefully, and on their own terms and find a unique way to make that partnership work. This book equips the field with advice and warnings that make these extended collaborative partnerships more likely to succeed.

You have in your hands a book that fits its times, that meets the field right where it needs most. Read this and you will surely emerge more knowledgeable and better equipped to join the rising tide of patients, clinicians, practice leaders, educators, researchers, policymakers, carriers, and purchasers whose lives, health, and welfare are improved by collaborative care.

Frank V. deGruy
Susan H. McDaniel

Acknowledgments

We cannot find the right words to adequately acknowledge the important influences of a diverse group of colleagues who have shaped this book—some in unintentional, simple ways, and others who were the backbone for this project. We want to recognize those who have sustained this project from an idea to a completed manuscript. The idea for this book came serendipitously when I (Mary) visited Maine and met pioneering integrated behavioral health care providers through MeHAF (Maine Health Care Access Foundation). Laura Ronan, a consultant at MeHAF, and I sparked up a conversation where we shared a secret about feeling like we were in a swirl of confusion in this field. She propelled the initial goal of this project—to provide some order to the chaos—and helped set guidelines for evaluating behavioral health initiatives. Laura, who has the talent for drilling down to the details, wanted to decipher the passion and vision conversations from the evidence-based practice statements. With her love of charts, she helped organize the "data" and helped define the common components of integrated behavioral health initiatives. By chance, Bill Gunn introduced me to Aimee Valeras who was able to walk onto this ambitious project as a coeditor in November of 2011. She brought to this project her strong clinical experience, keen critical analysis, and editorial skills.

The third serendipitous event was meeting CJ Peek at the CFHA annual meeting in 2010 and learning more about his efforts to form a lexicon for the stakeholders in integrated behavioral health. Without his tenacious efforts to organize the community, we would still be floundering. CJ Peek has an unassuming, approachable style with an engineer's sensibilities in his work. He has the knack for communicating sophisticated, robust concepts as if you were talking at the kitchen table. He is an expert at turning dry academic writing into something that has a narrative flow. We have turned to CJ at every juncture and impasse and he generously gave his time, detailed suggestions, and thoughtful revisions. He would pose questions to help us and other authors better articulate our subject. Without the lexicon and parameters, this book project would not be.

The last serendipitous event was the willingness of our stellar roster of authors who joined this endeavor. We were continually surprised whenever we approached experts in the field with their level of interest, openness, and investment in writing on their topic. Our regular conference calls with our authors were mini-tutorials that helped us connect the dots between a host of projects and perspectives from diverse groups around the USA. These authors devoted more time than they initially anticipated and shaped the way that we think about the breadth and depth of behavioral health and all of its nuances of meaning and reiterations of practices. We are thankful for the opportunity to have worked with such a talented group.

Lastly, we want to acknowledge the support of our institutions. I (Mary) have had the luxury of working within several family medicine residency programs that provided the rich experiences and support for integration of behavioral health—in particular Lorraine Stephens, MD, at Bethesda Family Medicine in Cincinnati, Ohio; Yvonne Murphy, MD, at MacNeal Family Medicine, Chicago; and Deb Edberg, MD, Lee Francis, MD, David Buchanan, MD, and Anuj Shah, MD, at Northwestern University–Erie Family Health Center's Family Medicine programs. I also want to acknowledge a few colleagues who have influenced my professional development over the years—Timothy Horton, Ph.D., Michael Floyd, Ed.D., Julie Schirmer, LCSW, Ed Shahady, MD, Randy Longenecker, MD, Cheryl Levine, Psy.D., and Scott Fraser, Ph.D. I (Aimee) have received unwavering support from the New Hampshire Dartmouth Family Medicine Residency and Leadership Preventive Medicine Residency housed at Concord Hospital Family Health Centers, in particular, Joni Haley, MS; Bill Gunn, PhD; Dominic Geffken, MPH, MD; Doug Dreffer, MD; Marie Wawziniack, RN; and Dan Eubank, MD. Angela Phillips, LICSW, David Twyon, LICSW, Lori Pelletier-Baker, LICSW, and Jeannine Ouelette, LICSW, regularly implement some of the most groundbreaking practices of integrated behavioral health care, and I learned from them and laughed with them throughout this process.

As coeditors, we want to acknowledge our simpatico relationship. We easily shared responsibilities, talked about our new discoveries, and relished in making connections between the evidence-based practices and our own experiences. Email, texting, conference calls, and in-person meetings became a regular part of our daily communication routines. It is rare to have such a mutually admiring relationship. We are finding more and more ways that our lives overlap and professional interests merge. We may have another book in us.

Lastly, our families have been the backbone of support throughout the process of editing this book.

My (Aimee) husband, Andy, was steadfast in his support of me joining Mary in this project. He inquired genuinely about the content and process of each chapter because he sincerely wanted to learn as much as he possibly could about integrated care. On a regular basis, I get the unique opportunity to work alongside him and partner together to put theory and evidence into practice. Together, and through the process of engaging with this book, he has helped me hone my skills as a social worker with a true biopsychosocial approach and he has earned a reputation as a physician who sees the whole person. During the life of this book, my days were packed with joy and love and energy, as my wonderful son, Alique, joined our family and my caring daughter, Ayanna, became a big sister. My two toddlers were patient with me when this book stole my attention, and they gave me the best possible reason to "get the work done."

If it weren't for my (Mary) husband, Thomas Dozeman, telling me that I had a book in me that I had to get out, I never would have taken this on. He was like my marathon coach balancing the messages "you can do it" with "just do it." My children, siblings, and parents have given me the rich balance in life that fuels my passion for a family-focused foundation for wellness and behavioral health.

Contents

Contributing Authors

Andrea Auxier, PhD, is a licensed clinical psychologist focused on the operational and policy aspects of behavioral health integration into primary care in a medical home model. She holds a B.A. from Cornell University, an M.A. from New York University, and an M.A. and Ph.D. from the University of Massachusetts Boston. As a Senior Clinical Information Strategist for the Colorado Community Managed Care Network, Dr. Auxier is responsible for implementing a strategic approach to clinical and financial outcome data. She is also a clinical consultant for Management Solutions Consulting Group, Inc, providing operational site visits and technical assistance for federally qualified health centers throughout the country. She also remains active in teaching and research: she is a senior clinical instructor at the University of Colorado Denver, Department of Family Medicine, an adjunct faculty member at the University of Denver, an associate editor for the Journal of Translational Behavioral Medicine, and serves on the Executive Board of the Collaborative Care Research Network.

Macaran (Mac) A. Baird, MD, MS, is professor and head of the University of Minnesota Department of Family Medicine and Community Health. In addition, he is board of directors' chair for UCare Minnesota, the fourth largest Minnesota HMO. Baird began his medical career in 1978 as a rural family physician in Wabasha, Minnesota. He has held academic positions in Oklahoma, New York, and Rochester, Minnesota. In addition to being a family physician, he is a family therapist.

Baird served on the Robert Wood Johnson Depression in Primary Care National Advisory Council and co-chaired the Institute of Medicine (IOM) Report on Health and Behavior. He was a member of a national panel of experts invited to work with the Carter Center in Atlanta, Georgia, to encourage government and insurers efforts to integrate behavioral health and prevention services into primary care. His research foci are integration of behavioral medicine into primary care, population-based health, family therapy, and improving the care of patients with chronic illness.

For the past 5 years, Baird has worked with a multidisciplinary team to develop the Minnesota Complexity Assessment Method©, currently being tested in collaboration with a variety of practices in Minnesota.

Jamie Banker, PhD, MFT, is the Director of Counseling Psychology Masters program and Assistant Professor at California Lutheran University in Thousand Oaks California. She has a special interest in integrated care and has worked in three integrated primary care practices. Now her focus is on training Marriage and Family Therapy students to work in integrated care sites.

Banker's current research is on understanding postpartum depression and disorders of the endocrine system for a biopsychosocial model.

John Bartlett, MD, MPH, is the senior adviser for the Carter Center's Mental Health Program activities. His focus is leading and coordinating the activities of the Mental Health Program's Primary Care Initiative, which is intended to identify policy levers to improve the coordination and cooperation between the mental health and substance abuse treatment sectors and primary care. Dr. Bartlett is a psychiatrist and former physician executive who specializes in quality and accountability issues for mental health, substance abuse, and chronic health care. Prior to working at The Carter Center, he was a principal partner at The Avisa Group, a policy, research, and consulting firm that specializes in behavioral health care. Dr. Bartlett also has served as the senior medical director and senior vice president for CIGNA Behavioral Health and as the executive vice president for clinical strategy for Charter/Magellan Health Services. He received his medical training at Yale University and completed his psychiatric residency at the UCLA School of Medicine, where, following his residency, he was a Robert Wood Johnson Clinical Scholar.

Joane G. Baumer, MD, is an active clinical practitioner that oversees the largest family medicine residency training program in the country and the JPS Physician Re-entry Program. She is an associate clinical professor at UTSW School of Medicine at Dallas. She serves on legislative committees with the State of Texas, the Board of the Society of Teachers of Family Medicine, Commission on Education of the AAFP, and the Steering Committee of the Forum on Behavioral Health. She has authored numerous presentations and publications on educational topics for clinicians.

Jerica M. Berge, PhD, MPH, LMFT, CFLE, is an assistant professor and behavioral health provider in the Department of Family Medicine and Community Health at the University of Minnesota's Medical School. Her research and clinical expertise focuses on using integrated health care models and community-based participatory research methods to create partnerships between health care providers, mental health clinicians, and families to address child health issues such as childhood obesity.

Larry A. Cesare, Psy.D., is a Clinical Health Psychologist who has served as an executive, clinician, professor, and consultant in the behavioral health field for over 30 years. With extensive experience in developing innovative care delivery systems, in integrating medical and behavioral services, and in optimizing health care operations via metrics-based performance improvement methods, evidence-based practices, and outcomes evaluation, he has played lead roles in (a) private sector managed care and insurance corporations providing at-risk health care services and

(b) not-for-profit organizations and delivery systems providing behavioral, medical, support, and housing services for Medicare, Medicaid, and other underserved populations. Dr. Cesare has been in direct service and executive roles within community behavioral health and social service organizations and has held positions as Vice President of Behavioral Health at Health Care Service Corporation in Richardson, Texas, Regional Quality Director for Magellan Behavioral Health in Columbia, Maryland, and Assistant Professor in the School of Professional Psychology at Wright State University in Dayton, Ohio.

William J. Doherty, PhD, LMFT, LP, is a Professor at the University of Minnesota (UMN) in the Department of Family Social Science and the Director of the UMN's Citizen Professional Center. His investigative interests center on creating and advancing community organizing approaches to working with families and promoting cultural change, and target a broad range of important social and medical content areas, including engaged and responsible fatherhood, overscheduled families, diabetes/obesity, and teen pregnancy.

James M. Fauth, PhD, received his doctorate in counseling psychology from the Pennsylvania State University in 2000. After graduation, he became an assistant professor in the Counseling and School Psychology program at the University at Buffalo. His initial clinical and research interests focused on psychotherapy process and training research, and he continues to publish and serve on several editorial boards (e.g., Journal of Counseling Psychology) in this area. Since coming to Antioch University New England (AUNE) in 2002 to direct the Center for Research on Psychological Practice, his scholarship has increasingly focused on the collaborative/integrated health care, participatory methods of evaluation and quality improvement in naturalistic settings, and the promotion of health and wellness in community settings.

Jennifer S. Funderburk, PhD, is a Clinical Research Psychologist for the Veteran's Administration Center for Integrated Health Care located at the Syracuse VA Medical Center. She is also an adjunct assistant professor at Syracuse University's Department of Psychology and an adjunct senior instructor at the University of Rochester's Department of Psychiatry. She has been either serving as a clinician or conducting research on integrated health care for the past 10 years. Her research interests focus on the implementation of integrated health care and the types of brief interventions providers can use within the primary care setting, especially those interventions targeting depression, alcohol misuse, and insomnia.

William B. Gunn, PhD, is a faculty member of the NH Dartmouth Family Medicine Residency in Concord, NH, and holds a clinical appointment at Dartmouth Medical School. He is a board member of the Collaborative Family Health Care Association. Bill is a co-author of *Models of Collaboration* (2006) and *The Collaborative Psychotherapist* (2009). He coordinates an integrated care "learning community" in New Hampshire, which meets regularly. He is co-chair with Nancy Ruddy of the Division 38 primary care subcommittee.

Tricia Hern, MD, is the Associate Program Director of the Community Health Network Family Medicine Residency Program and serves as the Medical Director of their Family Medicine Center. Dr. Hern attended Northwestern University Medical School, completed her residency at University of North Carolina in Chapel Hill, and was a Primary Care Faculty Development Fellow at Michigan State University. Dr. Hern's areas of interest include curricular redesign and innovation in residency training, Patient-Centered Medical Home transformation, and building and leading health care teams.

Jennifer Hodgson, PhD, LMFT, is a Professor in the Department of Child Development and Family Relations and has reappointed time in the Department of Family Medicine at East Carolina University. She received her doctoral degree from Iowa State University, specializing in marriage and family therapy, and completed a fellowship in medical family therapy at the University of Rochester, New York. She co-authored the nation's first doctoral program in medical family therapy. She is a clinical member of AAMFT, an AAMFT Approved Supervisor, Chair of the Commission on Accreditation for Marriage and Family Therapy Education, Chair of the NC Marriage and Family Licensure Board, and long time member and immediate past president of the Collaborative Family Health Care Association.

Christopher L. Hunter, PhD, ABPP, did his graduate work at the University of Memphis specializing in behavioral medicine. He is board certified in clinical health psychology and works for TRICARE Management Activity as the Department of Defense Program Manager for Behavioral Health in Primary Care. He has extensive experience as a staff member in Air Force and Navy psychology internships where he trained interns to work as behavioral health consultants in primary care. Dr. Hunter also has extensive experience working in outpatient behavioral health clinics and primary care settings treating common mental health conditions (e.g., depression) as well as tobacco dependence, obesity, sleep problems, and working with individuals who have chronic medical conditions like diabetes and chronic pain. In 2002 he received the Arthur W. Melton Early Career Achievement Award from Division 19 (Military Psychology) of the American Psychological Association for his work on integrated behavioral health in primary care service and training. He has published several research articles and book chapters and is the lead author on the book *Integrated Behavioral Health in Primary Care: Step-by-Step Guidance for Assessment and Interventions.*

Bethany M. Kwan, PhD, MSPH, is a senior instructor in the Department of Family Medicine at the University of Colorado Denver. She received her PhD in social health psychology from the University of Colorado at Boulder in 2010, where she studied physical activity promotion and depression. She currently works for a practice-based research network of safety net health care organizations, which conducts health services research in the domains of patient-centered medical home and collaborative care for patients with chronic disease.

Misty M. Mann, Psy.D., received her doctorate degree in clinical psychology (Psy.D.) from the Illinois School of Professional Psychology at Argosy University,

Chicago. She completed her pre-doctoral internship at MacNeal Hospital Family Medicine Residency program, and it was here she was introduced to collaborative care and primary care psychology. Currently, she is an Associate Director of Training at the Chicago School of Clinical Psychology where she assists clinical psychology graduate students in matters related to their clinical training. Additionally, she teaches graduate level courses which include group theory, seminar, and a research clerkship focused on primary care and health promotion programs.

Danna Mauch, PhD, is principal scientist/associate at ABT Associates Inc., a company that applies scientific research, consulting, and technical assistance expertise to a wide range of issues in social, economic, and health policy; international development; clinical trials; and registries. The focus of her work has been on integration of systems of care, financing, and management information to support clinical decisions and quality improvements toward excellent outcomes for children and adults with special health care needs. Dr. Mauch was a member of the SAMHSA National Advisory Council, the White House Conference, and the Surgeon General's Task Force on Mental Health. She is past board president and current vice president for clinical and educational outreach of the Massachusetts Association for Mental Health and a founding board member and committee chair of the MetroWest Community Health Care Foundation. She studied for her B.A. degree at Connecticut College and Wesleyan University and received her Ph.D. from Brandeis University.

Tai J. Mendenhall, PhD, LMFT, CFT, is an Assistant Professor at the University of Minnesota (UMN) in the Department of Family Social Science, the Associate Director of the UMN's Citizen Professional Center, and the co-Director of mental health teams within the UMN's Academic Health Center/Office of Emergency Response's Medical Reserve Corps (MRC). His investigative interests center on the use and application of community-based participatory research (CBPR) methods to target chronic illnesses in minority- and under-served patient and family populations.

Benjamin F. Miller, Psy.D., is an Assistant Professor in the Department of Family Medicine at the University of Colorado Denver School of Medicine where he is the Director of the Office of Integrated Health Care Research and Policy. He is a co-principal investigator and co-creator of the National Research Network's Collaborative Care Research Network and has been the principal investigator on several federal grants examining mental health and primary care integration.

Daniel J. Mullin, PsyD, is an Assistant Professor in the Center for Integrated Primary Care and the Department of Family Medicine and Community Health at the University of Massachusetts Medical School. He a clinician, educator, researcher, and consultant specializing in the integration of behavioral health and primary care services. Dr. Mullin completed his doctorate at Spalding University in Louisville, Kentucky, his internship in Primary Care Psychology in the Department of Family Medicine at the University of Colorado Health Sciences Center, and his fellowship in Primary Care Family Psychology in the Departments of Medicine, Psychiatry, and Family Medicine at the University of Rochester School of Medicine and Dentistry. He is also a member of the Motivational Interviewing Network of Trainers and conducts research, teaches, and provides consultation related to Motivational Interviewing in health care settings.

Donald E. Nease Jr., MD, is the Associate Vice Chair for Research in the Department of Family Medicine at the University of Colorado—Denver, School of Medicine. He also serves as the Director of Practice Based Network Research at the Colorado Health Outcomes Program at CU Denver. Dr. Nease completed his Family Medicine residency at the Medical University of South Carolina in Charleston following medical school at the University of Kansas. Dr. Nease has pursued extensive research on effective recognition and care for mental health problems in primary care and is also a leader in patient and relationship centered care through work with the American Balint Society and the International Balint Federation.

Kavita K. Patel, MD, MSHS, is a fellow in the Economic Studies program and managing director for clinical transformation and delivery at the Engelberg Center for Health Care Reform. Dr. Patel is also a practicing primary care internist at Johns Hopkins Medicine and served in the Obama administration as director of policy for the Office of Intergovernmental Affairs and Public Engagement in the White House. She received her medical degree from the University of Texas Health Science Center.

C.J. Peek, PhD, is an Associate Professor with the Department of Family Medicine and Community Health at the University of Minnesota Medical School, where he focuses on care system development, integration of behavioral and medical care, organizational effectiveness, and leadership development. He has facilitated multiple stakeholder dialogue in state and national meetings on the integration of behavioral and medical care, implementation of patient-centered medical home, and addressing behavioral risk factors in primary care. As a clinician in the mid-eighties, he helped integrate behavioral and medical care in a large system and has co-authored a book, book chapters, and articles on the integration of mental health and medical care, presenting regularly on these and other topics. He has worked on state and national projects to develop workable lexicons and conceptual systems for emerging health care subfields, such as integrated behavioral health care, palliative care, shared decision-making, and patient-centered medical home, and has applied these to the creation of research agendas. Dr. Peek speaks, writes, and consults on a practical blend of clinical, organizational, communication, and leadership topics. He earned a PhD in clinical psychology from the University of Colorado in 1976, where he studied with Dr. Peter G. Ossorio, founder of the discipline of Descriptive Psychology.

Genevieve Riebe, MD, attended medical school at the University of Washington and is currently a Family Medicine resident at the University of Arizona. She plans on working with underserved populations and continuing research in primary care.

Randall Reitz, PhD, LMFT, is the Director of Behavioral Sciences at the St Mary's Family Medicine Residency in Grand Junction, Colorado. He is also the Director of Social Media with the Collaborative Family Health Care Association. His research interests include collaborative care policy, collaboration with health information technology, and multiple role relationships in health care training settings.

John Rogers, MD, MPH, MEd, While President of the Society of Teachers of Family Medicine for 2007–2008, Dr. Rogers wrote a series of seven President's columns on the patient-centered medical home (PCMH) for Family Medicine as well as an invited editorial on the PCMH for the Journal of the American Board of Family Medicine. He was a guest co-editor for a special issue on the patient-centered medical home for *Families, Systems, & Health*, Vol 28(4), Dec 2010, and a dedicated issue on education and the PCMH for *Family Medicine*, Vol 43(10), November-December 2011. Dr. Rogers has been invited to speak on the medical home in eight US states, Canada, and China.

Mary R. Talen, PhD, is a licensed psychologist and the Director of Behavioral Health Primary Care at Northwestern University's Family Medicine Residency Program, Chicago, IL. She graduated with her masters and doctoral degree from Columbia University in New York City and she is certified in Family Therapy from Philadelphia Child Guidance Center. Dr. Talen has focused her research, teaching, and clinical practice in systems-based health care. She has taught family medicine residents, medical students, family nurse practitioners, and doctoral clinical psychology interns in behavioral health and multiprofessional health care. She has published and presented at national and international conferences in primary care psychology and integrative behavioral health. Her current research projects are in physician wellness, patient engagement, complexity care, and collaborative team practice.

George C. Tremblay, PhD, received his doctorate in clinical psychology from the University at Albany (SUNY) in 1996, following a pre-doctoral internship at the University of Mississippi and Veterans Affairs Medical Centers in Jackson, Mississippi. His early clinical and research interests focused on high conflict families and child maltreatment. Since then, he has become increasingly interested in promoting and evaluating community health and improving quality of care and access to health services.

Aimee Burke Valeras, PhD, LICSW, works with the NH Dartmouth Family Medicine Residency and the Leadership Preventive Medicine Residency and in the Behavioral Health Department at Concord Hospital Family Health Center. She received her undergraduate and Masters of Social Work degrees from Boston College and her Doctorate in Social Work from Arizona State University. Dr. Burke Valeras has presented nationally and internationally on the topics of integrating behavioral health and primary care, disability and illness identity, and qualitative research methodology.

Andrew Valeras, DO, MPH, is a faculty member of NH Dartmouth Family Medicine Residency. He received his undergraduate degree from Boston College, his Doctor of Osteopathy from Midwestern University, and training at NH Dartmouth Family Medicine Residency. Also a graduate of the Dartmouth Hitchcock Leadership Preventive Medicine Residency, Dr. Valeras currently seeks to integrate quality improvement and systems based thinking with the clinical practice and education of family medicine providers.

Part I
Essentials of Integrated
Behavioral Health Care

Chapter 1
Introduction and Overview of Integrated Behavioral Health in Primary Care

Mary R. Talen and Aimee Burke Valeras

Abstract The future vision for our health care system recognizes the importance of holistic patient care that stands firmly on a biopsychosocial foundation of prevention and primary care. Yet, weaving together the complex factors of biomedical and psychosocial systems, which have been long divided, is a perplexing and challenging enterprise. Even when policy makers, health care administrators, and clinicians have embraced the vision for wholistic health care, they often flounder in a web of diverse cultures, different languages, competing values, opposing structures, and conflicting resources. The purpose of this book is to organize the immense amount of information in this field, to provide a systematic analysis of the contributions and challenges of integrated care initiatives, and to develop a consumer's report for stakeholders on the foundational components of integrated behavioral health in primary care.

Introduction and Overview

Health care reform is on the lips of our national dialogue. State and local communities are struggling to design organizational systems for health care reform while securing funding and resources for evidence-based clinical practices. There are multiple stakeholders with competing agendas in health care debates; among them are the advocates, providers, and policy makers who are committed to weaving together our long divorced biomedical and psychosocial systems of care. There are a

M.R. Talen, Ph.D. (✉)
Northwestern Family Medicine Residency, Erie Family Health Center,
2570 W. North Ave. Chicago, IL 60647, USA
e-mail: mary.talen@gmail.com

A.B. Valeras, Ph.D., MSW
NH Dartmouth Family Medicine Residency, Concord Hospital Family Health Center,
250 Pleasant St., 03301, Concord, NH, USA
e-mail: aimeevaleras@gmail.com

M.R. Talen and A. Burke Valeras (eds.), *Integrated Behavioral Health in Primary Care:*
Evaluating the Evidence, Identifying the Essentials, DOI 10.1007/978-1-4614-6889-9_1,
© Springer Science+Business Media New York 2013

growing number of vested individuals and teams that are championing the development and dissemination of information about the merits of integrated behavioral health care models, as evidenced by the proliferation of books and articles on integrated and collaborative health care that have mushroomed in the past decade. This explosion of literature, however, has resulted in a cacophony of voices with an array of uniquely designed collaborative approaches to integrated care. We have been inundated with interesting and innovative pilot studies but few unifying themes, cohesive evidence-based factors, or sustainable organizational policies for implementing systems-based integrated behavioral health care initiatives. Consequently, as a community of providers with a shared biopsychosocial mission, we are struggling to find our grounding and a unified language to advance our vision of health care reform. We are limited by our local "dialects" with no overarching concepts or objective templates to evaluate the benefits and limitations of our various models.

The vision for tomorrow's health care system includes strengthening primary care using the Institute of Medicine's principles of safety, timeliness, efficiency, efficacy and patient-centeredness. This future vision recognizes the importance of holistic patient care that stands firmly on a biopsychosocial foundation of prevention and primary care. Yet, weaving together the complex factors of biomedical and psychosocial systems, which have been long divided, is a perplexing and challenging enterprise. Even when policy makers, health care administrators, and clinicians have embraced the vision for integrated health care, they often flounder in a web of diverse cultures, different languages, competing values, opposing structures, and conflicting resources (Peek, 2011). These all add layers of complexity and confusion in the advancement towards a new approach to health care.

Integrated behavioral health care principles can be traced to Dr. Engel's biopsychosocial model outlined in the 1960s, which has been used as a guiding conceptual model for the emerging fields of family medicine, family therapy, and integrated health care. Research and clinical practices using the biopsychosocial framework have emerged in health psychology, social work, alternative and complimentary medicine, and primary care (Doherty, McDaniel, & Baird, 1996; McDaniel, Campbell, & Seaburn, 1991). Some of the seminal work in the 1980s focused on the epidemiology of mental health needs of patients seen in primary care practices. Identifying the prevalence of the problem set the stage for research, such as PRIME-MED to develop reliable and valid ways to identify patients with mental health symptoms in primary care settings (Brody et al., 1998; Spitzer et al., 1994). Out of this empirical base, researchers and providers focused on treatments for targeted patient populations using mental health diagnostic criteria. Depression screening and treatment using the chronic disease model over the past decade has become the most prominent and public practice model that demonstrates the effectiveness of integrated behavioral health care (Von Korff, Gruman, Schaefer, Curry, & Wagner, 1997; Wagner, 1997). Other types of research, such as substance abuse screening and treatment (e.g., SBIRT) or counseling for smoking cessation (e.g., 5 As), have also gained traction for integrated behavioral health care within medical settings and have contributed more empirical support for integrated care (Addo, Maiden, & Ehrenthal, 2011; Babor et al., 2007; Bodenheimer, Wagner, & Grumbach, 2002).

More recently, the Four Quadrant Model has emerged as a robust conceptual model for describing integrated behavioral health care initiatives. Community mental health centers and the Department of Defense and the VA have used the Four Quadrant Model to develop a variety of integrated care initiatives. Championed by the National Council and SAMSA, the Four Quadrant Model offers a wide spectrum for depicting a continuum of care between mental health and primary care services. However, this is not an evidence-based approach that validates the effectiveness or efficacy of integrated behavioral health care practices. Currently, the focus of integrated behavioral health care is shifting from more traditional schemes of diagnosing mental health in primary care to the role of behavioral health in enhancing protective factors in patient functioning, promoting healthy behaviors, or preventing poor coping tendencies. The conversations about integrated behavioral health care have expanded from primarily mental health to a host of behavioral health approaches such as motivational interviewing, health behavior coaching, team-based care, group visits, self-management, health literacy, and patient activation strategies for "whoever comes to see a doctor." These developments may be forging our future pathway in integrated care and will need a systematic and organized foundation for evaluating this direction.

Before we spawn more innovative integrated care initiatives, we need to take stock of our collective efforts and build our community of collaborators, organize our research and evaluation systematically, and incorporate lessons learned and essential components into our future endeavors.

As providers and educators intimately involved in a variety of integrated behavioral health care initiatives, we have been struck by how often we would randomly hear about another locally grown integrated behavioral health project or about another organization or foundation with a stake hold in integrated behavioral health care agendas. Like looking at scattered puzzle pieces, we had difficulty fitting the pieces together into a meaningful whole or a site map of the territory. The variability between the plethora of integrated behavioral health care efforts has resulted in confusion and chaos that make it difficult to identify core concepts, themes, and elements in defining success or evaluating the essential components of an initiative. There are many stakeholders from providers to policy makers engaged in the development and dissemination of information about the merits of integrated health care models, but there are few organizing principles with which to systematically evaluate the benefits and limitations. The purpose of this book, therefore, has been to help organize the immense amount of information, to provide a systematic analysis of the contributions and challenges of these diverse approaches, and to develop a consumer's report for stakeholders on the foundational components of integrated behavioral health care.

In Part I, we provide an overview of integrated behavioral health care from a bird's eye view. CJ Peek sets the stage by presenting a unifying language and primary parameters of integrated behavioral health care efforts. The call of the Agency for Healthcare Research and Quality (AHRQ) for integrated behavioral health care proponents to organize and synthesize our work has been established to help give our voice a similar tone and more volume within the larger health care discussion.

Dr. Peek has led this process by organizing a community of key stakeholders to begin defining a lexicon or a common language and core components of integrated behavioral health care, similar to what has been done in other scientific communities. The lexicon and its companion template of parameters provide the unifying theme and focus of each chapter. Our hope is that applying this language and the parameters throughout the book will create a familiarity with these organizing categories and increase our ability to define and describe our local initiatives and coordinate our efforts for a larger network of integrated behavioral health care providers. This lexicon also provides the template to summarize the evidence from different projects and compare essential elements from these different initiatives. In this introductory section, we also set the stage of integrated behavioral health care within the larger Patient Centered Medical Home movement. Andrea Auxier, Ben Miller, and John Rogers have given a historical context for understanding how integrated behavioral health care fits into the larger agenda for health care reform and the credentialing and accountability processes for organizations invested in PCMH. They identify where integrated behavioral health care is part of the PCMH reform and where it lacks potency. Ben Miller, Mary Talen, and Kavita Patel review the larger national policy debates and outline key policy issues that have a significant impact on integration efforts.

In Part II, we focus on a mid-level perspective of health care systems. In this section, the authors address the organizational dynamics and dilemmas in implementing integrated behavioral health care. Bethany Kwan and Don Nease provide a rich analysis of the research efforts and evidence for integrated care. In this chapter, Drs. Kwan and Nease have taken on the challenging task of organizing our empirical base, describing where there is evidence (or lack of evidence) to support integrated behavioral health care and more importantly, describing the future research direction and agenda for integrated behavioral health care investigators. The following chapter is written by a team of providers and researchers who have focused on the macro community lens of integrated behavioral health care. This section offers a unique picture on how integrated behavioral health care extends to community partnerships and the importance of sustainable committed relationships between providers and neighbors to truly build culturally engaged community-based health care. Tai Mendenhall, Jerica Burke, William Doherty, James Fauth, and George Tremblay present the evidence and innovation for community-based collaborative care research. Chris Hunter describes the closed health care system model that has emerged within the Department of Defense and Veteran's Administration, which provides a wealth of both organizational guideposts and cautionary comments even when there is a unifying culture and single-payer approach. Danna Mauch and John Bartlett unravel the complexities of how some states have approached merging Federally Qualified Health Centers and State or locally funded Community Mental Health Systems. Drs. Mauch and Bartlett tackle the murky and unwieldy process of integrating cultures of care with diverse missions, clinical approaches, and structures. Jennifer Hodgson and Randall Reitz offer an overview of the shifting sands of funding streams for integrated behavioral health care and describe the historical funding sources in states that have found some success in sustaining integrated behavioral health care.

The third section zeros in on the clinical practices in integrated behavioral health care efforts. The lead chapter on team partnerships is meant to put front and center the essential components of relationship-centered care and teamwork in integrated behavioral health care practices. Without this base of coordinated teamwork, integrated behavioral health care resembles a parallel referral practice model. Tricia Hern, Aimee Valeras, Jamie Banker, and Genevieve Riebe use the integrated care parameters to interview functioning multi-disciplinary collaborating teams from diverse clinical settings to distill the core ingredients of team-based care. These authors define the roles, communication patterns and challenges of relationship dynamics to the sustainability of integrated care. The other clinically focused chapters—screening and identification, evidence-based clinical interventions, and complexity care—have organized direct clinical services within the five core parameters and lexicon of integrated behavioral health care. These chapters build on a stepped care perspective on integration—starting with routine standard care approaches to multi-dimensional complex strategies of patient care. Mary Talen and Aimee Valeras describe how to identify patient populations that would benefit from integrated behavioral health in primary care. Mary Talen, Joanne Baumer, and Misty M. Mann describe valid screening tools, but more importantly how screening tools need to be embedded within a population-focused system of care. Dan Mullin and Jen Funderburk focus on the evidence behind direct clinical interventions with a focus on the expertise of the health care team members and population-based approaches to practice management and quality improvement. The complexity care chapter describes integrated approaches to providing health care to complex patient populations, while building on all of the key parameters—team-based care, patient identification, clinical protocol development, and a review process for monitoring patient's health. Collaborators from Minnesota, Mac Baird and CJ Peek and colleagues in New Hampshire—William Gunn and Andrew Valeras, describe the process of managing patients through a complexity lens, embracing the biomedical and psychosocial worlds.

In the concluding section, Part V, we connect the information in the preceding sections to provide a coherent synopsis of the common themes and practices from the macro, mezzo and micro levels of care that foster successful integration of the medical and psychosocial systems. This last section ties together the lessons learned from the wealth of integrated care initiatives. We review the "take home" points from the organizational, clinical care systems, and partnership elements of integrated behavioral health care. Through this critique, we identify the unintended consequences of these initiatives and describe some of the rate-limiting obstacles of these projects and programs that have stifled or squashed the efforts of well intended and committed stakeholders. Planners, administrators, researchers, and clinicians employed by private and public behavioral (mental health and substance abuse) and primary health care organizations, as well as training programs for health care professionals, advocacy groups, foundation personnel and government agencies, stand to benefit from the collection of information gleaned from this skilled and expert group of authors. Overall, this book holds the potential to build resiliency in the integrated behavioral health care movement. Our goal is for integrated behavioral health care enthusiasts to be on message and align the vision and mission of important, evidence-based initiatives from multiple regions. Through this analysis, we hope to solidify the foundation and future directions for stakeholders, providers, and collaborators as integrated behavioral health care takes shape.

References

Addo, S. F., Maiden, K., & Ehrenthal, D. B. (2011). Awareness of the 5 A's and motivational interviewing among community primary care providers. *Delaware Medical Journal, 83*(1), 17–21.

Babor, T. F., McRee, B. G., Kassebaum, P. A., Grimaldi, P. L., Ahmed, K., & Bray, J. (2007). Screening, Brief Intervention, and Referral to Treatment (SBIRT): Toward a public health approach to the management of substance abuse. *Substance Abuse, 28*(3), 7–30. doi:10.1300/J465v28n03_03.

Bodenheimer, T., Wagner, E. H., & Grumbach, K. (2002). Improving primary care for patients with chronic illness: the chronic care model, Part 2. *Journal of the American Medical Association, 288*(15), 1909–1914.

Brody, D. S., Hahn, S. R., Spitzer, R. L., Kroenke, K., Linzer, M., deGruy, F. V., 3rd, et al. (1998). Identifying patients with depression in the primary care setting: a more efficient method. *Archives of Internal Medicine, 158*(22), 2469–2475.

Doherty, W. J., McDaniel, S. H., & Baird, M. A. (1996). Five levels of primary care/behavioral healthcare collaboration. *Behavioral Healthcare Tomorrow, 5*(5), 25–27.

McDaniel, S. H., Campbell, T., & Seaburn, D. (1991). Treating somatic fixation: A biopsychosocial approach: When patients express emotions with physical symptoms. *Canadian Family Physician, 37*, 451–456.

Peek, C. J. (2011). A collaborative care lexicon for asking practice and research development questions. One of three papers in: a national agenda for research in collaborative care: papers from the collaborative care research network research development conference. Agency for healthcare research and quality, Rockville MD. http://www.ahrq.gov/research/collaborativecare/.

Spitzer, R. L., Williams, J. B., Kroenke, K., Linzer, M., deGruy, F. V., 3rd, Hahn, S. R., et al. (1994). Utility of a new procedure for diagnosing mental disorders in primary care. The PRIME-MD 1000 study. *Journal of the American Medical Association, 272*(22), 1749–1756.

Von Korff, M., Gruman, J., Schaefer, J., Curry, S. J., & Wagner, E. H. (1997). Collaborative management of chronic illness. *Annals of Internal Medicine, 127*(12), 1097–1102.

Wagner, E. H. (1997). Managed care and chronic illness: health services research needs. *Health Services Research, 32*(5), 702–714.

Chapter 2
Integrated Behavioral Health and Primary Care: A Common Language

C.J. Peek

Abstract The field of integrated behavioral health has been around for decades, but until recently in the hands of pioneers in their own particular settings, using their own distinctive language and concepts. That work was generally successful and gathered around it considerable energy in this era of patient-centered medical home and primary care transformation. Mainstream application requires the field to coalesce enough in language and concept to be consistently understood by implementers, health systems, researchers, policymakers, purchasers—and of course patients themselves. Unifying a field with consistently understood concepts and definitions is a normal stage in the development of emerging fields. Inconsistently understood concepts and definitions—including what constitutes the essential functions of integrated behavioral health—have been a practical concern and source of confusion in the field. Even authors writing about different topics in the same book have encountered such ambiguities and confusions. The response to this practical problem was to employ published methods from the field of Descriptive Psychology to create a consensus lexicon or operational definition for behavioral health integrated in primary care. This work sponsored by the Agency for Healthcare Research and Quality—on behalf of the field—resulted in a lexicon described here and employed by chapter authors to move toward using consistently understood terms and functional descriptions of integrated behavioral health.

Most contents adapted from Peek (2011) and Peek and National Integration Academy Council (2013). These are projects and publications sponsored by the Agency for Healthcare Research and Quality (AHRQ).

C.J. Peek, Ph.D. (✉)
Department of Family Medicine and Community Health, University of Minnesota
Medical School, 6-240 Phillips-Wangensteen Building, MMC 381, 420 Delaware Street SE,
Minneapolis, MN 55455, USA
e-mail: cjpeek@unm.edu

M.R. Talen and A. Burke Valeras (eds.), *Integrated Behavioral Health in Primary Care:*
Evaluating the Evidence, Identifying the Essentials, DOI 10.1007/978-1-4614-6889-9_2,
© Springer Science+Business Media New York 2013

Introduction: "Why Should I Read a Lexicon?"

The purpose of this book is to provide a detailed snapshot of the state of integrated behavioral health initiatives (also known as collaborative care) and a "consumer's report" for stakeholders on the evidence and foundations and essential ingredients of integrated behavioral health. While the mission and vision for integrating physical and behavioral health propel the field forward, this book provides a critical analysis of risks, resources, and challenges of different models.

The field has evolved from a few isolated initiatives to many approaches spearheaded by diverse groups of professionals and organizations. The availability of descriptive information on the various models has not kept pace with the growth of this field, and few resources exist that compare and contrast integrated care models. The book is meant to provide a comprehensive digest for stakeholders who are new to these initiatives and a resource for those planners, administrators, researchers, and clinicians that are already invested.

This chapter aims to provide an overarching definitional template language for clinician implementers, patients, health care system administrators, researchers, and policymakers—a common language that chapter authors could use to describe and assess strengths and weaknesses of various integrated behavioral health models. Note the various phrases in the preceding paragraphs—*foundational components... essential ingredients...compare and contrast models*. These reveal an ambitious goal of making it possible for a broad range of audiences to orient themselves and navigate this emerging field by creating a framework of both its defining functions and its many legitimate variations.

But having a common definitional framework is a recent development. The field of integrated behavioral health has often not been clear about what is foundational, or even the meanings of commonly used terms. This chapter offers a standard language to discuss the essential elements of integrated care, the different forms it may take, and common definitions for the many terms used to describe its basics. Identifying the need to clarify concepts in use within the subject matter is a normal developmental stage of emerging fields (Miller, Kessler, Peek, & Kallenberg, 2011; Peek, 2011).

The rest of this chapter (1) tells the story of the practical need for development of this lexicon; (2) describes the method for reaching a consensus lexicon or operational definition of behavioral health integrated in primary care; (3) outlines the resulting lexicon; and (4) describes current and potential applications for such a lexicon.

The Story: The Practical Need for a Lexicon in Integrated Behavioral Health

This section is adapted, paraphrased, or quoted from similar sections in Peek (2011).

The Field Requires More Consistent Language Today Than in Earlier Times

Exploding interest in the concepts of "patient-centered medical home" (PCMH), "health care home," or "advanced primary care" (all synonyms) have brought increased attention to the 40 year-old subfield of improved integration of behavioral health and medical care. The field of integrated behavioral health at this stage of development is aiming for implementation on a meaningful scale, not just in pockets created by pioneers. But the subject matter called "integrated behavioral health and medical care" also goes by "collaborative care", "mental health integration," "integrated care," "shared care," "co-located care," "primary care behavioral health," "integrated primary care," or sometimes "behavioral medicine"—and this is just a start. Each of these terms encompasses a similar core of subject matter for implementation and study. But each of the names for that subject matter has emerged from different practice, intellectual, geographical or disciplinary traditions—as if dialects of a more general language loosely understood by insiders or "native speakers" in that field. To find a meaningful place in PCMH—broad implementation on a meaningful scale—the field of integrated behavioral health must not only show its effectiveness empirically, but must become a field more consistently and widely understood in language and practice by the public and by the practitioners themselves.

Such language must help everyone navigate the subject matter in a consistent and precise enough way to enable the practical work of (1) practice redesign—shaped by (2) performance evaluation and research—leading to (3) patient engagement, demand, and purchasing decisions—and sustained by (4) policy and business model change.

Consistent Understanding of Core Concepts Is Far from a Theoretical Concern

In planning an AHRQ-funded research development conference for the Collaborative Care Research Network (CCRN), in 2009 (Miller, Kessler, Peek, & Kallenberg, 2011), very practical concerns pointed to the need for a common language or lexicon. Research funders, policymakers, and those trying to redesign health care had become interested in integrated behavioral health (then referred to as "collaborative care") as a means of accomplishing the larger goals of primary care or of PCMH.

However, during conference planning, it became apparent that integrated behavioral health care clinicians and advocates seemed to stumble over language, even naming their field inconsistently. It was more like individual voices without a structure of shared concepts, rather than an organized group using a consistent framework of concepts and language for their subject matter. While policymakers and research funders remained persuaded by the *potential* value of integrated behavioral health care, they felt handicapped in advocating for it publicly or behind the scenes because of the perceived lack of consistency or rigor of the concepts in use. The composite message received leading up the conference was clear: "It would help if you all talked about the components and terms of your field in a much more consistent way than you do now."

Conference planners stumbled over language, with conference calls slowed down by observations such as, "I'm not sure we mean the same thing by that," or "I thought I understood where you were going five minutes ago, but now I don't think we meant the same thing by X," and "I wonder if what I call Y, you call Z, and if there is really any difference." In a starter list of research questions brainstormed by the committee, the terms "continuum of integration", "extent of collaborative care components," and "degree of collaborative care" appeared—along with a conversation about whether these are the same or not and whether anyone would know how to measure them. It became very difficult for the program committee to formulate an initial series of unambiguously understood integrated behavioral health care research questions that could be examined, refined, or replaced by the broad audience invited to the research conference. The following questions arose:

> Do we have a good enough *shared* vocabulary (set of concepts and distinctions) for asking research questions together across many practices? Do we mean similar enough things by the words we use or how we distinguish one form of practice from another, for purposes of investigating their effects? Do we have a shared view of the edges of the concepts we are investigating—the boundaries of the genuine article or the scope of our subject matter? If we don't share enough of that vocabulary, we will *think* we are asking the same research questions, using the same distinctions, doing the same interventions, or measuring the same things, but we won't be and we will confuse our network practices and our funding organizations…

Confusion over Language and Definitions Typically Takes Two Forms

Meaning of commonly used terms. What are the differences between mental health care and behavioral health care? What are the differences between collaborative care, integrated care, integrated primary care, integrated behavioral health, shared care, coordinated care, co-located care, and consultation/liaison? These and other common terms frequently stopped conversations while the group verified what each other meant by these. As a result of these conversations, a literature-based "family tree of common terms" was created (See Fig. 2.1—reproduced from Peek and the National Integration Academy Council (2013).

Integrated Care

Tightly integrated, on-site teamwork with unified care plan as a standard approach to care for designated populations. Connotes organizational integration involving social & other services. "Attitudes" of integration: 1) Integrated treatments, 2) integrated program structure; 3) integrated system of programs, and 4) integrated payments. (Based on SAMHSA)

Shared Care

Predominately Canadian usage — PC & MH professionals (typically psychiatrists) working together in shared system and record, maintaining 1 treatment plan addressing all patient health needs. (Kates et al, 1996; Kelly et al, 2011)

Patient-Centered Care

"The experience (to the extent the informed, individual patient desires it) of transparency, individualization, recognition, respect, dignity, and choice in all matters, without exception, related to one's person, circumstances, and relationships in health care"— or "nothing about me without me" (Berwick, 2011).

Collaborative Care

A general term for ongoing working relationships between clinicians, rather than a specific product or service (Doherty, McDaniel& Baird, 1996). Providers combine perspectives and skills to understand and identify problems and treatments, continually revising as needed to hit goals, e.g. in collaborative care of depression (Unützer et al, 2002)

Coordinated Care

The organization of patient care activities between two or more participants (including the patient) involved in care, to facilitate appropriate delivery of healthcare services. Organizing care involves the marshalling of personnel and other resources needed to carry out required care activities, and often managed by the exchange of information among participants responsible for different aspects of care" (AHRQ, 2007).

Co-located Care

BH and PC providers (i.e. physicians, NP's) delivering care in same practice. This denotes shared space to one extent or another, not a specific service or kind of collaboration. (adapted from Blount, 2003)

Integrated Primary Care or Primary Care Behavioral Health

Combines medical & BH services for problems patients bring to primary care, including stress-linked physical symptoms, health behaviors, MH or SA disorders. For any problem, they have come to the right place — "no wrong door" (Blount). BH professional used as a consultant to PC colleagues (Sabin & Borus, 2009; Haas & deGruy, 2004; Robinson & Reiter, 2007; Hunter etal, 2009).

Patient-Centered Medical Home

An approach to comprehensive primary care for children, youth and adults — a setting that facilitates partnerships between patients and their personal physicians, and when appropriate, the patient's family. Emphasizes care of populations, team care, whole person care — including behavioral health, care coordination, information tools and business models needed to sustain the work. The goal is health, patient experience, and reduced cost. (Joint Principles of PCMH, 2007).

Primary Care

Primary care is the provision of integrated, accessible health care services by clinicians who are accountable for addressing a large majority of personal health care needs, developing a sustained partnership with patients, and practicing in the context of family and community. (Institute of Medicine, 1994)

Behavioral Health Care

An umbrella term for care that addresses any behavioral problems bearing on health, including MH and SA conditions, stress-linked physical symptoms, patient activation and health behaviors. The job of all kinds of care settings, and done by clinicians and health coaches of various disciplines or training.

Mental Health Care

Care to help people with mental illnesses (or at risk) — to suffer less emotional pain and disability — and live healthier, longer, more productive lives. Done by a variety of caregivers in diverse public and private settings such as specialty MH, general medical, human services, and voluntary support networks. (Adapted from SAMHSA)

Substance Abuse Care

Services, treatments, and supports to help people with addictions and substance abuse problems suffer less emotional pain, family and vocational disturbance, physical risks — and live healthier, longer, more productive lives. Done in specialty SA, general medical, human services, voluntary support networks, e.g. 12-step programs and peer counselors. (Adapted from SAMHSA)

Fig. 2.1 A family tree of terms encountered in integrated behavioral health or collaborative care

Necessary components of integrated behavioral health. What actually has to be in place for a particular practice to be regarded as doing integrated behavioral health? This question posed the more difficult challenge, and is not fulfilled by the "family tree of terms." It is all too easy for a practice or clinician to say, "Integrated behavioral health—yes we already do that. We have a social worker in the hospital and a psychiatrist across town on our referral list." But for many, this would not count as a genuine instance of integrated behavioral health care. But on what basis? Who says? What is the package of functional components we all agree is necessary for a particular practice to be doing integrated behavioral health? This was important for many reasons—identifying genuine instances of integrated care in practice, enrolling practices in research, identifying differences between them—and of course knowing what you are buying and what functions you want to support if you are designing a system, payment model, or public policy.

Without common language for the subject matter and what counts as the genuine article, creating a national research agenda and other developmental tasks for the field would be difficult to accomplish. One of the conference tasks was to create a usable "lexicon" or system of concepts for this new (or newly rediscovered) field.

The 2009 conference experience led to a two-stage process to develop a lexicon or functional definition for behavioral health integrated in primary care. The first stage was to convene a subset of the planning committee to use a systematic lexicon development method to create a product for use only at that conference (Peek, 2011). The second stage was an AHRQ funded conference in 2012 to broaden and deepen that starter lexicon among members of the AHRQ National Academy Integration Council, a steering group for the Academy for Integration of Behavioral Health and Primary Care. Patient representatives were also included in this process.

Conceptual Confusion Is a Normal Stage of Development for Emerging Fields

The research conference committee decided it had to sharpen concepts and language if it was to successfully create a research agenda—the "deliverable" of the funded conference. And later, the AHRQ Integration Academy broadened and deepened the lexicon for its purposes—which included measures of integration (AHRQ, 2013), and workforce competencies—as well as to have a consistent way to portray the field via its website (http://integrationacademy.ahrq.gov).

All this was done without apology or sheepishness. All mature scientific or technical fields have lexicons (systems of terms and concepts) developed well enough to allow collaborative and geographically distributed scientific, engineering, or applications work to take place. Systematically related concepts have an esteemed place in the history of mature fields, such as electrical engineering, physics, and computer science, and have enabled them to become mature sciences or technologies with associated empirical triumphs. In many cases the definitional, conceptual or pre-empirical development of these fields was done so long ago that we take it for granted and now see only the concrete or empirical achievements. But it takes a generally understood system of concepts and distinctions to do good science. Here is one example of lexicon development from nineteenth century science:

> At the time of the first International Electrical Congress in Paris in 1881, "complete confusion had reigned in this field; each country had its own units". Multiple different units were in use across researchers and countries for electromotive force, electric current and resistance. At this first Congress, agreements were reached on the ohm and the volt—with ampere, coulomb and farad also defined, all done as one conceptual system. Governments saw that it had become necessary for commercial transactions to create an international system of definitions and to provide a forum of scientists, manufacturers, and learned societies to establish terminology for the whole field of scientific and technical concepts (du Couëdic, 1981).

Without this system of electrical concepts becoming community property with standing across all electrical researchers, the field could not have developed into the mature form of empirical science that we now witness. The effect was immediate:

> The first Congress of 1881 has borne good fruit. It has not only brought about a rapprochement between electricians of all countries, but it has led to the adoption of an international system of measurement which will be in universal use. (The Electrical Congress of Paris, 1884)

Conceptual Clarification Is Especially Important for Anything "Behavioral"

Historically, subject matters that include the terms "behavior," "mental health," "psychosocial" or "collaborative" in their names have stereotypically been seen as soft, subjective, or not as conducive to scientific investigation, despite the existence of extensive literature and research. Different published papers often employ disparate conceptual and language systems, and this can lead to a sense (especially as seen by those outside the field) that the field is "not quite worked out" or seems to be re-created anew by each author. As important as "behavior" is to contemporary health care and the PCMH, an impression remains that it is a fuzzy concept compared to traditional medical areas. The behavioral dimensions of health and health care not only entail studying immensely complex phenomena, but also may be earlier in their development as fields compared to their biomedical cousins. Creating a lexicon for integrated behavioral health puts at least a few things "behavioral" or "collaborative" as they relate to primary care on a more systematic and consistent conceptual consensus-based foundation that is accessible to anyone, including the authors of the chapters of this book. More on the need for widely accepted conceptual systems for use in behavioral fields and psychology appears in Peek (2011), Bergner (2006), and Ossorio (2006).

A Consensus-Based Method for Creating a Lexicon for Integrated Behavioral Health

This section is adapted or paraphrased from Peek (2011) *and Peek and National Integration Academy Council* (2013).

Requirements for a Lexicon Development Method

For a lexicon to become more than one person's invention for one limited study or application, it would have to serve the practical purposes of a broad range of people over a broad range of applications. This could not be created and published as an opinion by one person or small group in isolation, which is a common to proposing definitions and gives rise to the sense of cacophony that policymakers and researchers had noticed. Instead, a method for creating a lexicon with standing in the field should:

- Be consensual but analytic (a disciplined transparent process—not a political campaign)
- Involve actual implementers and users ("native speakers" of the field—those actually doing the work—not only observers, consultants and commentators)
- Focus on what functionalities look like in practice (not just on principles, values, goals, or visible "anatomical features")
- Portray both similarities and differences (specify both theme and legitimate variations)
- Refine and employ existing familiar concepts that are serviceable to the extent possible
- Be amenable to gathering around it an expanding circle of "owners" and contributors (not just an elite group with a declaration)

Fortunately methods for defining complex subject matters that meet these requirements exist in the published literature—"paradigm case formulation" and "parametric analysis"—as described by Ossorio (2006). The product, a lexicon for posing integrated behavioral health care research and practice development questions, is described in later sections.

About Definitions, Paradigm Case Formulation, and Parametric Analysis

Before describing the lexicon itself, we'll step back and contrast paradigm case formulation and parametric analysis with the usual approach to creating definitions. The usual approach is to create one or two sentences, such as "integrated behavioral health care is X, Y, and Z," often done pragmatically for the purposes of just one study or project. If done to structure the concepts for an entire field, a standard definition would

1. *Paradigm case:* A husband and his wife living with their natural children, who are a seventeen-year-old son and a ten-year-old daughter.

2. *Transformations:*

   T1. Eliminate one parent but not both.

   T2. Change the number of children to N, N > 0.

   T3. Change the sex distribution of children to any distribution other than zero boys and zero girls

   T4. Change the ages of the children to any values compatible with the ages of the parents.

   T5. Any combination from T1, T2, T3, and T4.

   T6. Add any number of additional parents.

   T7. Add adopted and other legally defined sons and/or daughters.

   T8. Eliminate the requirement of living together.

   T9. Change the number of children to zero if husband and wife are living together.

Fig. 2.2 Example—paradigm case formulation of "family" (Quoted from Ossorio, 2006; pp. 26–27)

attempt to identify genuine instances on the basis of uniformities in common across all instances. But integrated behavioral health care is characterized not only by uniformities (a common core), but also by many legitimate differences between instances of integrated behavioral health. The definitional challenge is to develop a consistent shared language for both commonalities and differences without devolving into either "a cookie cutter" or "anything counts." A simple one-sentence definition such as "integrated behavioral health care is X, Y, and Z" would likely be oversimplified, full of qualifications and exceptions, or considered wrong or incomplete by many.

Paradigm case formulation. For complex subject matters such as integrated behavioral health care, a paradigm case formulation is an improved device for creating a definition because it maps both similarities and differences at any level of detail desired. For example, the concept of "family" is a complex subject matter and would be very difficult to define in a single sentence that would satisfy everyone. The paradigm case formulation approach to "family" starts with one archetypal statement (the paradigm case) that no one could possibly disagree with—and then goes on to systematically describe what could be changed (transformations of the paradigm case) and still be "family" (see Fig. 2.2).

Note that constructing a paradigm case formulation calls for careful decisions and the exercise of judgment in regard to which cases to include or exclude. Disagreement may arise among different persons. For example, T6-T9 seem much more likely to elicit objections ("I wouldn't call that a family!") than T1-T5.

In this example, the paradigm case and its transformations *becomes* the "definition" of family. One can distill a one-sentence summary definition of the usual sort found in great diversity and abundance in dictionaries, in professional publications, and on the web. But the limitations of one-sentence definitions are why the paradigm case formulation method was employed for the integrated behavioral health lexicon.

If you go to the lumberyard and ask for a 2x4, the person behind the counter will ask three questions:

    A) How long?
    B) What grade?
    C) What species?

If you say, "I need an 8-foot, #2, fir", they will go back into the stacks and get one. There is little more to say to specify a 2 x 4. These three parameters are the finite ways 2x4's can differ from one another. The parameters and some of the possible values for each parameter are illustrated below.

Parameters Possible "settings" for each parameter

1. Length	4'	8'	12'	16'
2. Grade	# 1	#2	# 3	C Select
3. Species	Fir	Pine	Maple	Oak

Fig. 2.3 Example—parameters of 2 × 4's

Parametric analysis. A complementary device, parametric analysis, goes on to create a specific vocabulary for how one instance of integrated behavioral health in action might be the same or different from another instance across town. In the "family" example, two of the parameters would be "number of children" and "number of parents." Parametric analysis (understanding the dimensions of something) sounds exotic, but is commonplace in other fields. One extremely simple illustration is shown in Fig. 2.3—parameters of number 2 × 4's.

A scientific example of parametric analysis is in the specification and comparison of different colors employing the three parameters of color: brightness, hue, and saturation. Any color can be specified through supplying a "setting" (formally called a "value") on each of these parameters as expressed in the Munsell color chart (Ossorio, 2006; pp. 35–36). Parametric analysis is used routinely to fine tune product design and market competitiveness for industrial products and software because it allows the designer to measure the influence of all parameters (or design features) on the outcomes desired and the trade-offs between them (Thieffry, 2008).

Parametric analysis sets the stage for comparative effectiveness research in integrated behavioral health care, where one set of arrangements is tested against a different set of arrangements. The "arrangements" are expressed through the parameters.

Overview of the Consensus Process to Reach Paradigm Case and Parameters

The lexicon process began with a core group of CCRN program committee members in 2009 that consisted of Benjamin F. Miller, Gene Kallenberg, and Rodger Kessler

and this author. A larger circle of contributors included research conference participants and those attending a Collaborative Family Healthcare Association presentation
soon after. With this wisdom incorporated, the lexicon became the organizing system
for integrated behavioral health care research questions submitted to AHRQ (Miller,
Kessler, Peek, & Kallenberg, 2011). The lexicon shown here is a condensation of the
updated version (Peek and the National Integration Academy Council, 2013).

About the discussion process for creating a consensus definition. *(Adapted from
Peek, 2011).* An functional definition to serve practical purposes for a broad range
of people interested in integration of behavioral health and primary care could not
be created by one person or perspective alone. Doing so would increase the sense of
ambiguity or multiplying compatible but different definitions (usually without much
functional specificity) that implementers and patients had noticed, sometimes as
cacophony.

As described earlier, a "paradigm case formulation" is a vehicle for creating
a definition that maps both similarities and differences. A "parametric analysis"
builds on the paradigm case to create a specific vocabulary for how one instance
of integrated behavioral health practice might differ from another instance
across town.

The paradigm case and parameters amount to a set of interrelated concepts (like
an extended definition) that can be used in comparing practices, setting standards,
or asking research questions using a common vocabulary.

The consensus process is facilitated in two stages. (1) A core group draft was
done in this case by four people, followed by (2) a "second ring" review/contributor
group in this case of 20 people.

In each stage, the product contains parts A to C—progressively refined until
good enough to use:

A. *Create a* paradigm case *of integrated behavioral health in action:* "Here's a case
   of integrated behavioral health in action if ever there was one". One indisputable
   example—that is deliberately aspirational—not necessarily representative of
   what you find out there but would like to find. *This step maps out the uniformities in what we mean by integrated behavioral health.*
B. *Introduce* transformations *of this paradigm case.* The purpose of *transformations* is to identify additional cases that we as a group also believe qualify as
   integrated behavioral health—*"You could change X or delete Y and it would still
   be integrated behavioral health."* This step maps the differences. The paradigm
   case and transformations, when taken together is our "definition" of behavioral
   health integrated in primary care.
C. *Parameters: Dimensions for legitimate differences between practices.* This is a
   vocabulary for how one integrated behavioral health practice might be different
   from the one next door.

Facilitation details for this group consensus process were devised by CJ Peek,
and are beyond the scope of this chapter. Facilitation included individual feedback
via emailed documents and worksheets, a daylong intensive meeting, plus rounds of
follow-up input and editorial work.

The Product: A Lexicon for Integrated Behavioral Health Care

This section is a condensed version of the full lexicon that appears in Peek and National Integration Academy Council (2013), a project of Agency for Healthcare Research and Quality

Structure of this Lexicon

The summary (Fig. 2.4) starts with a general definition ("what"), followed by defining clauses ("how" and "supported by") and named parameters. The *defining clauses* are declarative statements of what genuine behavioral health integrated in primary care looks like in action—an extended definition—uniformities to be expected. *Read these numbered clauses as if one long run-on sentence.* The *parameters* are a vocabulary for how one instance of how one integrated care practice might legitimately differ from another one across town. *Read these as a typology of differences.*

The defining clauses and sub-clauses are spelled out, often with bullet points. Some defining clauses also include "transformations"—legitimate variations on the defining clause, e.g., "you can delete X, modify Y, or substitute Z and it's still a genuine case of integrated behavioral health". Where no transformations appear, the defining clause is required as stated. Defining clauses are a set of required functions, not specific ways of carrying them out. They represent fidelity to the definition of behavioral health integrated in primary care, but leave room (and require) a great deal of local adaptation such as specific workflows. *Read this as a pattern, not a "cookie cutter."*

The parameters are spelled out as a vocabulary for legitimate differences. Each parameter has a set of categories (in boxes) that represent legitimate differences between integrated behavioral health practices. Some parameters articulate *types*—different legitimate approaches or methods. Other parameters outline *levels* that might be regarded as developmental stages toward full aspiration. But there is no presumption that one of these variations is empirically proven best. Some parameters show grayed-in categories. These are not acceptable variations, shown only as context for the others.

In the lexicon, many fine-print annotations appear that define terms, refer to literature, or clarify concepts and balances. For simplicity, these details are omitted here in favor of figures (2.5, 2.6, 2.7, 2.8 and 2.9) that are excerpted from the Executive Summary of Peek and the National Academy Council (2013).

Applications for the Lexicon: What Good Can It Do for Whom?

As said at the outset of this chapter, a lexicon is not just an academic exercise. It is a response to practical problems for stakeholders in this field who often have an inconsistent understanding of the vocabulary for core functionalities of integrated

Lexicon for Behavioral Health and Primary Care Integration
At a Glance

What
The care that results from a practice team of primary care and behavioral health clinicians, working together with patients and families, using a systematic and cost-effective approach to provide patient-centered care for a defined population.
This care may address mental health and substance abuse conditions, health behaviors (including their contribution to chronic medical illnesses), life stressors and crises, stress-related physical symptoms, and ineffective patterns of health care utilization.

Defining Clauses	Corresponding Parameters
What integrated behavioral health needs to look like in action	*Calibrated differences between practices*
How	
1. A practice team tailored to the needs of each patient and situation	1. Range of care team function and expertise that can be mobilized
A. With a suitable range of behavioral health and primary care expertise and role functions available to draw from	2. Type of spatial arrangement employed for behavioral health and primary care clinicians
B. With shared operations, workflows and practice culture	3. Type of collaboration employed
C. Having had formal or on-the-job training	4. Method for identifying individuals who need integrated behavioral health and primary care
2. With a shared population and mission	
A panel of patients in common for total health outcomes	5. Protocols
3. Using a systematic clinical approach (and a system that enables the clinical approach to function)	A. Whether protocols are in place or not for engaging patients in integrated care
A. Employing methods to identify those members of the population who need or may benefit	B. Level that protocols are followed for initiating integrated care
B. Engaging patients and families in identifying their needs for care and the particular clinicians to provide it	6. Care plans
C. Involving both patients and clinicians in decision-making	A. Proportion of patients in target groups with shared care plans
D. Using an explicit, unified, and shared care plan	B. Degree to which care plans are implemented and followed
E. With the unified care plan and manner of support to patient and family in a shared electronic health record	7. Level of systematic follow-up
F. With systematic follow-up and adjustment of treatment plans if patients are not improving as expected	
Supported by	
4. A community, population, or individuals expecting that behavioral health and primary care will be integrated as a standard of care.	8. Level of community expectation for integrated behavioral health as a standard of care
5. Supported by office practice, leadership alignment, and business model	9. Level of office practice reliability and consistency
A. Clinic operational systems and processes	10. Level of leadership/administrative alignment and priorities
B. Alignment of purposes, incentives, leadership	
C. A sustainable business model	11. Level of business model support for integrated behavioral health
6. And continuous quality improvement and measurement of effectiveness	12. Extent that practice data is collected and used to improve the practice
A. Routinely collecting and using practice-based data	(Plus three auxiliary parameters)
B. Periodically examining and reporting outcomes	

Fig. 2.4 Summary

behavioral health. A consistent understanding and vocabulary can be especially difficult to establish across different stakeholder communities such as clinicians, purchasers, health plans, policymakers, and patients themselves. This lexicon is intended to provide a common language and functional definition across the communities listed below—and was created with representation from most of them.

The following sections list stakeholders, their basic need for a lexicon—or a sample of their applications for a lexicon. This is a list of what the lexicon can do for whom.

"How" Defining Clauses (1-3)

(Those functions that define what integrated behavioral health care looks like in action)

1. A practice team tailored to the needs of each patient and situation

A. *With a suitable range of behavioral health and primary care expertise and role functions available to draw from* — so team can be defined at the level of each patient, and in general for targeted populations. Patients and families are considered part of the team.

B. *With shared operations, workflows, and practice culture* that support behavioral health and medical clinicians and staff in providing patient-centered care
   - Shared physical space — co-location
     > ***Alternative(what could change):*** *Change "shared physical space—co-location" to "a set of working relationships and workflows between clinicians in separate spaces that achieves communication, collaboration, patient-centered operations, and practice culture requirements."*
   - Shared workflows, protocols, and office processes that enable and ensure collaboration — including one accessible shared treatment plan for each patient.
   - A shared practice culture rather than separate and conflicting behavioral health and medical cultures.

C. *Having had formal or on-the-job training* for the clinical roles and relationships of integrated behavioral healthcare, including culture and teamwork (for both medical and behavioral clinicians).

2. With a shared population and mission

With a panel of clinic patients in common, behavioral health and medical team members together take responsibility for the same shared mission and accountability for total health outcomes.
   > ***Alternative:*** *Change "a panel of clinic patients in common" to "any identifiable subset of the panel of clinic patients for whom collaborative, integrated behavioral health is made available."*

3. Using a systematic clinical approach (and system that enables it to function)

A. *Employing methods to identify those members of a population who need or may benefit* from integrated behavioral and medical care, and at what level of severity or priority.

B. *Engaging patients and families in identifying their needs for care,* the kinds of services or clinicians to provide it, and a specific group of health care professionals that will work together to deliver those services.

C. *Involving both patients and clinicians in decision-making* to create an integrated care plan appropriate to patient needs, values, and preferences.

D. *Caring for patients using an explicit, unified, and shared care plan* that contains assessments and plans for biological/physical, psychological, cultural, social, and organization of care aspects of the patient's health and health care. Scope includes prevention, acute, and chronic/complex care. (See full lexicon for elements)

E. *With unified care plan, treatment, referral activity, and manner of support to patient and family contained in a shared electronic health record* or registry, with ongoing communication among team members
   > ***Alternatives:***
   > *Change "unified care plan in shared medical record" to "problem list and shared plans are contained in provider notes or other records in same organization medical record which everyone reads and acts upon,"*
   > *Delete "electronic" in "shared electronic medical record" (interim, not desired final state).*

F. *With systematic follow-up and adjustment of treatment plans* if patients are not improving as expected. This is the "back-end" management of patients from "front-end" identification. (See full lexicon for specifics)

Fig. 2.5 The "How" defining clauses spelled out

Patients and Families

Questions:

"What should I expect from integrated behavioral health in my own doctor's office? How would I recognize the genuine article if I encountered it? How would I know whether the integrated care my family received was up to standard? Is there a standard?"

"Supported by" Defining Clauses (4-6)

(Functions necessary for the "how" clauses to become sustainable on a meaningful scale)

4. **A community, population, or individuals expecting that behavioral health and primary care will be integrated as a standard of care** so that clinicians, staff, and their patients achieve patient-centered, effective care.

5. **Supported by office practice, leadership alignment, and a business model**

   A. *Clinic operational systems, office processes, and office management* that consistently and reliably support communication, collaboration, tracking of an identified population, a shared care plan, making joint follow-up appointments or other collaborative care functions

      Alternative: Delete "consistently and reliably" (an interim state, not adesired final state).

   B. *Alignment of purposes, incentives, leadership, and program supervision within the practice.*

      Alternative: Substitue "Intention and process underway to align... " for "alignment of."

   C. *A sustainable business model* (financial model) that supports the consistent delivery of collaborative, coordinated behavioral and medical services in a single setting or practice relationship. .

      Alternative: Substitue "working toward sustainable business model" for "sustainable business model,"

6. **And continuous quality improvement and measurement of effectiveness**

   A. *Routinely collecting and using measured practice-based data* to improve patient outcomes—to change what the practice is doing and quickly learn from experience. Include clinical, operational, demographic and financial/cost data.

   B. *Periodically examining and internally reporting outcomes*—at the provider and program level—for care, patient experience, and affordability (The "Triple Aim") and engaging the practice in making program design changes accordingly.

Fig. 2.6 The "Supported by" defining clauses spelled out—those necessary for the clinical "how" to become sustainable on a meaningful scale

Applications:

One of the "supported by" defining clauses points to the need for patients to understand and expect better integrated care as a standard of practice. The functional definition of the lexicon can serve as the basis for simple orientations or conversations that help patients and families understand the potential value to them for integrated behavioral health.

For example, the author and a patient who participated in the lexicon development process used the lexicon to query a patient advisory council at the Institute for Clinical Systems Improvement in 2012. When these patients said they didn't know what "behavioral health" or "integrated behavioral health" was, the defining clauses clarified it. Then the conversation could quickly move to whether the group thought that patients would expect or demand it as a standard of practice.

Purchasers of Health Care Plans

Questions:

"What exactly am I buying if I add integrated behavioral health care to the benefits? What do I tell my employees (or other constituents) they can expect to encounter in this benefit—especially for any change in service or employee cost?"

Parameters 1-7 Related to the "How" Clauses
How one integrated practice might differ from another

Types of practice arrangements

1. Range of care team function and expertise that can be mobilized	Foundational functions for target population • Triage/identification for need for integrated BH • Behavioral activation/self management, community res. • Basic MH-SApsychological and pharmacologic interventions; psychological support/crisis intervention • Common chronic/complex illness care • Follow-up, monitoring for timely adjustment of care		Foundational plus others • Registry tracking & coordination • Specialized MH or pharmacologic therapies	Extended functions, add Specialized expertise in • Conditions, populations • School, vocational, spiritual, community

2. Type of spatial arrangement employed for BH and PC clinicians	Mostly separate space • Little time in same space • Patient sees providers in at least twobuildings	Co-located space • Different parts of same building; some but not all time in same space • Patient movesfrom PC to BH	Fully shared space • Share rooms in shared space • Typically, the clinicians see the patient in same exam room.

3. Type of collaboration employed	Referral-triggered periodic exchange--Minimally shared care plans or workflows	Regular communic. /coordination Separate systems and workflows, but significant care plan coordination	Full collaboration/ integration Treatment plans,documentation, communication,workflows

4. Method for identifying individuals for integrated BH	Patient or clinician Patient or clinician identification done in a non-systematic fashion	Health system indicators Demographic, registry, claims, or other system data	Universal screening or identification processes All or most patients identified or screened for being part of a target population

Levels of implementation of practice arrangements — from getting started to full implementation

5A. Protocols in place for engaging patients in integrated BH?	Protocols not in place Undefined or informal *(Not acceptable)*	Protocols in place Protocols and workflows for integrated BH are built into clinical system as a standard part of care process	

5B. Level that protocols followed for initiating integrated BH	Protocols followed less than 50% *(Not acceptable)*	Protocols followed more than 50% but less than 100% (an interim state)	Protocols followed nearly 100% (Standard work)

6A. Proportion of patients in target groups with shared care plans	Less than 40% *(Not acceptable)*	40% to nearly 100% (Meaningful proportion but less than full-scale)	Nearly 100% (Standard work)

6B. Degree care plans are implemented & followed	Less than 50% *(Not acceptable)*	More than 50%, less than 100% (An interim state, not final state)	Care plans followed nearly 100% (Standard work)

7. Level of systematic follow up*	Less than 40 % *(Not acceptable)*	40% to 75% (Significant but incomplete)	76% to 100% (Standard work)

*Follow upelements: A) At least one follow-up for those engaged in care; B) At least one follow-up in initial 4 weeks of care; C) Cases reviewed for progress on a regular basis (e.g., every 6-12 weeks); D) Receive treatment adjustments if not improving.

Fig. 2.7 Parameters corresponding to the "how" defining clauses—how one genuine integrated practice might differ from another one

Applications

When employers or other purchasers change the "product" or benefits for health care, they must also explain and set expectations—and what they expect the value to become. A clear functional description of a particular purchase of integrated behavioral health using language of the lexicon can help be more specific about what is being purchased and what the patients should expect for their own premium contributions.

Health Plans

Important questions:

"What specifically do I require clinical systems to provide to health plan members—and what will I specifically look at to see if they are providing it or not?"

Parameters 8-12 Related to the "Supported by" Clauses
Conditions needed for success of clinical action in the real world on a meaningful scale

8. Level of community expectation for integrated BH as standard of care	**Little or no understanding & expectation** *(Not acceptable)* Insufficient reach of understanding and expectation to enable integrated BH to start and function	**Expected as standard of care only in pockets** Partial but substantially incomplete community understanding and expectation	**Widely expected as standard of care** Community understanding & expectation for integrated BH health as a standard of care
9. Level of office practice reliability and consistency	**Non-systematic** *(Not acceptable)* Office processes are non-standard with unwarranted variation across clinicians and situations	**Substantially routinized** Standards set for most processes, but unwarranted variability and clinician preference still operate—not yet standard work	**Standard work** Whole team operates each part of the system in a standard expected way that improves reliability and prevents errors.
10. Level of leadership / administrative alignment and priorities	**Misaligned** *(Not acceptable)* Conflicts apparent with other priorities, resource allocations, incentives, habits, standards	**Partially aligned** Some alignment achieved, but unresolved tensions evident	**Fully aligned** Constructive balance achieved between priorities, incentives, and standards. Emerging conflicts routinely addressed
11. Level of business model support for integrated BH	**Behavior health integration not fully supported** The business model has not yet found ways to fully support the integrated behavioral health functions selected and built for this practice.		**Behavioral health integration fully supported** The business model has found ways to fully support the integrated behavioral health functions selected and built for this practice.
12. Scale of practice data collected & used For the integrated BH aspect of the practice	**Minimum:** **(less than 40% of patients)** *(A startup state—not desired final state)* Very limited system for collecting and using practice data to improve quality and effectiveness (of integrated BH)	**Partial:** **(40%-75% of patients)** *(An interim state, not a desired final state)* Significant but less than full collection and use of practice-based data for decision-making	**Full / standard work:** **76% -100% of patients** Routine data collection on most patients with integrated BH to improve effectiveness at the system, unit, population level

Fig. 2.8 Parameters corresponding to the "supported by" defining clauses—conditions needed for success of clinical action in the real world on a meaningful scale

Applications:
Health plans are not only insurance companies, but administrators of health care insurance across provider groups. Health plans set rules, policies, and are in a position to confirm that particular practices are providing the benefits described. A common functional framework for integrated behavioral health can help give structure to those administrative functions.

Clinicians and Medical Groups

Questions:
"What exactly do I need to implement—to count as genuine behavioral health integrated in primary care—and to advertise myself as doing integrated behavioral health? What are the core functions, and what is up to me to locally adapt?"

Applications:
First of all, sufficient shared language and definition for the field increases clinician confidence in talking with each other and other stakeholders. Clinicians do not like to stumble over basic terms or language that distinguishes the components and

Auxiliary Parameters

These may be useful for specific purposes, though not considered central to the full lexicon.

Target sub-population for integrated BH	**A. Setting**	Primary medical care		Specialty medical care		Specialty mental health care
	B. Life stage	Children	Adolescents	Adults/young adults	Geriatrics	End of life
	C. Type of symptoms targeted	Severe mental illness	Mental health or substance abuse conditions	Stress-linked or "medically unexplained" physical symptoms	Medical conditions; chronic illnesses, self-management	Complex blend, including social factors interfering with health and care
	D. Type of situations targeted	Patients with no health system contacts for problems or prevention	Diseases and conditions	Prevention, wellness	Acute life stresses	Health disparities	High risk and/or high cost cases

Degree that program is targeted to specific population or situation *(Blount, 2003)*	Targeted	Non-targeted
	Program designed for specific populations such as disease, prevention, at-risk, age, racial and ethnic minorities, social complexity, pregnancy or other	Program designed generically for any patient deemed to need collaborative care for any reason— "all comers"

Breadth of outcomes expected depending on program scale or maturity *(From Davis, 2001)*	Pilot scale	Project scale	Full-scale
	Limited expectations for a limited set of outcomes for a limited group of patients	Significant, but not full-scale outcomes expected, e.g., multiple pilots gathered together	Full-scale and broad-based outcomes expected for the entire population; no longer a project within a mainstream that hasn't changed

Fig. 2.9 Auxiliary parameters: These were used by chapter authors and may be useful to readers for specific purposes, though not considered central to the published lexicon

variations for integrated behavioral health. This is especially frustrating when communicating with policymakers, patients, or researchers. If clinicians talk with each other and those outside the field using common language they are likely to be more confident engaging others.

Second, the defining clauses and parameters of the lexicon can be translated into simple "checklists" with which a practice can inventory what it does or does not do by way of integrated behavioral health—and set development or improvement agendas. Multiple different practices can compare notes with each other on what they do and learn from others who are better at some parts of this than others. The field has lacked such a shared framework for self-description or self-evaluation—with each practice typically inventing its own. This makes it more difficult for practices to compare and collaborate on practice improvement or create local or regional shared improvement agendas. If the field is to develop as whole rather than in pockets, such a common framework for self-description and self-assessment is needed.

Policymakers and Business Modelers

Questions:

"If I am being asked to change the rules or business models to support integrated behavioral health, exactly what functions need to be supported?"

Applications:
Common language and functional description for integrated behavioral health in its various forms makes it easier for policymakers to answer important questions such as what exactly are people getting from "X" form of integrated behavioral health care—the product and benefits? What policies are needed to sustain the functions leading to those benefits? How much will people pay for that benefit (and those functions)? How do I justify that cost as a return on investment?

These are only basic questions, but if the lexicon is used across policymakers and longitudinally over time, it may bring more respectability to the field as seen through policymaker eyes.

Researchers and Program Evaluators

Questions:
"What functions need to be the subject of research questions on effectiveness? What functions require and form the basis for metrics? What terms will I use to ask consistently understood research questions across geographically distributed research networks?"

Applications:
The functional description of the lexicon can help researchers identify practices that qualify as doing integrated behavioral health for purposes of recruitment to a practice-based research network such as the Collaborative Care Research Network (Sieber et al., 2012). Moreover, the lexicon can help researchers (and the practices themselves) articulate (with sufficient definition) the comparisons to be made. For example, a research design might call for comparing different approaches to team composition and function, or look at which of the functions described in the lexicon account for what proportion of positive outcomes. Comparative effectiveness research requires clearly articulated comparisons to be made in real-world settings.

The papers resulting from the AHRQ-supported research conference framed the research questions using the vocabulary of the lexicon (Miller, Kessler, Peek, & Kallenberg, 2011). The lexicon can function as a consensus-based definitional reference for the terms and components listed in the research questions.

The lexicon provides distinctions for asking consistently understood practice development and research questions. But measurable indices (metrics) are also needed to serve as quantitative measures, or approximations of otherwise qualitative descriptions of integrated behavioral health care practice contained in the lexicon. Such data elements are needed for comparative effectiveness research (Kessler & Miller, 2011). Because of the variations in integrated behavioral health care practice, specific data elements and what should be expected to count as a successful outcome will vary. For example, what is reasonable to expect or measure depends in part on the target population under study. Exactly what data elements to include depends on whether the integrated behavioral health practice is aimed at children or adults, whether aimed at mental health conditions or chronic medical conditions or both, and whether it is aimed at a specific disease or subpopulation of some kind.

In addition, what is reasonable to expect or compare from practice to practice also depends on level of practice development (Davis, 2001). Some implementations may be limited startups or pilots, others are larger scale projects, and a few may be mainstream implementations within a larger organization or community. It would not be appropriate to compare results of limited pilots with mature large-scale projects or mainstream implementations because reasonable performance expectations for these will be different and the specific data elements available may be different.

The lexicon functional descriptions can also be converted to process measures—evaluation of processes that drive the performance that people ultimately care about. Each of the six defining clauses could become the basis for an internal process measure for practice self-evaluation and quality improvement.

Conclusion

A Vision for a Unified Set of Concepts and Language for Emerging Fields in Health Care

Other emerging fields are also important to PCMH. Program and planning committees also encounter definitional confusions and quibbles over the concepts in their subject matter. The examples below illustrate other examples where clarifying systems of definitions and functions were needed to build a foundation of support and understanding for patients, clinicians, health plans, policymakers, and researchers.

Palliative care. The Institute for Clinical Systems Improvement (ICSI) in Minnesota embarked on a community effort in 2009 to improve the availability and quality of palliative care among groups in the state. Similar patterns of confusion over language emerged. This author facilitated development of a consensus palliative care lexicon or operational definition—a joint product of the Institute for Clinical Systems Improvement (ICSI) and the University of Minnesota (2012). This lexicon is in use in Minnesota to give definition to palliative care in practice, along with derivative self-evaluation checklists.

Patient-centered medical home. The Institute for Clinical Systems Improvement (ICSI) has facilitated extensive Minnesota work on PCMH (called "health care home" in Minnesota) since 2007. Again, confusion over terms and "what is the genuine article" arose on phone calls. A consensus operational definition of health care home was developed first with a core group from four state systems and four private medical groups across the country, with contributions by a larger national review group of PCMH implementers—a joint product of the University of

Minnesota and Institute for Clinical Systems Improvement (Peek & Oftedahl, 2010). Observations about inconsistent understanding of PCMH for purposes of implementation and policymaking have been made by Stenger and Devoe (2010) and Stange et al. (2010).

Shared decision-making. In shared decision-making, patients and providers become active partners in clarifying acceptable options and helping the patient choose a course of care consistent with patient values and preferences and best available medical evidence. The Minnesota Shared Decision-Making Collaborative steering committee encountered similar definitional confusions and embarked on lexicon creation facilitated by the present author. This consensus lexicon or operational definition is a joint product of the Minnesota Shared Decision Making Collaborative, Institute for Clinical Systems Improvement, and the University of Minnesota (2012).

These lexicons are interlocking in some respects. For example, the health care home lexicon calls for integrated behavioral health. When someone asks, "what is integrated behavioral health?" it is now possible to go to the integrated behavioral health lexicon for specifics. The palliative care lexicon calls for shared decision making. Similarly, when someone asks, "what is shared decision making?" it is now possible to go to the shared decision making lexicon for specifics. And the health care home lexicon also calls for what amounts to palliative care functionality. Again, when a person asks, "What is palliative care exactly?" it is now possible to go to the palliative care lexicon for those specifics. Taken together these begin to clarify the conceptual and functional structure for these important emerging fields in health care.

A Generalized Need for Consistently Understood Concepts and Vocabulary in Emerging Fields

Steering groups in all these emerging fields experienced similar reasons to go through the painstaking process of developing a lexicon—a conceptual framework or operational definition. It became apparent when clearer and more consistent concepts and definitions for a field are needed:

1. Enough people are stumbling over language and what things mean—especially as encountered in practice, not only in theory or at the level of principles and values.
2. Enough people need clearer boundaries for an area X—what counts as "this is an example of X" for describing to the public, setting expectations, assigning insurance benefits, certifications, or saying how something is different than "usual" care.
3. People are asking, "What components are necessary for a given practice to really be X? What are the dimensions and milestones for practice improvement?"

4. Researchers want to ask quality or research questions more consistently and clearly—especially in geographically distributed research or QI networks
5. There is a felt need to improve the consistency or reputation of an area with "outsiders", e.g., policy-shapers, legislators, funders, and others not "native speakers" of the field.
6. When your field is being distorted or misunderstood by the public (or a vocal subset).
7. When practitioners themselves are unhappily inconsistent in the way they present their field to the outside world.

Lexicons are for practical communication across stakeholders who want to collaborate—to build the field while they improve their own implementations. Shared language is needed to ask questions and aggregate results or lessons learned. In one's own setting of course "we know what we mean by X". But the challenge of the field is to create enough [italicized] shared language for collaboration.

A journey has been underway to articulate and answer empirical research questions in integrated behavioral health and to help practices achieve the performance that everyone needs them to achieve. The necessary pre-empirical development of a basic conceptual system for this important subfield is being done—something that enables researchers, clinicians, and policymakers to talk to each other using a common vocabulary and an organized way of specifying the required components of integrated behavioral health care. The consensus-based approach described here avoids the debates and lack of uptake typically associated with a single author or elite group devising a conceptual system or vocabulary for one isolated purpose and proposing it in a journal article. Yet the lexicon described in this chapter is an evolving document to be shaped by succeeding groups as collective wisdom emerges on just what functions are required and the best ways to articulate them.

References

AHRQ Atlas of Integrated Behavioral Health Care Quality Measures (2013). http://integratio-nacademy.ahrq.gov/atlas

Bergner, R. M. (2006). An open letter from Isaac Newton to the field of psychology. In *Advances in descriptive psychology* (Vol. 8). Ann Arbor, MI: Descriptive Psychology Press.

du Couëdic, M. (1981). 1881—The Electrical Congress and Universal Exposition. IEC Bulletin Vol XV, No. 67—January 1981. (International Electrotechnical Commission).

International Electrical Commission—history. Accessed September, 2012 at www.iec.ch/zone

Kessler, R., & Miller, B. F. (2011). A framework for collaborative care metrics. One of three papers in: *A National Agenda for Research in Collaborative Care: Papers from the Collaborative Care Research Network Research Development Conference*. Rockville, MD: Agency for Healthcare Research and Quality. http://www.ahrq.gov/research/collaborativecare/

Miller, B. F., Kessler, R., Peek, C. J., & Kallenberg, G. (2011). Establishing a research agenda for collaborative care. One of three papers in: *A National Agenda for Research in Collaborative Care: Papers From the Collaborative Care Research Network Research Development Conference*. Rockville, MD: Agency for Healthcare Research and Quality. http://www.ahrq.gov/research/collaborativecare/

Ossorio, P. G. (2006). *The behavior of persons: The collected works of Peter G. Ossorio* (Vol. 5). Ann Arbor, MI: Descriptive Psychology Press.

Peek, C. J. (2011). A collaborative care lexicon for asking practice and research development questions. One of three papers in: *A National Agenda for Research in Collaborative Care: Papers From the Collaborative Care Research Network Research Development Conference*. Rockville, MD: Agency for Healthcare Research and Quality. http://www.ahrq.gov/research/collaborativecare/

Peek, C. J., & ICSI. (2012). *A parametric analysis or operational definition of palliative care*. A joint product of the University of Minnesota and the Institute for Clinical Systems Improvement (ICSI).

Peek, C. J., & National Integration Academy Council. (2013). *Lexicon for Behavioral Health and Primary Care Integration: Concepts and Definitions Developed by Expert Consensus*. AHRQ Publication No.13-IP001-1-EF. Rockville, MD: Agency for Healthcare Research and Quality. Available at: http://integrationacademy.ahrq.gov/lexicon

Peek, C. J., & Oftedahl, G. (2010). A consensus operational definition of patient centered medical home. A joint product of the University of Minnesota and the Institute for Clinical Systems Improvement (ICSI). http://www.icsi.org/health_care_home_operational_definition/health_care_home_operational_definition__.html

Sieber, W., Miller, B., Kessler, R., Patterson, J., Kallenberg, G., Edwards, T., et al. (2012). Establishing the collaborative care research network (CCRN): A description of initial participating sites. *Families, Systems, & Health, 30*(3), 210–223.

Stange, K. C., Nutting, P. A., Miller, W. L., Jaén, C. R., Crabtree, B. F., Flocke, S. A., et al. (2010). Defining and measuring the patient-centered medical home. *Journal of General Internal Medicine, 25*(6), 601–612.

Stenger, R., & Devoe, J. (2010). Policy challenges in building the medical home: Do we have a shared blueprint? *Journal of American Board of Family Medicine, 23*(3).

Thieffry, P. (2008). Parametric Analysis for evaluating a range of variables. *ANSYS Advantage, II*(1). www.ansys.com/magazine/issues/2-1-2008-rotating-machinery/12-analysis-tools.pdf

Chapter 3
Integrated Behavioral Health and the Patient-Centered Medical Home

Andrea M. Auxier, Benjamin F. Miller, and John Rogers

Abstract The current health care environment is characterized by reform initiatives that aim to improve quality while reducing costs through practice transformation. This chapter will introduce the reader to the Patient-Centered Medical Home concept, accreditation processes, and key findings from pilot demonstrations throughout the country. We will highlight the requirements for the provision of behavioral health services in primary care-based medical homes and will argue that the recent inclusion of behavioral health in the medical home is a promising start with much room for improvement.

Primary care, the largest platform of health care delivery, is witnessing yet another redesign through the evolution of Patient-Centered Medical Home (PCMH) (Green, Fryer, Yawn, Lanier, & Dovey, 2001; Nutting et al., 2009). Within this large multi-system process, there appear to be several innovative and unique opportunities to bend the cost curve while providing more efficient and effective health care. Nowhere is this more apparent than in the integration of behavioral health (BH).

A.M. Auxier, Ph.D. (✉)
Director of Integration Value Options, Inc. Colorado Springs, CO, USA

Senior Clinical Instructor, Department of Family Medicine,
University of Colorado, Denver, CO, USA
e-mail: andrea.auxier@valueoptions.com

B.F. Miller, Psy.D.
Director of the Office of Integrated Health Care Research and Policy Department of Family Medicine, University of Colorado Denver School of Medicine, Denver, CO, USA
e-mail: Benjamin.miller@ucdenver.edu

J. Rogers, M.D., MPH, MEd
Professor and Executive Vice Chair of Family and Community Medicine
Baylor College of Medicine, 3701 Kirby Dr., Suite 600, Houston, TX 77098, USA
e-mail: jrogers@bcm.edu

M.R. Talen and A. Burke Valeras (eds.), *Integrated Behavioral Health in Primary Care:*
Evaluating the Evidence, Identifying the Essentials, DOI 10.1007/978-1-4614-6889-9_3,
© Springer Science+Business Media New York 2013

It has been known for some time that behavioral health (BH) and primary care are inseparable (deGruy, 1996). Systematic reviews have concluded that integration of BH into primary care leads to improved health outcomes (Blount, 2003; Butler et al., 2008; Craven & Bland, 2006), and it has been recognized for decades that the primary care function of "comprehensively meeting all health needs" is a behavioral health issue (deGruy, 1996). The President's Commission on Mental Health has highlighted an unmet need for the linking data on the prevalence of mental disorders with national data on the use of mental health services. Provisional estimates indicate that at least 15 % of the US population is affected by mental disorders in one year (Kessler, Demler et al., 2005).

Because the vast majority of the public with a BH or substance use issue is seen only in primary care (Kessler, Berglund et al., 2005; Regier et al., 1993), the need to provide whole-person quality care to ever-growing numbers of patients has motivated primary care practices throughout the country to turn their attention and efforts toward integrating BH into their standard service-delivery (Blount, 1998; Blount & Bayona, 1994; Coyne, Schwenk, & Fechner-Bates, 1995). However, the profound fragmentation of the US health care system continues to present additional challenges for patients with multiple medical problems complicated by BH, substance use, and/or health behaviors (Hoffman, Rice, & Sung, 1996; Simon et al., 2001; Simon, VonKorff, & Barlow, 1995). Unfortunately, the forced division of BH from the rest of health care yields unsatisfying and expensive care, generating avoidable suffering and premature death (Lurie, Manheim, & Dunlop, 2009). The PCMH offers a critical opportunity to transform patient care, especially for patients who present with BH conditions in addition to their medical conditions (American Academy of Family Physicians (AAFP), American Academy of Pediatrics (AAP), American College of Physicians (ACP), & American Osteopathic Association (AOA), 2007; Kessler, Stafford, & Messier, 2009; Petterson et al., 2008; Rittenhouse & Shortell, 2009). This is particularly true for problems associated with chronic disease (Bodenheimer, Wagner, & Grumbach, 2002; Hwang, Weller, Ireys, & Anderson, 2001; Lurie et al., 2009; Moussavi et al., 2007).

Despite the potential benefits of the PCMH, the process involved in becoming a PCMH is a cumbersome one. The TransforMed National Demonstration Project (NDP) stated, "Creating a PCMH is much more than a sum of implementing discrete model components. Such transformation is exceedingly difficult, and those who attempt it are heroic" (Stewart, Jaen, Crabtree, Miller, & Stange, 2009). It is important to understand from the outset that the accreditation process is rigorous out of necessity. Practice transformation of this magnitude demands leadership, teamwork, and the participation of individuals from all levels of an organization. The scope of assessment is broad, requiring attention to clinical considerations, practice workflows, data collection and tracking, and information technology.

There are currently several recognition programs with similar philosophies but slightly different emphases. All focus on benchmarking and performance measurement regardless of whether the medical home is a medical practice or community mental health center that provides medical services. They currently include the National Committee for Quality Assurance (NCQA), the Accreditation Association for

Ambulatory Health Care (AAAHC), the Joint Commission (JCAHO), and the Utilization Review Accreditation Committee (URAC). The National Quality Forum (NQF) offers a survey tool developed by NCQA and JCAHO. Since JCAHO and NQF are based on NCQA standards, this chapter will review NCQA, AAAHC, and URAC.

Background of the Medical Home Model

The following section will summarize the history of the PCMH concept with an emphasis on key developments that have driven its evolution. In addition, selections from the Patient Protection and Affordable Care Act (PPACA) will be offered as examples of where the PCMH approach fits in current health care policy and in the national debate on health.

In 1967, The Council on Pediatric Practice of the American Academy of Pediatrics (AAP) released its Standards of Child Care report, stating: "For children with chronic diseases or disabling conditions, the lack of a complete record and a 'medical home' is a major deterrent to adequate health supervision. Wherever the child is cared for, the question should be asked, 'Where is the child's medical home?' and any pertinent information should be transmitted to that place" (Sia, Tonniges, Osterhus, & Taba, 2004).

The AAP's definition was refined in 1992: "The AAP believes that the medical care of infants, children, and adolescents ideally should be accessible, continuous, comprehensive, family centered, coordinated, and compassionate. It should be delivered or directed by well-trained physicians who are able to manage or facilitate essentially all aspects of pediatric care. The physician should be known to the child and family and should be able to develop a relationship of mutual responsibility and trust with them. These characteristics define the 'medical home' and describe the care that has traditionally been provided by pediatricians in an office setting" (Sia et al., 2004).

In 2004, the American Academy of Family Physicians (AAFP) released its Future of Family Medicine report. The report described a "change in orientation from the traditional model of family medicine to the New Model" that included enhanced patient access to care with the goal of securing a personal medical home for every American. The personal medical home was intended to serve as the "focal point through which all individuals—regardless of age, sex, race, or socioeconomic status—receive a basket of acute, chronic, and preventive medical care services." Care was envisioned as "not only accessible but also accountable, comprehensive, integrated, patient-centered, safe, scientifically valid, and satisfying to both patients and their physicians" (Future of Family Medicine Project Leadership Committee, 2004).

In 2006, the American College of Physicians (ACP) highlighted the longitudinal intent of the medical home philosophy by proposing the Advanced Medical Home: "The advanced medical home acknowledges that the best quality of care is provided not in episodic, illness-oriented, complaint-based care—but through patient-centered, physician-guided, cost-efficient, longitudinal care that encompasses and values both the art and science of medicine. An attribute of the advanced medical home is promotion of continuous healing relationships through delivery of care in a variety of care settings according to the needs of the patient and skills of the medical provider" (Barr & Ginsburg, 2006).

One year earlier, the US technology company, IBM, had begun to question the very foundation of the health care it was buying, and had reached a significant conclusion: when compared to other industrialized countries, US health care fails to deliver comprehensive primary care because of the way primary care is financed. Noting that primary care is the only entity charged with the longitudinal care of the whole patient, and that it is the primary care relationship that has the most profound effect on health care outcomes, IBM, together with several other large national employers, helped create the Patient-Centered Primary Care Collaborative (PCPCC) in 2006.

The PCPCC's primary objective was to reach out to the ACP, the AAFP, and other primary care physician groups in order to (1) facilitate improvements in patient-physician relations, and (2) create a more effective and efficient model of health care delivery (PCPCC, 2011). Since then, the PCPCC has become one of the major developers and advocates of the PCMH model in the USA. Its membership includes a number of large national employers, most of the major primary care physician associations, health benefits companies, trade associations, profession/affinity groups, academic centers, and health care quality improvement associations. The PCPCC has created an open forum where health care stakeholders freely communicate and work together to improve the future of the American health care system. It has also developed model language for inclusion in health reform proposals to include the PCMH concept, and acts as a key source for the continued education of congressional representatives, federal and state governments, and individual practices on the PCMH model as a "superior form of health care delivery" (PCPCC).

In 2007, the American Academy of Family Physicians (AAFP), American Academy of Pediatrics (AAP), American College of Physicians (ACP), and American Osteopathic Association (AOA) released the Joint Principles of the patient-centered medical home: "The Patient-Centered Medical Home (PCMH) is an approach to providing comprehensive primary care for children, youth and adults. The PCMH is a health care setting that facilitates partnerships between individual patients, and their personal physicians, and when appropriate, the patient's family" (AAFP, 2007). The Joint Principles are described in Table 3.1.

The Joint Principles of the PCMH are a natural extension of the foundational features of primary care: "Important functions of primary care include serving as the first point of contact for all new health needs and problems; delivering long-term, person-focused care; comprehensively meeting all health needs except those whose rarity renders it impossible for a generalist to maintain competence in them; and coordinating care that must be received elsewhere" (Blount, 1998). According to Blount, these functions parallel the original definition of the modern family physician: "The central elements of this definition were that a modern family physician would do the following: (1) serve as the patient's personal physician and provide entry to the health care system, (2) provide a comprehensive set of evaluative, preventive, and general medical services, (3) maintain continuing responsibility for the patient,

Table 3.1 Joint Principles of the patient-centered medical home (AAFP, 2007)

Principle 1: Personal Physician
Each patient has an ongoing relationship with a personal physician trained to provide first contact, continuous and comprehensive care

Principle 2: Physician-Directed Medical Practice
The personal physician leads a team of individuals at the practice level who collectively take responsibility for the ongoing care of patients

Principle 3: Whole-Person Orientation
The personal physician is responsible for providing for all the patient's health care needs or taking responsibility for appropriately arranging care with other qualified professionals. This includes care for all stages of life: acute care; chronic care

Principle 4: Care is Coordinated and/or Integrated
- Across all elements of the complex health care system (e.g., subspecialty care, hospitals, home health agencies, nursing homes) and the patient's community (e.g., family, public and private community-based services)
- Care is facilitated by registries, information technology, health information exchange, and other means to assure that patients get the indicated care when and where they need and want it in a culturally and linguistically appropriate manner

Principle 5: Quality and Safety
- Practices advocate for their patients to support the attainment of optimal, patient-centered outcomes that are defined by a care planning process driven by a compassionate, robust partnership between physicians, patients, and the patient's family
- Evidence-based medicine and clinical decision-support tools guide decision-making
- Physicians in the practice accept accountability for continuous quality improvement through voluntary engagement in performance measurement and improvement
- Patients actively participate in decision-making and feedback is sought to ensure patients' expectations are being met
- Information technology is utilized appropriately to support optimal patient care, performance measurement, patient education, and enhanced communication
- Practices go through a voluntary recognition process by an appropriate nongovernmental entity to demonstrate that they have the capabilities to provide patient-centered services consistent with the medical home model
- Patients and families participate in quality improvement activities at the practice level

Principle 6: Enhanced Access
Available through systems such as open scheduling, expanded hours and new options for communication between patients, their personal physician, and practice staff

Principle 7: Payment
- Should allow for separate fee-for-service payments for face-to-face visits. (Payments for care management services that fall outside of the face-to-face visit, as described above, should not result in a reduction in the payments for face-to-face visits.)
- Should recognize case mix differences in the patient population being treated within the practice
- Should allow physicians to share in savings from reduced hospitalizations associated with physician-guided care management in the office setting
- Should allow for additional payments for achieving measurable and continuous quality improvements

including necessary coordination of care and referral, (4) practice in a manner both sensitive and responsive to community concerns and needs, and (5) provide care appropriate to the patient's physical, emotional, and social needs, in the context of family and community" ((Blount, 1998). In January 2011, the Joint Principles for the Medical Education of Physicians as Preparation for Practice in the Patient-Centered Medical Home were released. The principles will guide medical school curricula in ensuring that all physicians, regardless of their specialty choice, will have the expertise to practice in a "reformed health care delivery system based on the patient-centered medical home" (AAFP, 2007).

In 2010, the Patient Protection and Affordable Care Act (PPACA) further established the medical home as the model for primary care in health care reform, defining the medical home as one that includes:

- Personal physicians or other primary care providers
- Whole-person orientation
- Coordinated and integrated care
- Safe and high quality care through evidenced informed medicine, appropriate use of health information technology, and continuous quality improvements
- Expanded access to care and
- Payment that recognizes added value from additional components of patient-centered care (Goodson, 2010)

PPACA also established a number of initiatives aligned with the medical home concept: providing coverage through a qualified direct primary care medical home plan, ensuring quality of care, rewarding quality through market-based incentives, establishing community health teams, supporting primary care training, and establishing a primary care extension program. Moreover, it commented specifically on issues relevant to this book, supporting "patient-centered medical home, team management of chronic disease, and interprofessional integrated models of health care that incorporate transitions in health care settings and integration of physical and mental health provision" (Kessler, Demler et al., 2005). Integration of physical and behavioral health care in the medical home, as promoted in PPACA, is consistent with prior efforts to improve care for mental health problems, since only 28 % of individuals suffering from psychiatric disorders seek care from mental health specialists (Hoffman et al., 1996).

Accreditation

National Committee for Quality Assurance (NCQA)

In 2003, the NCQA initiated the Physician Practice Connections (PPC) Recognition Program with support from The Robert Wood Johnson Foundation, the Commonwealth Fund, and Bridges to Excellence. The purpose of the program was to use "systematic process and information technology to enhance the quality of patient care" (National Committee for Quality Assurance [NCQA], 2010). In 2008, the ACP, the AAFP, the AAP, and the AOA joined forces to inform the creation of the PPC-PCMH standards. The standards were based on the Joint Principles outlined earlier in this chapter, and delineated specific requirements for recognition. The standards were intended to operationalize the core values of the PCMH in a way that could be captured and demonstrated through IT-driven practice-management

Table 3.2 Timeline of key events leading up to PCMH 2011 standards

2003: PPC Recognition Program

NCQA program to identify practices that use systematic processes and information technology to enhance the quality of patient care

2005: AAFP creates TransforMED

Creates funding opportunities for primary care centers to develop PCMH practices

2008: PPC-PCMH Standards

A standardized way to categorize primary care practices and how closely they align with the PCMH

2008: NQF Report

25 % of 514 endorsed standards apply to primary care. NCQA PCMH recognition requires reporting on at least 10 of these measures

2009: ARRA

Included $20 billion for health care information technology

2009: HITECH Act

Signed into law to promote adoption and meaningful use of health information technology

2010: CMS Final Rule

Outlined meaningful use requirements that reward clinicians for using HIT to improve health care quality

2011: PCMH 2011 Standards (New Draft Standards)

Updated PCMH standards better reflecting aspects of health care delivery other than HIT

efforts. Financial incentives were offered through various health plans and employers, and pilot projects were sponsored at both federal and state levels. Sustainability for these projects would ultimately depend on the ability to measure and demonstrate cost and quality outcomes as well as patient and provider satisfaction through formal evaluation processes (Stanek & Takach, 2010).

In 2011, the PPC-PCMH standards were revised to align with other health care developments evolving simultaneously (NCQA, 2011). The first of these was Meaningful Use (MU), a movement that grew out of the National Quality Forum's (NQF) 2008 report that identified a set of national priorities focused on performance improvement in health care (National Quality Forum [NQF], 2011). The priorities identified were: patient engagement, reduction of racial disparities, improved safety, increased efficiency, coordination of care, and improved population health. In 2009, the Health Information Technology for Economic and Clinical Health (HITECH) Act highlighted the centrality of using electronic health record (EHR) data and functionality to track and report data elements considered to be demonstrative of these principles for the purposes of continuous quality improvement and improved patient health (Health Information Technology for Economic and Clinical Health Act, 2011). This initiative became known as "meaningful use (MU)." Also in 2009, the Centers for Medicare and Medicaid Services (CMS) implemented the American Recovery and Reinvestment Act (ARRA, 2011). The act provided incentive payments to eligible providers for adopting and demonstrating meaningful use of EHR technology certified through the Certification Commission for Health Information Technology (CCHIT, 2011). In mid-2010, CMS released a Final Rule detailing MU requirements that reward clinicians for using Health Information Technology (HIT) to improve quality (Centers for Medicare and Medicaid Services [CMS], 2011). Table 3.2 summarizes the timeline for these developments.

Table 3.3 2011 and 2008 PCMH standards

Standard	2011 PCMH standards	2008 standards (PPC-PCMH)
1	Enhance Access & Continuity	Access & Communication
2	Identify & Manage Patient Populations	Patient Tracking & Registry Function
3	Plan and Manage Care	Care Management
4	Provide Self-Care Support & Community Resources	Patient Self-Management Support
5	Track and Coordinate Care	Electronic Prescribing
6	Measure and Improve Performance	Test Tracking
7		Referral Tracking
8		Performance Reporting Improvement
9		Advanced Electronic Communications

The 2011 original nine standards have been reduced to six and differ from the pre-2011 standards in significant ways. In addition to aligning with CMS and MU requirements, they emphasize integrating behavioral health care and care management, include patient surveys, and emphasize the involvement of patients and families in quality improvement. The clause, "to integrate behaviors affecting health, mental health and substance abuse" has been added to the goals and specified through PCMH Standard 1 (depression screening for adolescents and adults), PCMH Standard 3 (one of three clinically important conditions identified by the practice must be a condition related to unhealthy behaviors or a mental health or substance abuse condition), and PCMH Standard 5 (track referrals and coordinate care with mental health and substance abuse services) (NCQA, 2011). Table 3.3 lists both the 2008 and 2011 standards.

Practices must provide defined standards or policies and demonstrate performance monitoring against the standards they have defined. Each of the six standards contains a Must-Pass Element, defined earning a score of 50 % or higher on each element and passing all six elements, to achieve NCQA recognition. Some of the elements contain critical factors, identified as those that are "central to the concept being assessed within a particular element" (NCQA, 2011). Critical factors must be met in order for practices to receive any score on the element.

Practices receive a final ranging from 0 to100, with Levels of recognitions based on those scores as follows:

Level 1	35–59 points and all six must-pass elements
Level 2	60–84 points and all six must-pass elements
Level 3	85–100 points and all six must-pass elements

However, simply passing the Must-Pass Elements only adds up to 29 points, so practices must also pass other elements in order to qualify for recognition. Once granted, recognition is valid for three years.

As stated earlier, the 2011 standards of PCMH align with CMS MU specifications. These contain a core set of 15 requirements and five of 10 menu requirements that must include the capability to submit electronic data to immunization registries/

Table 3.4 PCMH 2011 elements targeting behavioral health

PCMH 2: Identify and Manage Patient Populations	Examples of Behavioral Health and PCMH 2011 Principles
PCMH 3: Plan and Manage Care Element A: Implement Evidence-Based Guidelines through point of care reminders for patients with: 3. The third condition, related to unhealthy behaviors or mental health or substance abuse *To receive a 50 % or 100 % score, at least one identified condition must be related to #3 (obesity, smoking, drug addiction, alcoholism, depression, anxiety, ADHD)* **PCMH 4: Provide Self-Care Support and Community Resources** Element B: Provide Referrals to Community Resources 3. Arranges or provides treatment for mental health and substance abuse disorders	It is Mrs. P's fourth visit in the month. Complaints include insomnia, fatigue, and vague chest pain. As part of her routine care, Mrs. P has also been screened for depression, with negative results. This time, in addition to inquiring about her physical symptoms, Dr. M requests an intervention from the behavioral health provider (BHP). The BHP administers a screening for posttraumatic stress disorder, which is positive. The BHP encourages Mrs. P to follow up for continued treatment. At the end of the visit, Mrs. P suddenly reveals that she is currently in an abusive relationship. After taking reasonable steps to ensure Mrs. P is in no imminent danger, the BHP refers her to the Domestic Violence Crisis Center for housing assistance and legal services. In addition, he schedules an appointment for the following week for further assessment of Mrs. P's trauma symptoms.

information systems or the capability to submit electronic surveillance data to public health agencies. Although NCQA added the integration of behaviors affecting health, mental health, and substance abuse to its stated goals in the 2011 standards, it is worth noting that none of the must-pass elements focus on behavioral health. Behavioral health is addressed in some of the non-must-pass elements, however, as detailed in Table 3.4.

Of the 152 possible factors listed, only 6 specifically target behavioral health (Element 2C, Factors 6–9; Element 3A, Factor 3; and Element 4B, Factor 3). Of these, Element 3A, Factor 3 is arguably the most significant since it requires practices to: (a) identify a behavioral health, substance abuse, or an unhealthy behavior condition as its "third important condition" and (b) design care management services targeting that condition. In other words, if a practice chooses depression as its behavioral health condition, it would also have to comply with Element 3C (Care Management), a Must-Pass Element that calls for practice to demonstrate management of at least 75 % of the patients identified in Element 3A (third important condition) as well as 3B (high-risk patients). As a Must-Pass Element, at least three of the seven factors must be present to achieve PCMH status. While behavioral health can theoretically satisfy the requirements of other elements and factors such as Element 3B or Element 1E, Factor 1 (coordinating patient care across multiple settings), a behavioral health emphasis, is not necessary. (For more detailed information on the operational requirements for the third most important condition and high-risk/complex patient groups, please see Appendix A.)

Application fees to become a PCMH are determined by the number of providers in a practice. Survey Tool Licenses include an $80 flat fee and Application Fees range

Table 3.5 AAAHC accreditation criteria

Standards	Definitions
Relationships	Including communication, understanding, and collaboration between the patient and physician, or the physician-directed health care team
Continuity of Care	Including the requirement that more than 50 % of a patient's visits are with the same physician/physician team
Comprehensiveness of Care	Including preventive, wellness, and end-of-life care in addition to acute and chronic care services
Accessibility	Including written standards to support patient access, routine assessment of patients' perceptions of access, on-call coverage and patient information on how to obtain medical care at any time
Quality of Care	Including care that is physician directed, incorporates evidence-based guidelines and performance measures in the delivery of clinical services

from \$450 for a solo practice to \$2,700 + \$10/number>100 for practices with more than 100 providers. A 20 % discount is offered to applicants sponsored by health plans, employers, and other programs. The discount applies when practices have fewer than 15 physicians and the sponsor has 10 or more applications in a market area within a 12-month period. Practices with a Level 1 or Level 2 designation can apply for an add-on survey discounted at the 50 % level of the standard application fees. Multi-site group survey pricing is also available for qualifying practices.

Accreditation Association for Ambulatory Health Care (AAAHC)

The AAAHC is private, nonprofit organization formed in 1979 that "develops standards to advance and promote patient safety, quality, and value for ambulatory health care through peer based accreditation processes, education, and research" (Accreditation Association for Ambulatory Health Care [AAAHC], 2011). It is currently the only agency to offer on-site certification surveys for PCMH. Standards are delineated in the Medical Home On-site Certification Handbook, and applicants must contact the Assistant Director of Accreditation Services before completing application. As defined by the Accreditation Association standards, a medical home is the primary point of care for patients. Organizations that choose to include medical home accreditation as part of their survey will be assessed according to the criteria in Table 3.5.

Utilization Review Accreditation Committee (URAC)

URAC is an independent, nonprofit organization founded in the late 1980s to "promote continuous improvement in the quality and efficiency of health care management through processes of accreditation and education." URAC defines a

Patient-Centered Health Care Home (PCHCH) as one that "provides comprehensive and individualized access to physical health, behavioral health, and supportive community and social services, ensuring patients receive the right care in the right setting at the right time." It offers over twenty-five accreditation and certification programs and has recently developed a series of three Program Toolkits based on ten guiding PCHCH Principles (URAC, 2011).

1. Patient-centered care culture
2. Appropriate access to care
3. Individualized care planning
4. Effective and timely care coordination and follow-up
5. Eliminating health care disparities
6. Promoting care quality and continuous quality
7. Stewarding the cost-effective use of health care resources
8. Excellence in customer service
9. Commitment to transparency
10. PCHCH infrastructure and operations

While not technically a recognition program, the toolkits include practice assessment standards, performance measures information resources, and survey information resources designed to help practices transform themselves into health care homes.

Summary of PCMH Research

In 2010, the PCPCC published a report summarizing the results of the reviewed evidence from controlled patient-centered medical home initiatives throughout the country that contained outcome data on service utilization and costs (Grumbach & Grundy, 2010). The main findings are summarized in Table 3.6.

In 2010, TransforMED led the country's first National Demonstration Project (NDP) by comparing facilitated and self-directed implementation approaches in a group randomized clinical trial utilizing 36 family practices located in 25 states over a 26-month evaluation period (Crabtree et al., 2010). Practice sizes ranged from solo to greater than seven primary care physicians. Adoption of model components during the NDP was associated with improved access for patients, with better prevention, Ambulatory Care Quality Alliance (ACQA), and chronic disease care scores. Despite these successes, there was no improvement in patient-rated outcomes for health status, satisfaction with service relationship, patient empowerment, comprehensive care, coordination of care, personal relationship over time, or global practice experience. The authors noted that implementing a PCMH model might actually worsen patients' perception of care: "Amidst the substantial practice, personal, and financial challenges practices face, it is easy to lose the patient at the center of the PCMH" (p. S81). Overall, the results of the NDP indicated that transformation into a PCMH will take time, and must include attention to improved communication among practice members, leadership, and an intense amount of resource allocation.

Table 3.6 Summary of 2011 PCPCC report findings on PCMH project outcomes

Type of collaborative health care system	Health care systems	Outcomes
Integrated Delivery Systems		
	WA: Group Health Cooperative	➢ $10 PMPM reduction in total costs
		➢ 16 % reduction in hospital admissions
		➢ $14 PMPM reduction in inpatient hospital costs
		➢ 29 % reduction in ER use
	PA: Geisinger Health System Proven Health Navigator PCMH Model	➢ $4 PMPM reduction in ER costs
		➢ 18 % reduction in hospital admissions
		➢ 7 % reduction in total PMPM costs
	MN, IA, ND, SD, NE: VA & VA Midwest Health Care Network	➢ $593 PP cost savings using CDM model versus UC
		➢ 27 % lower hospitalization and ER visits for CDM model
	MN: HealthPartners Medical Group BestCare PCMH Model	➢ 39 % decrease in ER visits
		➢ 24 % decrease in hospital admissions per enrollee
	MN, IA, ND, SD, NE: VA & VA Midwest Health Care Network	➢ Enrollee costs decreased from 100 % to 92 % of state average
		➢ Reduced hospitalizations 31.8 % versus 34.7 % for controls
		➢ Among diabetics, 30.5 % versus 39.2 % for controls
		➢ $640 reduction PPPY, $1,650 among highest risk patients
Private Payer Sponsored		
	BlueCross BlueShield of South Carolina-Palmetto Primary Care Physicians	➢ 10.4 % reduction in inpatient hospital days per 1,000 enrollees per year
		➢ Inpatient days 36.3 % lower
	BlueCross BlueShield of North Dakota-MeritCare Health System	➢ 6 % reduction in hospital admissions
		➢ 24 % reduction ER visits; Increase of 45 % and 3 %, respectively, in control group
		➢ Total annual expenditures per PCMH went from $5,661 to $7,433 versus from $5,868 to $10,108 for controls

FL: Metropolitan Health Networks-Humana
➤ Hospital days per 1,000 enrollees dropped by 4.6 % compared to 36 % increase for controls
➤ Hospital admissions per 1,000 enrollees dropped by 3 % with readmissions 6 % below Medicare benchmarks
➤ ER expenses rose 4.5 % versus 17.4 % for controls
➤ Pharmacy expenses rose 6.5 % versus 14.5 % for controls
➤ Diagnostic imaging expense decreased by 9.8 % versus 10.7 % increase for controls
➤ Overall medical expense rose 5.2 % compared to 26.3 % for controls

Medicaid Sponsored

Community Care of North Carolina
➤ Cumulative savings of $974.5 million over 6 years
➤ 40 % decrease in hospitalizations for asthma
➤ 16 % reduction in ER visit rate

Colorado Medicaid and SCHIP
➤ Lower costs for PCMH children, $785 versus $1,000
➤ $2,275 versus $3,404 in children with chronic conditions

Other Programs

MD: Johns Hopkins Guided Care PCMH model
➤ 24 % reduction in total hospital inpatient days
➤ 15 % fewer ER visits
➤ 37 % reduction in skilled nursing facility days

MI: Genessee Health Plan
➤ 50 % decrease in ER visits
➤ 15 % fewer inpatient hospitalizations
➤ Total hospital days 26.6 % lower than competitors

NY: Erie County PCMH Model
➤ Estimated savings of $1 million per 1,000 enrollees due to decreased duplication of services and tests, and lowered hospitalization rates

IN: Geriatric Resources for Assessment and Care of Elders
➤ Lower ER utilization and hospitalization

PMPM per member per month, *PPPY* per patient per year, *PP* per patient, *CDM* chronic disease management, *UC* usual care

The authors also point out the inherent contradiction in PCMH philosophy, namely, that while the PCMH envisions collaborative team-based care, its physician-directed principle continues to maintain the status quo. The whole-person orientation principle states that the personal physician is responsible for providing all of the patient's health care needs or for arranging care with other qualified professionals (AAFP, 2007). This is less constraining than the original clause that read, "The physician-led team is responsible for providing all the patient's health care needs, and, when needed, arranges for appropriate care with other qualified physicians" (NCQA, 2010). Having a physician to be responsible for the management of these patients in this fashion is an impossible standard. How feasible is it for one physician to provide for all of a patient's health care needs or to arrange for such care in the absence of an organizational structure that supports and facilitates such care? The authors of the NDP report also emphasize that most PCMH models do not explicitly include behavioral health even though the continued separation of mental from physical contradicts the core values PCMH is designed to espouse. Of the 31 practices providing data on the subject, 16 had some degree of behavioral health care available to patients at baseline. By the end of the NDP, only three of the 12 remaining sites had implemented behavioral health care (Nutting et al., 2010). Although the 2011 standards make some progress in this direction by incorporating mental health and substance abuse, they do not explicitly mention behavioral health providers for the provision of these services. The language remains physician centered by directing physicians to provide the treatment themselves or to arrange for its provision, even though studies show that most patients receiving referrals to specialty mental health do not follow through with the referrals (Cunningham, 2009; NCQA, 2011; Smith et al., 2003).

In addition to the NDP, individual states, recognizing the potential for health care reform, have begun using the PCMH as a platform for redesign. With an eye on bending the cost curve, many states have considered the role that a medical home can have in providing higher quality care at a lower cost. States leading the way with their medical home innovation include Vermont and North Carolina (Bachman et al. (2006); Mechanic (1999).

Governor Douglas formally launched the Vermont Blueprint for Health in 2003 in an attempt to decrease the cost of individuals with chronic disease. The Blueprint has expanded over the years where an increasing number of practices are designated as patient-centered medical homes (known as Advanced Primary Care Practices or APCPs in Vermont). The APCPs are the centers of the Blueprint's health care delivery. Building off the principle that primary care should be the center of a system that coordinates care seamlessly, the Blueprint has placed significant emphasis on practices achieving NCQA designation as a patient-centered medical home.

In addition to becoming a PCMH, the Blueprint asks practices to form Community Health Teams (CHT), a group of multidisciplinary teams, responsible for helping patients in their respective communities work on their health care. The CHTs operate as extensions to the APCPs. The end goal for the Blueprint is comprehensive, coordinated care whereby patients can have all their needs met in their medical home. Results from the Blueprint have been impressive, and can be found in the 2011 Vermont Blueprint for Health Annual Report.

Similar to Vermont, North Carolina has also developed several activities around the PCMH. Community Care of North Carolina, the North Carolina Center of Excellence for Integrated Care, and I-3 are working examples of health care innovation in the state.

Both Vermont and North Carolina have recently been included in the federal government's investigation of the PCMH. In 2010, CMS offered states the opportunity to apply for the Multi-Payer Advanced Primary Care Practice Demonstration project. The purpose of this demonstration was to evaluate whether the advanced primary care practice (read patient-centered medical homes), when supported by Medicare, Medicaid, and private health plans, will (1) reduce unjustified variation in utilization and expenditures; (2) improve the safety, effectiveness, timeliness, and efficiency of health care; (3) increase the ability of beneficiaries to participate in decisions concerning their care; (4) increase the availability and delivery of care that is consistent with evidence-based guidelines in historically underserved areas; and (5) reduce unjustified variation in utilization and expenditures under the Medicare program. Eight states—Maine, Vermont, Rhode Island, New York, Pennsylvania, North Carolina, Michigan, and Minnesota—were selected to participate in this Multi-Payer Advanced Primary Care Practice Demonstration ultimately leading to approximately 1,200 medical homes serving up to 1 million Medicare beneficiaries. While this program has just recently begun, it is another opportunity to see the PCMH in action and how states choose to address or not address mental health.

In May, 2011, the Department of Health and Human Services invited Federally Qualified Health Centers (FQHCs) throughout the Country to participate in the Medicare Federally Qualified Health Center Advanced Primary Care Practice Demonstration (FQHC APCP) Project announced by President Obama in 2009. The three-year demonstration will evaluate the effect of the PCMH model on Medicare beneficiaries served by FQHCs. CMS and HRSA will provide technical assistance to participating practices, and HRSA will provide a fee for each eligible Medicare beneficiary.

Summary

The goal of this chapter was to offer the reader an introduction to the Patient-Centered Medical Home and the importance of understanding the principles, accreditation criteria, and research efforts that provide its infrastructure. As the functionally transformative redesign of primary care, the PCMH provides a unique opportunity to address behavioral health in a more coordinated and comprehensive way. While there are several ways to measure the PCMH, they all remain consistent in their recognition that a more tightly coordinated primary care system is needed. Additionally, with the passage of the Patient Protection and Affordable Care Act, there is more of an impetus to place primary care at the front and center of any and all conversations pertaining to health care. The medical home without attention to the inseparable nature of mind and body will simply perpetuate fragmentation of the health care system, and will remain a house under construction.

Appendix A. NCQA Important Conditions and High-Risk/Complex Patient Groups

PCMH 3: Plan and Manage Care
Element A: Implement Evidence-Based Guidelines
The practice implements evidence-based guidelines through point-of-care reminders for patients with: 1. The first important condition * 2. The second important condition 3. The third condition, related to unhealthy behaviors or mental health or substance abuse
Element B: Identify High-Risk/Complex Patients
1. Establishes criteria and a systematic process to identify high-risk or complex patients 2. Determines percentage of these in its population

Important conditions and high-risk/complex patients are those identified for the Medical Record Review. It requires the following for the three important and high-risk/complex patient groups:
 	
    ➤ PCMH 3, Element C: Care Management (MUST PASS)
    ➤ PCMH 4, Element A: Self-Care Process (MUST PASS)

Element C: Care Management
The care team performs the following for at least 75% of the patients identified in Element A (important conditions) and B (high-risk/complex patients): 1. Previsit preparations. 2. Collaborative treatment plan including treatment goals updated at each relevant visit. 3. Gives patient/family written plan of care. 4. Assesses and addresses barriers when treatment goals are not reached. 5. Clinical summaries given to patient at each relevant visit. 6. Ientifies patients/families who might benefit from additional care management support. 7. Follows up with patients/families who have not kept important appointments.

Element D: Medication Management

The practice manages medications in the following ways:

1. Reviews and reconciles medications with patients/families for more than 50% of care transitions.**
2. Reviews and reconciles medications with patients/families for more than 80% of care transitions.
3. Provides information about new prescriptions for more than 80% of patients/families.
4. Assesses patient/family understanding of medications for more than 50% of patients.
5. Assesses patient response to medications and barriers to adherence for more than 50% of patients.
6. Documents over-the-counter medications, herbal therapies and supplements for more than 50% of patients/families, with the date of updates.

PCMH 4: Provide Self-Care and Community Resources
Element A: Support Self-Care Process

The practice conducts activities to support patients/families in self-management for patients identified in PCMH 3, Elements A (Important Conditions) and B (High-Risk/Complex):

1. Educational resources for at least 50% of patients.
2. Uses an EHR to identify patient-specific education resources and provide them to more than 10% of patients.
3. Develops and documents self-management plans and goals in collaboration with at least 50% of patients/families.
4. Documents self-management abilities for at least 50% of patients/families.
5. Provides self-management tools to record self-care results for at least 50% of patients/families.
6. Counsels at least 50% of patients/families to adopt healthy behaviors.

*Core Meaningful Use Requirement

**Menu Meaningful Use Requirement

References

Accreditation Association for Ambulatory Health Care. (2011). AAAHC. Retrieved February 22, 2011, from http://www.aaahc.org/eweb/dynamicpage.aspx?site=aaahc_site&webcode=about_aaahc

American Academy of Family Physicians (AAFP), American Academy of Pediatrics (AAP), American College of Physicians (ACP), & American Osteopathic Association (AOA). (2007). *Joint principles of the patient-centered medical home*. Retrieved August 13, 2009, from http://www.medicalhomeinfo.org/Joint%20Statement.pdf

American Recovery and Reinvestment Act. (2011). ARRA. Retrieved February 10, 2011, from http://frwebgate.access.gpo.gov/cgi-in/getdoc.cgi?dbname=111_cong_bills&docid=f:h1enr.pdf

Bachman, J., Pincus, H. A., Houtsinger, J. K., & Unutzer, J. (2006). Funding mechanisms for depression care management: opportunities and challenges. [Research Support, N.I.H., Extramural Research Support, Non-U.S. Gov't]. *General Hospital Psychiatry, 28*(4), 278–288. doi:10.1016/j.genhosppsych.2006.03.006.

Barr, M., & Ginsburg, J. (2006). *The advanced medical home: A patient-centered, physician-guided model of health care.* Retrieved April, 25, 2011, from http://www.acponline.org/advocacy/where_we_stand/policy/adv_med.pdf

Blount, A. (Ed.). (1998). *Integrated primary care: The future of medical and mental health collaboration.* New York: Norton.

Blount, A. (2003). Integrated primary care: Organizing the evidence. *Families, Systems & Health, 21*(2), 121–133.

Blount, A., & Bayona, J. (1994). Toward a system of integrated primary care. *Families Systems Medicine, 12,* 171–182.

Bodenheimer, T., Wagner, E. H., & Grumbach, K. (2002). Improving primary care for patients with chronic illness: The chronic care model, Part 2. *JAMA: The Journal of the American Medical Association, 288*(15), 1909–1914. doi:10.1001/jama.288.15.1909.

Butler, M., Kane, R. L., McAlpin, D., Kathol, R. G., Fu, S. S., Hagedorn, H., et al. (2008). *Integration of mental health/substance abuse and primary care* No. 173 (Prepared by the Minnesota Evidence-based Practice Center under Contract No. 290-02-0009.) AHRQ Publication No. 09-E003. Rockville, MD: Agency for Healthcare Research and Quality.

Centers for Medicare and Medicaid Services. (2011). *Electronic health record incentive program; final rule.* Retrieved February 22, 2011, from http://edocket.access.gpo.gov/2010/pdf/2010-17207.pdf

Certification Commission for Health Information Technology. (2011). CCHIT. Retrieved February 10, 2011, from http://www.cchit.org/

Coyne, J. C., Schwenk, T. L., & Fechner-Bates, S. (1995). Nondetection of depression by primary care physicians reconsidered. [Research Support, U.S. Gov't, P.H.S.]. *General Hospital Psychiatry, 17*(1), 3–12.

Crabtree, B., Nutting, P. A., Miller, W. L., Stange, K. C., Stewart, E., & Jaen, C. R. (2010). Summary of the national demonstration project and recommendations for the patient-centered medical home. *Annals of Family Medicine, 8*(S1), S80–S90.

Craven, M., & Bland, R. (2006). Better practices in collaborative mental health care: An analysis of the evidence base. *Canadian Journal of Psychiatry, 51,* 7S–72S.

Cunningham, P. J. (2009). Beyond parity: Primary care physicians' perspectives on access to mental health care. *Health Affairs, 28*(3), w490–w501.

deGruy, F. (1996). Mental health care in the primary care setting. In M. S. Donaldson, K. D. Yordy, K. N. Lohr, & N. A. Vanselow (Eds.), *Primary care: America's health in a new era.* Washington, DC: Institute of Medicine.

Future of Family Medicine Project Leadership Committee. (2004). The future of family medicine: A collaborative project of the family medicine community. *Annals of Family Medicine, 2,* S3–S32. doi:10.1370/afm.130.

Goodson, J. D. (2010). Patient Protection and Affordable Care Act: Promise and peril for primary care. *Annals of Internal Medicine, 152,* 742–744. doi:10.1059/0003-4819-152-11-201006010-00249.

Green, L. A., Fryer, G. E., Jr., Yawn, B. P., Lanier, D., & Dovey, S. M. (2001). The ecology of medical care revisited. *The New England Journal of Medicine, 344*(26), 2021–2025.

Grumbach, K., & Grundy, P. (2010). *Outcomes of implementing patient-centered medical home interventions: A review of the evidence from prospective evaluation studies in the United States.* Retrieved January 22, 2011, from www.pcpcc.net/content/pcmh-outcome-evidence-quality

Health Information Technology for Economic and Clinical Health Act. (2011). Retrieved February 10, 2011, from http://hipaasurvivalguide.com/hitech-act-text.php

Hoffman, C., Rice, D., & Sung, H. Y. (1996). Persons with chronic conditions: Their prevalence and costs. *Journal of the American Medical Association, 276,* 1473–1479.

Hwang, W., Weller, W., Ireys, H., & Anderson, G. (2001). Out-of-pocket medical spending for care of chronic conditions. *Health Affairs, 20*(6), 267–278.

Kessler, R. C., Berglund, P., Demler, O., Jin, R., Merikangas, K. R., & Walters, E. E. (2005). Lifetime prevalence and age-of-onset distributions of DSM-IV disorders in the National Comorbidity Survey Replication. *Archives of General Psychiatry, 62*(6), 593–602. doi:10.1001/archpsyc.62.6.593.

Kessler, R. C., Demler, O., Frank, R. G., Olfson, M., Pincus, H. A., Walters, E. E., et al. (2005). Prevalence and treatment of mental disorders, 1990 to 2003. *The New England Journal of Medicine, 352*(24), 2515–2523. doi:10.1056/NEJMsa043266.

Kessler, R., Stafford, D., & Messier, R. (2009). The problem of integrating behavioral health in the medical home and the questions it leads to. *Journal of Clinical Psychology in Medical Settings, 16*(1), 4–12. doi:10.1007/s10880-009-9146-y.

Lurie, I. Z., Manheim, L. M., & Dunlop, D. D. (2009). Differences in medical care expenditures for adults with depression compared to adults with major chronic conditions. *The Journal of Mental Health Policy and Economics, 12*(2), 87–95.

Mechanic, D. (1999). *Mental health and social policy – the emergency of managed care.* Englewood Cliffs, NJ: Prentice Hall.

Moussavi, S., Chatterji, S., Verdes, E., Tandon, A., Patel, V., & Ustun, B. (2007). Depression, chronic disease, and decrements in health: Results from the World Health Surveys. *Lancet, 370*, 851–858.

National Committee for Quality Assurance. (2011). *Patient-centered medical home 2011 standards and guidelines.* Retrieved April 14, 2011, from http://www.ncqa.org/tabid/631/default.aspx

National Committee on Quality Assurance. (2010). NCQA. *Patient-Centered Medical Home (PPC-PCMH). A new model of care delivery. Patient-Centered Medical Homes Enhance Primary Care Practices.* Retrieved January 11, 2011, from http://www.ncqa.org/Portals/0/PCMH%20brochure-web.pdf

National Quality Forum. (2011). *National priorities and goals: Executive summary.* Retrieved Feburary 22, 2011, from http://www.nationalprioritiespartnership.org/uploadedFiles/NPP/About_NPP/ExecSum_no_ticks.pdf

Nutting, P. A., Crabtree, B. F., Stewart, E., Miller, W. L., Palmer, R., Stange, K. C., et al. (2010). Effect of facilitation on practice outcomes in the national demonstration project model of the patient-centered medical home. *Annals of Family Medicine, 8*(S1), S33–S44.

Nutting, P. A., Miller, W. L., Crabtree, B. F., Jaen, C. R., Stewart, E. E., & Stange, K. C. (2009). Initial lessons from the first national demonstration project on practice transformation to a patient-centered medical home. *Annals of Family Medicine, 7*(3), 254–260. doi:7/3/254 [pii]10.1370/afm.1002.

PCPCC. (2011). *History of the collaborative.* Retrieved January, 15, 2011, from http://www.pcpcc.net/content/history-collaborative

Petterson, S., Phillips, B., Bazemore, A., Dodoo, M., Zhang, X., & Green, L. A. (2008). Why there must be room for mental health in the medical home. *American Family Physician, 77*(6), 757.

Regier, D. A., Narrow, W. E., Rac, D. S., Manderscheid, R. W., Locke, B., & Goodwin, F. (1993). The de facto US mental health and addictive disorders service system: Epidemiologic catchment area prospective. *Archives of General Psychiatry, 50*, 85–94.

Rittenhouse, D. R., & Shortell, S. M. (2009). The patient-centered medical home: Will it stand the test of health reform? *JAMA: The Journal of the American Medical Association, 301*(19), 2038–2040. doi:10.1001/jama.2009.691.

Sia, C., Tonniges, T. F., Osterhus, E., & Taba, S. (2004). History of the medical home concept. *Pediatrics, 113*, 1473–1478.

Simon, G. E., Katon, W. J., VonKorff, M., Unutzer, J., Lin, E. H., Walker, E. A., et al. (2001). Cost-effectiveness of a collaborative care program for primary care patients with persistent depression. [Clinical Trial Comparative Study Randomized Controlled Trial Research Support, U.S. Gov't, P.H.S.]. *The American Journal of Psychiatry, 158*(10), 1638–1644.

Simon, G. E., VonKorff, M., & Barlow, W. (1995). Health care costs of primary care patients with recognized depression. [Research Support, U.S. Gov't, P.H.S.]. *Archives of General Psychiatry, 52*(10), 850–856.

Smith, R., Lein, C., Collins, C., Lyles, J., Given, B., Dwamena, F., et al. (2003). Treating patients with medically unexplained symptoms in primary care. *Journal of General Internal Medicine, 18*, 478–489.

Stanek, M., & Takach, M. (2010). *Evaluating the patient-centered medical home: Potential and limitations of claims-based data*. National Academy for State Health Policy Briefing 2010. Retrieved January 11, 2011, from http://www.nashp.org/sites/default/files/EvalMedHomes Final-9-10-10.pdf

Stewart, E., Jaen, C. R., Crabtree, B., Miller, W. L., & Stange, K. C. (2009). *Evaluators' report on the National Demonstration Project (NDP) to the board of directors of TransforMED*. Retrieved December 4, 2009, from http://www.transformed.com/evaluatorsReports/report5.cfm

URAC. (2011). URAC. Retrieved November 18, 2011, from https://www.urac.org/about/ Utilization and Review Committee

Chapter 4
Advancing Integrated Behavioral Health and Primary Care: The Critical Importance of Behavioral Health in Health Care Policy

Benjamin F. Miller, Mary R. Talen, and Kavita K. Patel

Abstract The increased recognition of the importance of mental health, behavioral health, and substance use in primary care creates opportunities for helping better achieve a more efficient and effective health care system. Redesigning primary care through the Patient-Centered Medical Home has opened up new avenues for health care policy discussion; however, what remains unclear is the role behavioral health will play in this significant redesign.

Introduction

Ongoing fragmentation in health care between medical and behavioral health at the clinical, operational, financial, and training levels have restrained attempts to integrate policies and procedures for combining these two historically disparate systems of care. However, new health reform policies may offer opportunities for better

B.F. Miller, Psy.D. (✉)
Department of Family Medicine, University of Colorado
Denver School of Medicine, Aurora, CO, USA
e-mail: Benjamin.miller@ucdenver.edu

M.R. Talen, Ph.D.
Northwestern Family Medicine Residency, Erie Family Health Center,
2570 W. North Ave. Chicago, IL 60647, USA
e-mail: mary.talen@gmail.com

K.K. Patel, M.D., MSHS
BROOKINGS, 1775 Massachusetts Ave, 20036 NW Washington, DC, USA
e-mail: kpatel@brookings.edu

M.R. Talen and A. Burke Valeras (eds.), *Integrated Behavioral Health in Primary Care:*
Evaluating the Evidence, Identifying the Essentials, DOI 10.1007/978-1-4614-6889-9_4,
© Springer Science+Business Media New York 2013

behavioral health integration with primary care. While the past three decades have brought changes to the discipline and practice of behavioral health, the field has found itself in a place where it is viewed as a series of often disconnected and difficult to access specialty services. The implications of this for health care reform is that behavioral health disciplines are often overlooked and seen as another specialty vying for scarce financial resources. Efforts to integrate behavioral health into the larger health care milieu could not be more critical and are often fraught with challenges due to the fragmentation and territorial protection within mental health professions. However, behavioral health stakeholders from a variety of disciplines (e.g., social work, counseling, psychology, and psychiatry) have the opportunity to be connected to national health care policy through legislation such as: (1) the Patient Protection and Affordable Care Act; (2) Local, State, and Federal policies for medical and behavioral health billing; and (3) mental health parity legislation. These policy changes can better position the behavioral health field to advance beyond a specialty line of care and become more seamlessly integrated across health care systems.

The Patient Protection and Affordable Care Act

The Patient Protection and Affordable Care Act (PPACA) passed in 2010 is the most significant piece of health care policy legislation in decades (Goodson, 2010). PPACA presented several opportunities for those in the behavioral health field to be more involved in larger health care efforts. There are many important tenets of this Act, but health insurance expansion, increased access and primary care have received the most attention. The key components of the legislation that overlap with integrated behavioral health are as follows:

Key Patient Protection and Affordable Care Act: Legislation for Integrated Behavioral Health

Title II Subtitle I	Sec. 2303—Payment	See Amendment by Reconciliation Act below
	Sec. 2703. State option to provide health homes for enrollees with chronic conditions	Provides States with the option of enrolling Medicaid beneficiaries with chronic conditions into a "health home." Health homes are composed of a team of health professionals and are designed to provide a comprehensive set of medical services, including care coordination
From H.R. 3590 Patient Protection and Affordable Care Act	Sec. 2706. Pediatric Accountable Care Organization demonstration project	Establishes a demonstration project that allows qualified pediatric providers to be recognized and receive payments as Accountable Care Organizations (ACO) under Medicaid. The pediatric ACO would be required to meet certain performance guidelines. Pediatric ACOs that met these guidelines and provided services at a lower cost would share in those savings
Title III	Sec. 3021. Establishment of Center for Medicare and Medicaid Innovation within CMS	Establishes within the Centers for Medicare and Medicaid Services (CMS) a Center for Medicare & Medicaid Innovation. The purpose of the Center will be to research, develop, test, and expand innovative payment and delivery arrangements to improve the quality and reduce the cost of care provided to patients in each program. Dedicated funding is provided to allow for testing of models that require benefits not currently covered by Medicare. Successful models can be expanded nationally. Section 10306 adds payment reform models to the list of projects for the Center to consider, including patient-centered medical homes
	Sec. 3022. Medicare Shared Savings Program	The shared savings program, which is the fundamental payment reform for ACOs, has helped to define the various new models of care including those that try and integrate behavioral health services. Ultimately ACOs are designed to bring about high quality and efficient service. Under PPACA's shared savings programs, groups of providers and suppliers meeting certain criteria specified by CMS may work together to manage and coordinate care, through ACOs, for Medicare fee-for-service beneficiaries
Title V	Sec. 5301. Training in family medicine, general internal medicine, general pediatrics, and physician assistantship	Provides grants that aim to develop and operate training programs, provide financial assistance to trainees and faculty, enhance faculty development in primary care and physician assistant programs, and that establish, maintain, and improve academic units in primary care. Priority is given to programs that educate students in team-based approaches to care, including the patient-centered medical home

These new policies place primary care as the nation's largest platform of health care delivery, and the center of a substantial health care redesign. The principles and policies of Accountable Care Organizations focus on the implementation of three key issues for behavioral health: (1) team-based care; (2) quality improvement; and, (3) cost containment. A prominent means of redesign is through the patient-centered medical home (PCMH), which offers unique opportunities for innovation for behavioral health (Barr & Ginsburg, 2006; Green, Fryer, Yawn, Lanier, & Dovey, 2001). The PCMH is both an organizational model and certification process (see Chap. 3 on PCMH). PPACA policies are influencing the goals of the PCMH as a conceptual model for redesigning primary care. PCMH emphasizes the treatment of the whole person by a team of health care professionals who address a patient's primary health care needs in one setting (deGruy & Etz, 2010; McDaniel & Fogarty, 2009). National health care policy and health care reforms align with these PCMH concepts [(American Academy of Family Physicians (AAFP), American Academy of Pediatrics (AAP), American College of Physicians (ACP), & American Osteopathic Association (AOA), 2007; Barr & Ginsburg, 2006; Ferrante, Balasubramanian, Hudson, & Crabtree, 2010)].

Supported By: Continuous Quality Improvement and Effectiveness

In the area of quality improvement, behavioral health could have an important role in measuring what constitutes quality health care indicators. Patient factors such as quality of life, patient engagement, depression and/or anxiety or other healthy lifestyle behaviors have a significant impact on health outcomes. But these measures are marginalized as quality indicators for patient care. Acknowledging and advocating for the role of behavioral health metrics is an open door for advancing policy initiatives in quality improvement metrics, which include integrated behavioral health factors. Currently, these behavioral health metrics are in short supply, except for screening tools such as PHQ-9, and they are rarely incorporated into quality improvement systems. The potential to add behavioral health metrics as meaningful use measures through the PPACA policy holds promise. Providers and administrators from medical and mental health contexts need to become educated on how to best incorporate and implement these measures into quality improvement efforts.

How: Team-Based Care

The area of PPACA policy centers on team-based care. Most medical administrators tend to focus on the multidisciplinary team of physicians, mid-level providers, nurses, medical assistants, and other medical support staff. However, behavioral health providers and care managers have an opportunity to be included as integral members of these teams. They play a noteworthy role and have a significant contribution in not only direct clinical care for patients, but also in helping teams work more effectively. The teams could benefit from behavioral health providers' training and skills in group dynamics and group facilitation. These are new and untapped areas for behavioral health providers to expand and contribute to PCMH initiatives and the policy intentions of PPACA organizations.

Supported By: Business Model and Cost Containment

The third area of focus for PPACA policies is cost containment. Health care systems that integrate behavioral health have shown some gains in containing expenses in care delivery. The prevalence of behavioral health issues among patients (e.g., adherence, healthy life style) in the primary care setting is well established, as is the impact of mental health comorbidities on medical outcomes (Katon & Schulberg, 1992; Kessler & Stafford, 2008; Kessler et al., 2005; Unutzer, Schoenbaum, Druss, & Katon, 2006). And the evidence for having integrated behavioral health within a primary care system has demonstrated a positive outcome on managing acute, chronic, and preventative health care needs (Butler et al., 2008; Green et al., 2001; Starfield, 1998). However, policies are often not consistent with the evidence of the importance of behavioral health in cost containment. Behavioral health is not on the forefront of cost-cutting factors in health care policy debates and standards. Currently, policies are more prohibitive of integrating care than in support of it. For example, financially sustaining integrated behavioral health care is problematic due to antiquated reimbursement policies that force behavioral health and physical health into separate billing silos (Kathol, Butler, McAlpine, & Kane, 2010; Mauch, Kautz, & Smith, 2008). These payment policies do not acknowledge an integrated team, but rather pay for "behavioral health" or "physical health" codes or services.

Another area of policy that has created confusion has been in reimbursement regulations. Policies and regulations on state and local levels can undermine integrated behavioral health care practices. For example, state policies that limit same-day billing for medical and mental health treatment have interfered with medical and mental providers working in tandem with a patient to provide more seamless care. Policy regulations often limit continuity and collaboration, and contribute to patients' experience of obstacles in following through with behavioral health treatments. A number of states have addressed this by allowing for same-day billing, but it continues to be a complication throughout the country. When same-day billing policies are in place, behavioral health providers are able to provide psychotherapy services and receive reimbursement for same-day billing; however, the patient must have a mental health diagnosis (http://www.samhsa.gov/healthreform/index.aspx). When behavioral health providers use health and behavior codes (e.g., CPT 95801-4) on the same day as a medical visit to address the patient's engagement in health-related behavior change, many times these services cannot be reimbursed if billed on the same day of service. For example, if a physician sees an obese patient who could benefit from motivational interviewing to enhance their commitment to engaging in behavior changes for exercising, the patient would need to come back on another day rather than be seen on that same day. This policy significantly limits the continuity, efficiency, and collaboration of patient-centered care for the majority of primary care patients.

It is important to note that these payment and billing problems (same-day billing and health and behavior assessment codes) are workarounds and do not fundamentally address the problem at the heart of integration—behavioral health cannot be separated from overall health. To this end, payment schemes that continue to pay providers to only deliver their service line inadvertently perpetuate fragmentation. Global budgets and global payments may be more supportive of a truly integrated health care system and allow integrated behavioral health to flourish.

An untapped area of policy that may have an impact on reimbursement and practice is the Federal legislation that promoted parity between medical and mental health or substance abuse services. In 2008, the Paul Wellstone and Pete Domenici Mental Health Parity and Addiction Equity Act was signed into law and requires group health insurance plans (those with more than 50 insured employees) that offer coverage for mental illness and substance use disorders to provide those benefits in a way that is no more restrictive than all other medical and surgical procedures covered by the plan. The Mental Health Parity and Addiction Equity Act does not require group health plans to cover mental health (MH) and substance use disorder (SUD) benefits but, when plans do cover these benefits, MH and SUD benefits must be covered at levels that are no lower and with treatment limitations that are no more restrictive than would be the case for the other medical and surgical benefits offered by the plan (http://www.samhsa.gov/healthreform/parity/). This new legislation, which went into effect in January 2011, effectively puts mental health and substance abuse treatments on par with medical treatment. This policy can help health care systems merge medical and mental health care systems since the reimbursement practices need to be consistent. This practice of inequality has kept individuals with untreated SUD and MH disorders from receiving critically important treatment services. By providing parity, insurance covers treatment for SUD and MH disorders in a way that is equal to treatment coverage for other chronic health conditions, such as diabetes, asthma, and hypertension. The lack of health insurance coverage for MH and SUD treatment has contributed to a large gap in treatment services. Improving coverage of MH and SUD services will help more people get the care they need (http://www.samhsa.gov/healthreform/parity/).

Policy Challenges for Integrating Behavioral Health in Primary Care: Gaps Between Research and Policy

The relationship between health care policy and research on effective health care outcomes is often disconnected. There is a significant body of evidence that supports that behavioral health and primary care need to be integrated and attempts to separate and polarize the two systems puts health care delivery on a pathway to inferior patient care (Butler et al., 2008; deGruy, 1996). Research that supports best practices, however, may not trickle down into relevant policy debates, decisions, or regulations. There is a significant gap between effective patient-centered health care practices and policies that support and regulate integrated behavioral health. For example, if there is established evidence that better integrated treatment for mental health issues, such as depression and anxiety, improves outcomes, decreases cost, and improves patient and provider satisfaction, why would not these integration practices be adopted in policy? The answer to this question is found in the historical separation of behavioral health from physical health.

Likewise, policymakers may be hesitant to advance policies that may appear to "dictate" best practices and/or interfere in the science of medicine. What policymakers want to do is provide the environment for research that informs policy questions. For example, the Patient Centered Outcomes Research Institute (PCORI) was created to emphasize the need for patient-centered outcomes, especially in the context of clinical comparative effectiveness research. Behavioral health providers, administrators, and advocates within primary care settings need to actively build relationships with policymakers and organizations to better disseminate and translate research findings to policymakers and to raise the questions about the role of behavioral health to make it part of the discussion. Research has had a limited impact on the policy-making process and policymakers often do not understand the issues of integrated behavioral health care. Policymakers might erroneously assume that we have a health system that includes behavioral health care. This only points to the knowledge gap between those that draft the policy regulations and those that practice in primary care. Consequently, we need to connect the dots between the research in integrated behavioral health and what policymakers understand about this research and then what they can do to support it (Miller, 2010; Miller, Kessler, Peek, & Kallenberg, 2011). Behavioral health advocates, on the other hand, are often uninformed about the role and focus of policymakers. Behavioral health supporters need to know that policymakers have three essential roles: (1) approve additional monies for the Medicare Trust Fund, which could be used to support Center for Medicare and Medicaid Services (CMS) initiatives, (2) direct government entities to do something in a certain time frame (e.g., test new models of payment reform that include behavioral health), and (3) mandate aspects of the delivery of health care through rules and regulations in the public programs of Medicare, Medicaid, Veterans Affairs, Department of Defense, or through the Federal Employee Health Benefits Program. In addition policymakers can have a significant impact on the private sector through changes in regulations such as HIPAA and ERISA. Understanding this process may help advance and give voice in influential venues to the issues related to integrating behavioral health into our larger medical system.

Lack of Representation and Advocacy Within Integrated Behavioral Health Groups

While primary care behavioral health advocates from diverse professional backgrounds should continue to push for a larger clinical involvement in the PPACA initiatives and PCMH redesign, we need to better address and draft the policies that support behavioral health professions in primary care. While health care reform initiatives are moving toward having whole-person integrated care, only a small fraction of behavioral health providers currently work in integrated primary care practices and most of these providers are in public health settings (e.g., CHCs, FQHCs, CMHCs). We need an active, engaged leadership who can give voice and direction from the behavioral health point of view to legislators on local, state, and federal levels. Behavioral health providers, for the most part, are not educated, coached, or mentored in ways to participate in this legislative process. Consequently, the contributions of behavioral health has had limited impact in important policy decisions.

Some ways that behavioral health advocates have been involved with organizations that are advancing an agenda that integrates behavioral health include associations like the Collaborative Family Healthcare Association (CFHA). CFHA is a national not-for-profit association committed to multidisciplinary, patient, and family-centered integrated health care. Prior to each CFHA conference, the association hosts a policy summit that brings together stakeholders from across the state and has them work together on changing policy to accommodate integrated behavioral health (www.cfha.net).

The Agency for Healthcare Research and Quality (AHRQ) has also helped support integrated behavioral health by creating a national resource on integration—the Academy for Integrating Behavioral Health and Primary Care (http://integrationacademy.ahrq.gov/). This effort aims to unite the field and those interested in integrated behavioral health by providing resources for integration in one location. This effort is led by a National Integration Academy Council, which consists of leaders from the integrated behavioral health field. These leaders represent all aspects of the field including researchers, clinicians, policymakers, payers, patients, and actuaries.

The National Council for Community Behavioral Healthcare (National Council) is the unifying voice of America's behavioral health organizations. It has 1,950 member organizations, and its mission is to provide comprehensive, high-quality care that affords every opportunity for recovery and inclusion in all aspects of community life. The National Council advocates for policies that ensure that people who are ill can access comprehensive health care services. The National Council operates the SAMHSA-HRSA Center for Integrated Health Solutions to provide nationwide technical assistance in integrating primary and behavioral health. (http://www.thenationalcouncil.org/cs/about_us)

The Substance Abuse and Mental Health Services Administration (SAMHSA) and Health Resources and Services Administration (HRSA) have helped create the SAMHSA-HRSA Center for Integrated Health Solutions (http://www.integration.samhsa.gov/) another resource for the community interested in behavioral health and integration.

The National Institutes on Health (NIH) also has a dedicated institute for mental health, which has incorporated some aspects of behavioral and integrated health, but in a very limited interpretation and often without any concrete, stable source of funding.

Despite an increase in resources for integrated behavioral health, there remains an important need to address health care policy. For the field to move forward there must be a move beyond educating policymakers to action and implementation. In the context of health care policy reform and parity regulations, there are more opportunities to integrate behavioral health evidence and the strong interconnection between physical and mental health. Now, more than ever before, the field of integrated behavioral health should be uniting to take advantage of the opportunities within health care policy to integrate health care once and for all.

References

American Academy of Family Physicians (AAFP), American Academy of Pediatrics (AAP), American College of Physicians (ACP), & American Osteopathic Association (AOA). (2007). *Joint principles of the patient-centered medical home*. Retrieved August 13, 2009, from http://www.medicalhomeinfo.org/Joint%20Statement.pdf.

Barr, M., & Ginsburg, J. (2006). *The advanced medical home: A patient-centered, physician-guided model of health care*. Retrieved April 25, 2011, from http://www.acponline.org/advocacy/where_we_stand/policy/adv_med.pdf.

Butler, M., Kane, R. L., McAlpin, D., Kathol, R. G., Fu, S. S., Hagedorn, H., et al. (2008). *Integration of mental health/substance abuse and primary care no. 173.* Prepared by the Minnesota Evidence-Based Practice Center under Contract No. 290-02-0009 (AHRQ Publication No. 09-E003). Rockville, MD: Agency for Healthcare Research and Quality.

deGruy, F. (1996). Mental health care in the primary care setting. In M. S. Donaldson, K. D. Yordy, K. N. Lohr, & N. A. Vanselow (Eds.), *Primary care: America's health in a new era*. Washington, DC: Institute of Medicine.

deGruy, F. V., & Etz, R. S. (2010). Attending to the whole person in the patient-centered medical home: The case for incorporating mental healthcare, substance abuse care, and health behavior change. *Families, Systems & Health, 28*(4), 298–307.

Ferrante, J. M., Balasubramanian, B. A., Hudson, S. V., & Crabtree, B. F. (2010). Principles of the patient-centered medical home and preventive services delivery. *Annals of Family Medicine, 8*(2), 108–116. doi:10.1370/afm.1080.

Goodson, J. D. (2010). Patient Protection and Affordable Care Act: Promise and peril for primary care. *Annals of Internal Medicine, 152*, 742–744. doi:10.1059/0003-4819-152-11-201006010-00249.

Green, L. A., Fryer, G. E., Jr., Yawn, B. P., Lanier, D., & Dovey, S. M. (2001). The ecology of medical care revisited. *The New England Journal of Medicine, 344*(26), 2021–2025.

Kathol, R. G., Butler, M., McAlpine, D. D., & Kane, R. L. (2010). Barriers to physical and mental condition integrated service delivery. *Psychosomatic Medicine, 72*(6), 511–518. doi:10.1097/PSY.0b013e3181e2c4a0.

Katon, W., & Schulberg, H. (1992). Epidemiology of depression in primary care. *General Hospital Psychiatry, 14*(4), 237–247.

Kessler, R. C., Demler, O., Frank, R. G., Olfson, M., Pincus, H. A., Walters, E. E., et al. (2005). Prevalence and treatment of mental disorders, 1990 to 2003. *The New England Journal of Medicine, 352*(24), 2515–2523. doi:10.1056/NEJMsa043266.

Kessler, R., & Stafford, D. (Eds.). (2008). *Primary care is the de facto mental health system*. New York: Springer.

Mauch, D., Kautz, C., & Smith, S. A. (2008). *Reimbursement of mental health services in primary care settings*. Rockville, MD: Center for Mental Health Services, Substance Abuse and Mental Health Services Administration.

McDaniel, S. H., & Fogarty, C. T. (2009). What primary care psychology has to offer the patient-centered medical home. *Professional Psychology: Research and Practice, 40*(5), 483–492. doi:10.1037/a0016751.

Miller, B. F. (2010). Collaborative care needs a more active policy voice. *Families, Systems & Health, 28*(4), 387–388.

Miller, B. F., Kessler, R., Peek, C. J., & Kallenberg, G. A. (2011). *A national research agenda for research in collaborative care*. Papers from the Collaborative Care Research Network Research Development Conference, (AHRQ publication no. 11-0067). Retrieved June 12, 2012, from http://www.ahrq.gov/research/collaborativecare/.

Petterson, S., Phillips, B., Bazemore, A., Dodoo, M., Zhang, X., & Green, L. A. (2008). Why there must be room for mental health in the medical home. *American Family Physician, 77*(6), 757.

Phillps, R. L., Miller, B. F., Petterson, S. M., & Teevan, B. (2011). Better integration of mental health care improves depression screening and treatment in primary care. *American Family Physician, 84*(9), 980.

Starfield, B. (1998). *Primary care: Balancing health needs, services, and technology*. New York: Oxford University Press.

Unutzer, J., Schoenbaum, M., Druss, B. G., & Katon, W. J. (2006). Transforming mental health care at the interface with general medicine: Report for the president's commission. *Psychiatric Services, 57*, 37–47.

Part II
Review of Integrated Systems of Care Initiatives

Chapter 5
The State of the Evidence for Integrated Behavioral Health in Primary Care

Bethany M. Kwan and Donald E. Nease Jr.

Abstract Integrated behavioral health care is a complex, multifaceted healthcare delivery approach that is geared towards addressing mental and behavioral health concerns in primary care. There are a number of different models for integrated behavioral health care, with components that can be conceptualized as structures of care, processes of care, or principles of care. Common models include the IMPACT model (care management for depression), the three-component model (care management, enhanced mental health support, and a prepared practice), and the primary mental health care model of colocated integrated behavioral health care (on-site mental health specialists who collaborate with primary care providers), among others. Meta-analysis has shown that integrated behavioral health care improves health outcomes, although the extant evidence primarily pertains to depression. It is not well known which components of integrated behavioral health care are either necessary or sufficient for improving outcomes. There are many evidence gaps in integrated behavioral health care, including implementation and dissemination and the effects of integrated behavioral health care on disease contexts other than depression, behavioral medicine (e.g., lifestyle change in primary care), diverse populations, and cost and sustainability outcomes. Multiple methodologies should be deployed to address these gaps, including quasi-experimental, mixed methods (quantitative and qualitative), and observational designs.

Introduction

Integrated behavioral health care for mental and behavioral health in primary care settings is a general healthcare delivery concept that encompasses many complex multifaceted systems and practice models. These models are many and varied, but

B.M. Kwan, Ph.D., MSPH (✉) • D.E. Nease Jr., M.D.
Department of Family Medicine, University of Colorado Denver, Aurora, CO, USA
e-mail: Bethany.kwan@ucdenver.edu; Donald.Nease@ucdenver.edu

M.R. Talen and A. Burke Valeras (eds.), *Integrated Behavioral Health in Primary Care: Evaluating the Evidence, Identifying the Essentials*, DOI 10.1007/978-1-4614-6889-9_5, © Springer Science+Business Media New York 2013

generally include the following basic elements: a collaborative team comprised of mental/behavioral health and medical providers; protocols for identifying, triaging, treating, and tracking mental health concerns from within primary care; and supporting information technology infrastructure (Peek, 2011). The primary goal is to improve patient health outcomes (e.g., quality care); additional goals may include reducing costs and increasing efficiency (e.g., high-value care) and enhancing patient and provider satisfaction (e.g., the Triple Aim; Berwick, Nolan, & Whittington, 2008). The status quo in the US healthcare delivery system is that mental and behavioral health concerns are largely addressed by separate and distinct specialty mental health and private care settings (or not addressed at all). Such a system is often described as "fragmented" and difficult for both patients and providers to navigate.

In order to justify wide-scale system changes towards integrated behavioral health care, conclusive and consistent evidence is needed to convince policy and decision makers (including payers) of the value of collaborative care compared to the status quo. Such evidence includes an understanding of the models and their attributes that are feasible, sustainable, affordable, and effective. Such convincing evidence can only be the result of rigorous research and systematic evaluation designed to compare outcomes in integrated versus usual care settings. While the evidence base is fairly well established in some domains (e.g., primary care-based management of depression), in others it is quite sparse. Additionally, much of the research that has been done has been focused on the implementation of specific care protocols that feature aspects of integrated care, often targeted to particular chronic diseases or populations, with few evaluations of efforts to more globally transform the organizational aspects of practices into an integrated model. Mental and behavioral health providers in collaborative care models are positioned not only to aid in the treatment of specific mental disorders, but to enhance self-management of health through behavior change (e.g., motivational interviewing). The scope of the promise of integrated behavioral health care is as yet unrealized, and a key focus of future research should include both mental and behavioral health care.

The purpose of this chapter is therefore to describe the current evidence base (including reviews and meta-analyses), to identify evidence gaps, and to describe a range of research objectives and methodologies needed to fill these gaps. To facilitate interpretation of the evidence and identification of research gaps, the first step is to define integrated behavioral health care, with all of its complexities and variations. There are many terms used to represent this concept, including collaborative care, mental health integration, integrated care, integrated mental health and integrated behavioral health. We follow the standard adopted for this volume and use integrated behavioral health to refer generally to these models; however, when referring to specific projects or reviews, we use the authors' original terms. A number of attempts have been made to distill the concept of integrated care for the purposes of evaluation and comparison of the existing evidence (Blount, 2003; Butler et al., 2008; Collins, Hewson, Munger, & Wade, 2010; Doherty, McDaniel, & Baird, 1996). For instance, Blount (2003) described several key dimensions of the various models of integrated primary care: the relationship between mental health and primary care services (coordination, colocation, and integration), the populations served (targeted to patients with specific mental health needs vs. non-targeted), and the specificity of treatment modalities (a particular treatment protocol is specified vs. unspecified treatment that is essentially "provider's choice"). In a recent report from the Agency for Healthcare Research and Quality (AHRQ), the key dimensions outlined concerned systematic screening, integrating providers, and integrated care/proactive follow-up (Butler et al., 2008). Level of integration of the care process has been said to consist of ten elements (Butler et al. 2008, 2011), including (1) screening, (2) patient education/self-management, (3) medication, (4) psychotherapy, (5) coordinated care, (6) clinical monitoring, (7) assessment of medication adherence, (8) standardized follow-up, (9) formal stepped care, and (10) supervision. Level of integration of provider roles consists of degree of shared decision making between primary care and mental health providers (consensus, coordinated, or PCP principal responsibility), colocation of primary care and mental health, shared medical records, and communication links (such as e-mail or phone; Butler et al., 2008).

Most recently, Peek (2011) compiled a set of parameters to define a paradigm case for integrated behavioral health care, along with acceptable variations. According to Peek, an integrated behavioral health care practice has "a team with a shared population and mission, using a clinical system supported by an office practice and financial system and continuous quality improvement and effectiveness measurement." While this may represent the ideal or "paradigm" case for integrated behavioral health care, the forthcoming review of the evidence will reveal that little to none of the research conducted to date relates to something truly meeting this definition. Thus, this chapter will describe the variations on the theme of integrated behavioral health care and the evidence (or lack thereof) in support of each. We will then note the many gaps in this literature, especially concerning research on models consistent with the AHRQ report on integrated behavioral health care parameters and acceptable variations, and models consistent with what healthcare organizations are implementing in the real world.

Integrated Behavioral Health Models: Identifying Structural Features and Clinical Processes

As first proposed by Donabedian (1988), it is useful to consider healthcare delivery system models' structure and processes, which then can be examined in terms of their impact on specific outcomes. Integrated behavioral health care can be conceptualized as a set of structural features (clinical, operational, and financial) intended to help address mental health concerns as part of primary care. Research and evaluation can be designed to test the effects (across a range of outcomes) of these features individually, or, more realistically, as part of a comprehensive model. Indeed, it has been argued that integrated care is more than the sum of its parts, and thus we cannot easily evaluate the unique impact of any given component of an intervention or process change (Miller, Mendenhall, & Malik, 2009). Additionally, integrated care could be conceptualized as a set of processes expected to address a range of populations and health concerns, and targeted to particular outcomes. These processes could be performed under any number of different structural models, some of which may be more feasible or effective for achieving good outcomes in certain contexts. In addition to clinical outcomes, Blount (2003) suggested that attention to a broader array of nonclinical, process-oriented outcomes (e.g., patient and provider satisfaction, adherence to treatment regimens and evidence-based guidelines, and cost-effectiveness/cost-offsets) would facilitate comparison of various models. Access to care, detection, and treatment of mental and behavioral health concerns, practice-level improvement over time, and sustainability are likely all critical outcomes (Miller et al., 2009).

Going beyond Donabedian, a third component of integrated behavioral health care may be the overarching principles or attitudes towards mental health, the need to address it in primary care, and the practice of integrated behavioral health care itself that are embodied by healthcare organizations and their leaders, health care providers, and patients. Research on integrated behavioral health care could be conducted or interpreted based on any of these perspectives.

Structural Features of Integrated Behavioral Health

What happens in an integrated care delivery model? Who delivers care, where, and in what manner? What tools, resources, and infrastructure are needed to support the delivery of care? Table 5.1 represents a conceptual organization of the wide range of structural features of integrated behavioral health care, compiled based on descriptions of both research-based and real-world models of collaborative care, in order to identify gaps in the evidence.

Integrated Behavioral Health Care Processes

The structural features listed above comprise the practice and organizational infrastructure designed to provide mental health care to primary care patients (or vice versa). Ultimately, it may not matter what exactly this infrastructure looks like as long as it enables the provision of certain services. That is, the essential processes (Table 5.2) of an integrated behavioral health care infrastructure for any given setting are those that enhance access to care, detection, and treatment of mental health concerns, facilitate practice-level improvement over time, and are sustainable in terms of resources (Miller et al., 2009). While the structural features are the necessary but not sufficient tools for providing integrated care, these processes define the work done in an integrated behavioral health care setting. At a high level, these

Table 5.1 Structural features of integrated behavioral health care

Structural features	Possible components
Care delivery team	Medical care providers
	Mental/behavioral health providers (e.g., doctoral and masters level therapists, psychiatrists, social workers)
	Supporting nursing staff
	Supervising providers
	Care managers
	Clinical pharmacists
	Patients and families
Physical space	Dedicated space in a practice for mental and behavioral health care providers to interact privately with other providers *or* with patients both individually and in groups
	Practice location (freestanding clinic, part of larger hospital system, etc.)
Information technology	Computers and telephones
	Electronic medical records
	E-mail
	Registries
	Dashboards and portals for tracking outcomes
	Telemedicine (e.g., video conference)
	Mobile health technology
	Triage and clinical decision support
	Data collection and use (e.g., for quality improvement)
Office management policies and protocols	Established leadership (organizational and practice level) who have developed:
	Practice mission and values
	Time and effort protocols (how much time spent consulting with other providers vs. seeing patients)
	Provider access to patient records
	Privacy policies
	Billing and coding policies and protocols
	Incentives and organizational support for collaboration across disciplines
	Data collection and analysis policies and infrastructure (e.g., patient and staff satisfaction, measurement of processes and outcomes)
	Quality improvement models, teams, and procedures (e.g., Plan-Do-Study-Act [PDSA], Six Sigma, Continuous Quality Improvement [CQI])
Clinical care policies and protocols	Screening and population identification protocols
	Risk stratification and algorithms for determining appropriate level of care
	Diagnosis and Assessment Protocols
	Treatment protocols (e.g., use of evidence-based guidelines, stepped care)
	Monitoring and follow-up protocols
	Referral protocols
Education and training	Training programs (e.g., Primary Care Psychology Fellowships)
	Continuing education
	In-services
	Resources for attending conferences
	Informal consultation
	Practice preparation for change
	Team-building exercises

Table 5.2 Integrated behavioral health care processes

Process to enhance or optimize	Services routinely provided to patients and processes designed to enhance quality and value of care
Access	On-site mental/behavioral health
	Lists of local providers
	Helping people sign up for insurance
	Carve-ins versus carve-outs
	Matching with insurance coverage
	Navigation and care coordination services
	Connecting patients to community programs
Detection	Diagnosis and assessment
	Psychological testing
	Systematic mental health screening
	Systematic tracking and follow-up (primary prevention/at risk or at risk of relapse)
Treatment	Care management
	Evidence-based treatment
	Medication
	Psychotherapy and counseling (individual, group, couples, family)
	Shared/collaborative medical visits
	Patient education and skills building
	Counseling and support for patient self-management/behavior change/engagement/activation (e.g., motivational interviewing)
Practice improvement	Quality improvement processes
	Appropriate investment of resources to enhance quality and value of care
	Workforce development
Cost/sustainability	Processes for ensuring appropriate allocation of resources (utilizing community resources, leveraging less expensive personnel such as trainees)
	Securing funding (fund-raising, grant writing, advocacy, and building partnerships with payers to adapt reimbursement strategies and change policy)
	Ensuring receipt of payment for billable services
	Offering services for which patients are willing to pay out of pocket

processes include effective communication within the care delivery team and with patients and families, and monitoring change over time, with respect to the provision of services, appropriate resource allocation, and patient health status.

Principles and Attitudes Towards Integrated Behavioral Health Care

The most successful integrated behavioral health care systems are likely exemplary not only in terms of adequate staffing and resource allocation, but also embody certain attitudes, principles, and policies indicative of organizational value of integration. This includes principles such as the inseparation of physical and mental health, and the importance of the mind-body connection and caring for the whole person. Attitudes towards other care team members, the value of mental and behavioral health care, and the respective roles of mental and behavioral health versus medical care providers in primary care may also be relevant. If the structural features are the tools and the processes are the work, then the principles and attitudes are the energy compelling the investment of resources and the effort. These principles and attitudes are those held by the providers themselves, by organizational leadership, and by patients and families, and could directly impact the quality of the collaborations, relationships among mental health and primary care providers and patients and families, and ultimately both clinical and financial outcomes. This, however, has not been tested empirically, and most existing work is qualitative.

A number of the structures and processes described above are meant to support the development of positive attitudes and relationships within the care team and with practice management (e.g., education and training). Furthermore, the endorsement of such pro-integrated behavioral health care attitudes may facilitate implementation of practice changes. Positive provider attitudes (e.g., endorsement of the biopsychosocial model) and sensitivity to patient beliefs and preferences, including cultural competence, are said to enhance patient engagement (Beck & Gordon, 2010). At the organizational or administrative level, leadership must recognize the inherent challenges associated with change, and take care to engage practices in and adequately prepare them for the change process. According to Oxman and colleagues (Oxman, Dietrich, Williams, & Kroenke, 2002), a prepared practice is one in which providers have received education on how to follow new practice protocols. Feeling confident in one's abilities to follow new procedures is widely known to facilitate behavior change. Beyond knowledge about guidelines, skills, and communication protocols, however, team-building exercises, including the sharing of training backgrounds, perspectives on care, and strategies for collaboration and shared decision making, would be valuable. Chapter 10 discusses in further detail the relationship factors that are essential for successful collaboration.

Empirical Evidence for Integrated Behavioral Health Care

As mentioned above, much of the early work on integrated behavioral health care focused on depression. This grew directly from the work of Regier and others (Katon & Schulberg, 1992; Regier, Goldberg, & Taube, 1978; Schulberg, 1991) that identified primary care as the source of much mental health care. Subsequent studies examined the quality of care and efforts to improve screening (IMPACT, PRIMeMD, increasing use of the PHQ-9 to screen for depression), leading up to the landmark Agency for Health Care Policy and Research (AHCPR; now the AHRQ) depression guideline (Depression Guideline Panel, 1993). Subsequent work was then focused on trying to improve care once depression was identified. These focused, protocol-driven research projects have been essential for improving the way we attend to mental health in primary care. Increasingly, as our understanding of depression as a comorbid condition with other chronic diseases has grown, our conceptualization of integrated behavioral health care has transformed into something more broadly concerned with a range of mental health and behavioral health concerns in primary care populations. The systems and tools that have been developed—the use of care managers, integrated information systems, screening tools, protocols, and algorithms for providing the right level of evidence-based treatment, colocated mental/behavioral health providers and training programs—can be adapted to cover this broad range of care. This description of the evidence will start with coverage of the existing systematic reviews and meta-analysis, which are necessarily focused on the more classic models of integrated behavioral health care. A discussion of the classic models (care management for depression) and the contemporary models (integrated behavioral health care systems addressing a range of need) will ensue, including presentation of select research evidence. We will briefly mention how these integrated behavioral health care models have been used to facilitate patient self-management and behavioral health.

Systematic Reviews and Meta-analysis

Previous reviews of the literature support the conclusion that integrated care leads to better clinical outcomes—especially in terms of the treatment of primary care patients with depression. In their 2006 review of collaborative care for depression, Gilbody and colleagues (Gilbody, Bower, Fletcher, Richards, & Sutton, 2006) performed a meta-analysis of both short-term and long-term outcomes of 37 randomized controlled trials for the treatment of depression using a collaborative care approach. They defined collaborative care as "a multifaceted intervention involving combinations of three distinct professionals working collaboratively working within the primary care setting: a case manager, a primary care practitioner, and a mental health specialist." Compared to usual care, collaborative care for depression led to better depression outcomes at six months (standardized mean difference [SMD]=0.25, 95 % CI: 0.18–0.32) and longer term (1–5 years; SMD range 0.31 at one year to 0.15 at five years post-intervention, all confidence intervals excluded zero). The effect size was related to medication compliance and the professional background and supervision method of case managers, such that effects were larger for case managers with mental health training and regular, planned supervision. While considerable heterogeneity in effects was observed for earlier studies (in the 1980s and 1990s), as of 2006, the post-2000 evidence demonstrated more stable estimates of the effectiveness of collaborative care for managing depression. Of note, the authors concluded that further research would likely not reverse the conclusions that collaborative care for depression is effective.

In a systematic review, Oxman, Dietrich, and Schulberg (2005) described the research on collaborative care models as representing a third generation of research on the treatment of depression in primary care, following a first generation of multifaceted, collaborative care interventions and a second generation grounded in the principles of the chronic care model and guideline-based care. In this third generation (including the PRISM-E, IMPACT, PROSPECT, and RESPECT-D studies), there was increased emphasis on effectiveness rather than efficacy in the context of translation, dissemination, and sustainability (especially concerning system and practice redesign), and attention to aging populations. An enhancement of "consultation-liaison skills" and better relationships between primary care clinicians and mental health specialists was considered an important advancement in the field. While it was concluded that referral to specialty mental health care would likely lead to better outcomes at an individual level, it was also acknowledged that overall population health would be best improved with the more limited care made available from within primary care because of increased access. In another review, Katon and Seelig (2008) noted that a population-based approach that coordinates the care of depression from within primary care should be particularly effective for reducing overall prevalence of depression. They suggest that three activities well suited to primary care are key to secondary prevention of depression: improved diagnosis (including screening for risk factors and early evidence of minor depression), preventing chronicity, and preventing relapse/recurrence by virtue of more frequent contact and opportunities for tracking and monitoring symptomology.

Recently, the AHRQ published an in-depth report on mental health integration in primary care (Butler et al., 2008). The primary conclusion of this comprehensive review was that while there did not appear to be a relationship between level of integration and effects on clinical outcomes, the purported benefits of integrated care for managing both depression and anxiety were supported by the evidence. Similar methods later applied to the literature on integrated care for depression alone reached the same conclusion—integrated care improves depression outcomes, but level of integration (e.g., degree of shared treatment decision making or extent of colocation) in the care process or in provider roles was not associated with better outcomes (Butler et al., 2011). In both cases, the model with the most support for its effectiveness (in terms of symptom severity but not treatment response or remission rates, which did not differ among the various models) was the IMPACT model. However, it was noted that a continuing limitation in this literature is an inability to separate the effect of specific elements of integrated care on better outcomes from the overall effect of more attention to mental health problems as a result of integration. There are indeed many ways of conceptualizing integrated care, and attempts to quantify a global level of integration rather than distinct elements of the various models that can be independently evaluated have not yielded any increased understanding of how or under what circumstances integrated care is effective. As has been noted in meta-analysis (e.g., Gilbody, Bower, Fletcher, et al., 2006), there is heterogeneity in the effects of integrated care on depression—which therefore suggests that there is *some other variable or set of variables* related to how integrated behavioral health care is implemented (in what context, in what population, using which evidence-based treatments, by whom, with what mindset, in what permutations) that differentially influences outcomes.

Past attempts have been made to determine "active ingredients" of integrated care. In a review from the Canadian Collaborative Mental Health Initiative (CCMHI), Craven and Bland (2006) reached conclusions supporting several elements of integrated care as key factors in improving outcomes, including practice preparation, colocation, collaboration (especially when paired with treatment guidelines), systematic follow-up, patient education, sensitivity to patient preference, and counseling to promote treatment engagement and adherence. In a meta-analysis and meta-regression of specific intervention content, eight aspects of these interventions that varied across 34 studies on collaborative care for depression were tested as predictors of depression outcomes (Bower, Gilbody, Richards, Fletcher, & Sutton, 2006). These variables included setting (USA vs. non-USA), recruitment method, patient population, primary care physician training, case manager background, case management sessions, case manager supervision, and case management content. Of these, four were at least marginally significant predictors of depression symptoms in multivariate analyses—setting (in favor of non-USA studies), recruitment method (in favor of systematic identification through screening rather than referral by clinicians), case manager background (in favor of those with mental health expertise), and case manager supervision (in favor of those receiving regular/planned supervision). Notably, no aspects of intervention content predicted antidepressant use. While the heterogeneity in effect sizes for depression symptoms was reduced when considering these particular aspects of intervention content, as above, it appeared that there were as yet unmeasured intervention features or aspects of study context or setting influencing results. It may be that these unmeasured features are organizational aspects related to the principles and attitudes towards integrated care as described above.

More supporting evidence for these conclusions is emerging. While difficult to separate from other aspects of multifaceted interventions, care management does appear to be an important factor in depression care (Williams et al., 2007). However, care management is a role that functions in different ways across different contexts, and it is therefore not clear which are the most effective components of care management, which background or training is needed for care managers, or whether ongoing supervision of care managers is truly necessary. In a more recent meta-analysis of studies evaluating the effects of interactive communication between primary care clinicians and specialists—defined as "direct, personal interaction with specialists… such as curbside consultations" (Foy et al., 2010, p. 247)—randomized trials involving collaboration between primary care clinicians and psychiatrists on average exhibited a small to medium effect size for mental health outcomes in favor of collaboration. This is consistent with recent findings of a Congressional Budget Office review of Medicare Demonstration Projects, which found that in-person interactions between care managers, providers, and patients were uniquely associated with programs that demonstrated improved outcomes (Nelson, 2012). Continued investigation into the effectiveness of various elements of collaborative care, especially outside the context of depression care, is warranted. Next, we discuss exemplary and prototypical models of integrated behavioral health care, and research and evaluation of instances of these models.

Specific, Exemplar Studies of Integrated Behavioral Health Care Interventions

There are several models of integrated behavioral health care that have been tested using randomized trial designs, still considered to be the gold standard for establishing clinical effectiveness. Many of these models were designed specifically for depression, but the guiding principles and structural features of the care delivery system would presumably apply to other mental illnesses (with some evidence, described below, supporting this supposition). These models share various versions of care/case managers who act as intermediaries or partners with primary and specialty care, with differences in the specific protocols and degree to which care managers and specialty care is embedded within individual primary care clinics. A sampling of the models that have been subject to research and formal evaluation and major conclusions from this work are described here. Others have compiled detailed reviews of the evidence, including a deconstruction of the randomized trials of integrated behavioral health care and/or related interventions for mental health in primary care (Butler et al., 2008; Craven & Bland, 2006; Williams et al., 2007), and thus we will not repeat this work; we will, however, describe the major models of integrated behavioral health care and exemplar research on each.

IMPACT. The IMPACT model of collaborative care was originally conceptualized as a chronic disease management program for older adults with depression (Unutzer et al., 2001, 2002). This model involves a team-based approach to managing depression from within primary care. The care team includes a trained depression care manager, a primary care provider, and a consulting psychiatrist. The team uses a stepped-care approach to managing depression, with a three-step evidence-based treatment algorithm used to guide care advancement. At each step, psychiatric consultation is considered if clinically indicated, and care plans are discussed with the PCP and the consulting psychiatrist. Patients receive routine screening for depression. The acute and maintenance phases of depression are tracked by the care manager, a nurse, or psychologist who provides education, care management, and medication support or psychotherapy, with regular telephone follow-up for a year (weekly at first, and then less frequent as depression lessens). Treatment options include antidepressant medication or brief psychotherapy (Problem-Solving Treatment in Primary Care).

The IMPACT model has very good empirical support (http://impact-uw.org/about/research.html), across a number of health care settings and populations. In the initial grant-supported, multisite randomized trial, those in the intervention group had higher rates of depression treatment (odds ratio [OR] = 2.98 [2.34, 3.79], $p < 0.001$) and experienced significantly greater odds of 50 % reduction in depression symptoms than those in the usual care group (OR = 3.45 [2.71, 4.38], $p < 0.001$; (Unutzer et al., 2002). Usual care patients were also screened for depression and could receive treatment for depression through all existing channels. Evidence also suggested that the intervention led to lower health care costs over a four-year period (Unutzer et al., 2008). More than fifty publications have resulted from research on the IMPACT model (http://impact-uw.org/files/IMPACTPublicationsList.pdf), with overall favorable results. Having demonstrated the effectiveness of this model, research on IMPACT has shifted towards more complex populations (e.g., patients with comorbid mental health and physical health concerns) and wide-scale implementation and dissemination research, such as the DIAMOND project.

The "Depression Improvement Across Minnesota, Offering a New Direction" (DIAMOND) project is intended to incorporate the IMPACT collaborative care model for depression management in primary care practices throughout the state of Minnesota, using a new payment mechanism agreed upon by participating payers. In contrast to the original IMPACT studies, DIAMOND was designed to evaluate a structure of collaborative care that includes specific elements, rather than a specific care protocol that features collaborative care. An NIH-funded "T3" implementation study was designed to evaluate DIAMOND using a staggered implementation, multiple baseline design based on methods for practical clinical trials (Solberg et al., 2010). There are six components of collaborative care that have been implemented in DIAMOND: depression screening using the PHQ-9, tracking and monitoring with a patient registry, stepped care for depression, relapse prevention planning, care management, and psychiatric consultation and supervision. Within the quasi-experimental evaluation design, implementation of collaborative care and the corresponding changes in reimbursement is staggered in five sequences over 3 years, with 10–20 new clinics implementing the intervention during each sequence (a total of up to 85 clinics in 16 separate healthcare organizations). Patients are identified and data are collected weekly for thirty-seven months in all sites, before and after implementation of the intervention. Sites therefore serve as their own control, with multiple preimplementation scores on key outcomes for each site. Outcomes include use of evidence-based practices for depression (e.g., Institute for Clinical Symptoms Improvement's guidelines for treatment of depression in primary care (Trangle et al., 2012), depression symptoms, health care cost, and work productivity. Using the RE-AIM framework, outcomes related to translation and dissemination will also be evaluated. Among the benefits of this approach are the implications for generalizability to diverse patient populations and practice settings, as well the potential to evaluate questions of reach and organizational context. However, as might be expected in this sort of innovative natural experiment, challenges and tensions between the need to adhere to a study protocol and the practical goals of the overarching initiative have been reported. Results have not yet been reported in the peer-reviewed literature.

Various other integrated care interventions have been based on variations on the theme of care management. The Prevention of Suicide in Primary Care Elderly: Collaborative Trial (PROSPECT) study utilized care managers who used a protocol-based intervention to monitor depression treatment adherence and response and provide guidelines-based recommendations to physicians, the sole decision makers (Bruce et al., 2004). The care managers were nurses, social workers, and psychologists. Patients were offered citalopram as a first course treatment, or interpersonal psychotherapy (IPT) delivered by the care managers if they declined antidepressant medication. PCPs could also recommend other medication or other forms of psychotherapy. Twenty participating practices were randomized at the practice level to prevent contamination effects. Compared to usual care, the intervention led to increased access to depression care, greater declines in suicidal ideation, earlier treatment response, and higher rates of remission at 4, 8, and 24 months (Alexopoulos et al., 2005, 2009).

Three-component model. Another model is the three-component model (TCM), characterized by care management, enhanced mental health support, and a prepared practice (Oxman et al., 2002). In this model, care management can be either centralized in an organization or localized within a practice, with a spectrum of services such as telephone calls and limited psychotherapy. Important goals of care management include patient education, counseling for self-management and adherence, assessment of treatment response, and communication with other clinicians involved in a patient's care. A psychiatrist is another important component—he or she supervises and provides guidelines for the care manager, provides consultation services to the PCP, and facilitates appropriate use of additional mental health resources. The psychiatrist also plays an important role in preparing a practice to implement the model (primarily providing psychiatric education regarding diagnosis, risk assessment, and care plans) and providing ongoing reinforcement of this education.

The Re-Engineering Systems for Primary Care Treatment of Depression (RESPECT-D) project was a cluster randomized trial of an intervention based on the three-component model (Dietrich et al., 2004). Intervention patients had approximately double the odds of achieving a 50 % reduction in depression symptoms as well as remission at three and six months. The project was supported by training manuals and quality improvement resources, rather than research protocols and grant funding—potentially making this a more sustainable approach (Lee, Dietrich, Oxman, Williams, & Barry, 2007). The implementation and evaluation of RESPECT-D in the military setting (RESPECT-Mil) for the treatment of service members with post-traumatic stress disorder and depression showed that the three-component model was feasible, acceptable, and led to clinically significant improvement in that context (Engel et al., 2008).

Colocated collaborative care. The Strosahl (1998) primary mental health care model of colocated collaborative care is distinguishable from the aforementioned care management models because mental health specialists (e.g., masters and doctoral level psychotherapists, or "primary care psychologists") are located onsite in a primary care clinic and provide services to patients of that clinic, often in collaboration with a primary care clinician. However, as noted by Blount (2003), colocated does not necessarily mean collaborative. While care managers (even those with mental health backgrounds) often provide limited psychotherapy and consultant psychiatrists can provide periodic guidance and advice (often by telephone or e-mail), colocated mental health specialists can provide more traditional psychotherapy regimens (e.g., cognitive behavioral therapy) as well as "curbside" consultation for primary care clinicians from within the primary care clinic. Another key feature of this model is triage, in which level of care is increased depending on patient need, risk, or severity, ranging from behavioral health consultation, to specialty consultation, to fully integrated care. Appropriate training (and retraining of expectations) is also critical for both mental health and medical care providers. While widely adopted as a collaborative care model, there is limited empirical evidence on this model, with a few exceptions. In the Primary Care Research in Substance Abuse and Mental Health for the Elderly (PRISM-E) study, colocated mental health and primary care for mental health/substance abuse was compared to enhanced referral to specialty mental health care (Levkoff et al., 2004). In PRISM-E, there was evidence demonstrating that integrated care led to increased access to mental health and substance abuse services compared to enhanced referral (Bartels et al., 2004). However, clinical outcomes were generally comparable across the two conditions (Areán et al., 2008; Krahn et al., 2006), although enhanced referral to specialty mental health appeared to be superior for patients with major depression (Krahn et al.).

The US Veterans Health Administration (VA) has embraced integrated behavioral health care, and has implemented a variety of models involving the integration of mental health into primary care, including care management models targeted to depression (Felker et al., 2006) and other mental health conditions (Oslin et al., 2006), and a blended model (colocation plus care management) in a number of their practices across the country (Pomerantz et al., 2010). Nearly 25 years ago, the VA first colocated psychologists and psychiatrists in their primary care clinics. Today, the VA's White River Model incorporates comprehensive mental and behavioral health care into primary care, with colocated behavioral health providers (therapists and psychiatrists) as part of the care team, information technology to support assessment and tracking, care management, and chronic disease management. Screening and triage are also important processes of care. Patients can receive brief or long-term individual psychotherapy or group psychotherapy for a number of mental disorders, including depression, anxiety, stress/anger management, post-traumatic stress disorder, and substance use. Based on "before-after" study designs, this model appears to have led to improvements in access to care, patient and provider satisfaction, and adherence to evidence-based guidelines for depression treatment, and decreased cost of mental health care in the context of this capitated single-payer system (Pomerantz, Cole, Watts, & Weeks, 2008; Watts, Shiner, Pomerantz, Stender, & Weeks, 2007). Furthermore, in a comparison with VA facilities that had VA not implemented this model, facilities with mental health integration showed greater increases in rates of detection of mental health disorders (Zivin et al., 2010). This model has been sustained for over six years. (Further discussion of the approaches to integrated behavioral health care can be found in Chap. 9.)

The 6P framework. The Depression in Primary Care program (supported by the Robert Wood Johnson Foundation) was based on the "6P" conceptual framework incorporating the perspective of six groups of stakeholders—(1) patients/consumers, (2) providers, (3) practice/delivery systems, (4) plans, (5) purchasers, and (6) populations/policies. These programs were designed to promote the use of evidence-based chronic care models for depression (Pincus, Pechura, Keyser, Bachman, & Houtsinger, 2006). A unique focus to this framework is the inclusion of economic considerations and innovative financial incentive arrangements, and the encouragement of collaborations between care providers and payers. Additionally, this framework explicitly invites the use of clinical information systems to assist in link-ing stakeholders, enabling clinical decision support, and monitoring and tracking outcomes. While not a model of integrated care per se, the program did define a number of key components as a "blueprint" for treating depression in primary care. These components included a leadership team, decision support to enhance adher-ence to evidence-based treatment guidelines, delivery system redesign (e.g., use of patient registries), clinical information systems, patient self-management support, and community resources. The program funded a number of demonstration projects in eight states to encourage implementation of a chronic care model for depression in primary care. There was wide variety in how integrated care was implemented across these demonstration projects, consistent with the planned flexibility of the 6P conceptual framework.

As a recipient of one of the Depression in Primary Care grants, Intermountain Health care in Utah developed a model of mental health integration (MHI) that com-bines evidence-based treatment algorithms (based on degree of patient and family need—low, moderate, high) with innovative informatics tools (e.g., electronic health records, registries, electronic clinical decision support) for tracking patient progress and navigation of the system (Reiss-Brennan, 2006). The goal is to enhance care in three ways: 1) detection, monitoring, and management of mental health conditions, 2) patient and family engagement to support adherence and self-management, and 3) treatment matching and adjustment. In Intermountain's model of risk stratification, progressively more intensive treatment is provided as risk level (severity and nonre-sponse) increases or persists, with universal screenings for and continued diagnostic assessment of those at risk (Babor et al., 2007). The explicit focus on multiple stake-holder perspectives—including payers and health plans—is intended to promote sus-tainability. The MHI program at Intermountain was evaluated in terms of patient and provider satisfaction, patient and family health, functioning and productivity, and cost neutrality, using cohort and cost-trend analysis to show changes over time in outcomes in the system (Reiss-Brennan, Briot, Daumit, & Ford, 2006). In a quasi-experimental, retrospective cohort study comparing 73 out of 130 clinics that had implemented the MHI program with those that had not, patients in the treatment cohort had a lower rate of increase in costs than those in usual care—especially for those with depression and at least one other comorbidity (Reiss-Brennan, Briot, Savitz, Cannon, & Staheli, 2010). Intermountain has reported that other analyses from the MHI evaluation showed improvements in satisfaction and depression severity.

In contrast, the University of Michigan's Depression in Primary Care project relied on primary care clinicians to selectively refer patients to care management, in which care managers were remotely based, but assigned to specific clinics (Klinkman et al., 2010). Results showed improved rates of remission in the intervention prac-tice patients at six months (43.4 % vs. 33.3 %, $p=0.11$), 12 months (52.0 % vs. 33.9 %, $p=0.012$), and eighteen months (49.2 % vs. 27.3 %, $p=0.004$).

Reverse integration. Reverse integration models support bringing primary health care to patients with severe mental illness in specialty mental health settings, either through colocated primary care providers or care coordination. The VA system has also been the context for several reverse integration models (Druss, Rohrbaugh, Levinson, & Rosenheck, 2001; Druss et al., 2010; Saxon et al., 2006). For instance, the Primary Care Access, Referral, and Evaluation (PCARE) study is a randomized trial of primary care management for patients with severe mental illness being cared for in a community mental health center (Druss et al., 2010). In this study, nurse care managers performed two major roles—encouraging patients to seek medical care for their medical conditions through patient education and motivational interviewing, and assisting patients with accessing and navigating the primary care system through advocacy and addressing system-level barriers such as lack of insurance. At the PCARE 12-month follow-up, intervention patients were significantly more likely than usual care patients to have received recommended preventive services (58.7 % vs. 21.8 %), to have experienced greater improvements in mental health status, based on the SF-36 (8 % improvement vs. 1 % decline), and to have lower cardiovascular risk, based on Framingham Cardiovascular Risk scores (Druss et al., 2010).

Telemedicine. Circumstances may exist that prevent on-site mental health services—but innovation in the field of health information technology (HIT), especially mobile HIT, may present new opportunities for integration, especially in rural settings where on-site mental health is not feasible. A number of telemedicine models have been subject to research and evaluation (Rollman et al., 2009; Simon, Ludman & Rutter, 2009). These models include antidepressant consultation with an off-site psychiatrist via video conference (Fortney et al., 2006), telephone-based care management for depression in patients recovering from coronary artery bypass graft (Rollman et al., 2009), telephone care management plus cognitive behavioral psychotherapy for patients taking antidepressant medication (Ludman, Simon, Tutty, & Von Korff, 2007; Simon et al., 2009; Simon, Ludman, Tutty, Operskalski, & Von Korff, 2004). The use of telemedicine for delivering mental health services has been popular in rural Australia in recent decades (Lessing & Blignault, 2001), predominantly for assessment and consultation rather than psychotherapy, with trends over time showing increased access to care.

The TEAM (Telemedicine Enhanced Antidepressant Management) intervention (Fortney et al., 2006) consisted of annual screening for depression using the PHQ-9 and a depression care team that provided a stepped-care model of depression treatment to patients screening positive for depression. This model was essentially a variation on the theme of IMPACT, but with telepsychiatry rather than on-site psychiatry, using interactive video technology. The team was comprised of an on-site primary care physician, a consulting psychiatrist available via teleconference, and off-site nurse depression care managers, clinical pharmacists, and supervising psychiatrists. The stepped-care treatment included (1) watchful waiting or treatment with antidepressant medication (ADM), with symptom monitoring by the care manager; (2) given nonresponse to the initial ADM, the psychiatrist, PCP, and clinical pharmacist consulted (generally via an electronic progress note in the medical record) to make further recommendations; (3) given further nonresponse, a telepsychiatry consultation was recommended; (4) a final step was referral to specialty mental health at the parent VA medical center. Usual care patients were also screened for depression, had their depression scores entered in to the EMR, and had interactive video equipment available at the point of care for specialty mental health consultation. The results of this randomized trial (randomized at the practice level but analyzed at the patient level due to low intraclass correlations at the practice level) demonstrated no difference in rate of prescription of ADM; however the intervention led to significantly higher odds of experiencing a 50 % improvement in depression severity at six months, and significantly higher odds of remitting at twelve months (Fortney et al., 2007). This rural telemedicine collaborative care intervention was, however, more expensive than its urban, on-site counterparts (Pyne et al., 2010).

Evidence Gaps in Integrated Behavioral Health Care

Despite the number of studies performed on various models and protocols of integrated behavioral health care, there remain many gaps in our knowledge. The existing research covers many of the structural features of integrated behavioral health care, especially members of the care delivery team, screening and treatment protocols, and education and training for practice personnel for specific protocols. The evidence is more limited for other structural features (information technology, training programs, practice management policies, and physical space considerations). Similarly, some processes of care are well covered in the literature, especially access, detection, and treatment of depression. There are increasing reports of cost and sustainability issues, as more research and evaluation concerns real-world implementation of integrated behavioral health care models that are not solely supported by grant funds. More evidence is needed for business models and practice improvement in integrated behavioral health care models, or principles and attitudes towards integrated care, from the perspectives of organizations, providers, and patients. There continues to be a predominant focus on clinical trial methodology, which may not result in knowledge that is easily translatable or sustainable outside well-controlled, resource-rich settings. The more rigorous research tends to be protocol driven and often disease and population specific, rather than focused on care delivery systems in general. The practical barriers to large-scale care delivery systems research are notable, however, and this gap will not be easily filled; such research may never be amenable to the gold-standard randomized trial design. Additionally, despite more recent work done in comorbid conditions such as diabetes and asthma, the broader impacts of multimorbidity and integrated behavioral health care processes and outcomes remain largely unknown. Finally, studies focused on implementation and dissemination remain less common, and results are just beginning to emerge.

Recently, the AHRQ published a research agenda (Miller, Kessler, Peek, & Kallenberg, 2011) for integrated behavioral health care, in which they prioritized the following broad research questions: (1) In what ways (according to what models or adaptations thereof, and for what populations) are real-world practices implementing collaborative care? (2) Which aspects of these real-world collaborative care models are effective, and for whom? Addressing these broad questions and the others noted above will involve evaluating effectiveness of structures, processes, and attitudes towards integrated behavioral health care in the following contexts, using a variety of complementary methodologies.

Disease Contexts

Empirical research (especially randomized controlled trials) on integrated behavioral health care has typically been conducted in the context of a single disease state (or a specific combination of disease states), such that outcomes are tied directly to the amelioration of these particular conditions (rather than a range of mental health conditions). The main body of evidence is not only disease specific but most often concerns the management of depression, a pervasive and burdensome illness but by no means the only mental health problem confronted in primary care. Limited evidence exists in other mental health domains, such as panic disorder (Roy-Byrne, Katon, Cowley, & Russo, 2001), substance abuse and addiction (Alford et al., 2011; Areán et al., 2008), and bipolar disorder (Kilbourne et al., 2009). In the Netherlands, a collaborative stepped-care RCT for the treatment of panic disorder and generalized anxiety disorder in primary care is currently underway (Muntingh et al., 2009).

Much of the most recent literature on integrated care involves management of multiple psychiatric and/or physical comorbidities. The care delivery system features adopted as part of integrated mental health care (e.g., care management, interdisciplinary collaboration, clinical monitoring and follow-up, stepped care) reflect an instantiation of Wagner's chronic care model and can be used to comanage multiple chronic diseases. It is also thought that treating mental illness may have direct and/or indirect effects on other illnesses, possibly because of physiological, social, cognitive, and/or behavioral factors common to the comorbid conditions (Rustad, Musselman, & Nemeroff, 2011). In a pilot study of a patient-centered depression care management intervention characterized by several elements of integrated care (e.g., education and adherence monitoring), elderly adults with comorbid depression and hypertension were found to have lower depression scores, lower blood pressure, and greater medication adherence at six weeks (Bogner & de Vries, 2008).

Based on the IMPACT model, the Multifaceted Diabetes and Depression Program (MDDP) targets comorbid diabetes and depression in a low-income, predominantly Hispanic population (Ell et al., 2010). MDDP incorporates several IMPACT-like features, with diabetes depression clinical specialists (DDCSs) serving in the care manager capacity, stepped care for depression, supervision by a PCP, and an available consultant psychiatrist. In addition, MDDP involved "sociocultural enhancements" (e.g., addressing social stigma towards mental health), education and counseling in self-management of both depression and diabetes, and patient navigation services. Consistent with the results of other combined depression-and-diabetes collaborative care interventions (Katon et al., 2004) and subgroup analyses of patients with diabetes in the original IMPACT study (Williams et al., 2004), MDDP resulted in improved depression, functioning, and financial status and reduced symptom burden for both depression and diabetes—but there were no objective effects on diabetes control (e.g., change in HgA1c).

It therefore remains a question as to whether the effective treatment of mental illness (in the context of integrated care) can lead to improved outcomes for comorbid chronic diseases. Longer term follow-up and/or the addition of more intensive chronic disease-specific intervention content may be required to observe an effect on these other outcomes. For instance, the Stepped Care for Affective Disorders and Musculoskeletal Pain (SCAMP) study implemented a 12-week antidepressant therapy intervention in sequence with a six-session pain management intervention (followed by a six-month continuation phase) in patients with comorbid depression and musculoskeletal pain (Kroenke et al., 2009). Not only did patients in the intervention experience significantly greater improvements in depression than those in usual care, they also experienced significantly greater improvements in pain severity and interference. Note that as the intervention involved treatment algorithms coordinated by nurse care managers in primary care settings, who were supervised by a physician depression specialist, SCAMP qualifies as an integrated care investigation, akin to IMPACT.

The results of the TEAMCare intervention, focusing on patients with diabetes or coronary heart disease or hyperlipidemia and depression at Group Health Cooperative, have recently been reported (Lin et al., 2012). The TEAMCare intervention utilized nurse case managers with specialist consultation working with primary care physicians in an attempt to increase adherence to medication and other self-care behaviors for both depression and comorbid physical illnesses (McGregor, Lin, & Katon, 2011). The TEAMCare intervention failed to demonstrate significant effects on medication adherence, but led to significant changes in provider prescribing behavior (Lin et al., 2012).

An early implication of these findings is that treating mental illness may aid in improving coping skills (e.g., emotion coping) and self-regulation/self-management, which have subsequent salutatory effects on stress and pain, which helps to improve functioning and quality of life—even if short-term effects on medical illnesses are not observed. Testing for indirect effects of integrated care interventions on comorbidity outcomes via changes in coping and self-regulatory skills may be a fruitful area of future research.

A broader focus on general mental health across a range of mental health needs, including basic psychosocial needs, health behavior modification, and the myriad mental health conditions presenting in primary care (Ansseau et al., 2004), is much less common in the research literature. When broadly focused models are evaluated, the designs are generally less rigorous, the outcomes are generally more process oriented (rather than clinical), and the conclusions are less generalizable outside the context in which the evaluation took place. The primary exception to this rule is that reverse integration models often seek general medical care (e.g., not just for diabetes) for a range of patients cared for in specialty mental health (e.g., not just patients with schizophrenia). By design, necessity, and/or default, these broad health-focused models are concerned with process and system capacity, such as defining and expanding the roles of health care professionals (e.g., advanced practice nurses; Asarnow & Albright, 2010).

Behavioral Medicine

In practice, the term "behavioral health" (and associated "behavioral health providers") appears to be commonly used to refer globally to mental health (the assessment, diagnosis, and treatment of mental health conditions, representative of psychopathology) as well as a range of other social, environmental, and psychological processes pertaining to human behavior in the domain of health, both clinical and nonclinical. Primary care patients may be in need of assistance with health behavior change (e.g., diet, physical activity, smoking cessation, sleep), stress management, chronic disease coping and self-management, infectious disease prevention behaviors (e.g., vaccination), and enhanced social support and health education, at the individual, family, or group level. Health psychologists, typically trained as masters and doctoral clinical psychologists, are capable of providing psychoeducation and intervention services across this range of what is called "behavioral medicine." Although there is a plethora of research demonstrating the effectiveness of behavioral medicine interventions in primary care settings (e.g., Etz et al., 2008; Pronk, Peek, & Goldstein, 2004) and compelling literature on how to integrate behavioral health into primary care (Martin, 2012), the research on integrated behavioral health care as a care delivery system is largely silent on the structures, processes, and attitudes pertaining to this potentially invaluable role of behavioral health specialists in primary care settings (although see Ray-Sannerud et al., 2012). As psychosocial and behavioral factors are implicated in a rather large proportion of the preventable causes of death in the United States and worldwide (Mokdad, Marks, Stroup, & Gerberding, 2004, 2005), investment in the development of an evidence base on the implementation, dissemination, and sustainability of behavioral medicine structures and processes in primary care is warranted. This may influence policy decisions, as training programs and reimbursement for behavioral medicine services (where it exists at all) fail to recognize the level of training required to effectively deliver behavioral medicine interventions.

Other Specific Populations

There is a good evidence base for older and middle age adults, veterans, and patients cared for HMO settings, although limited to the disease contexts previously noted. Both IMPACT and PROSPECT focused primarily on geriatric populations. In contrast, there is only limited evidence on integrated care for children and adolescents. The Youth Partners-in-Care (YPIC) study was an RCT of the effects of a care management quality improvement intervention compared to enhanced usual care, in youth ages 13–21 with depression (Asarnow et al., 2005). Although generally consistent with standard care management duties, YPIC care managers were masters or doctoral level psychotherapists who delivered cognitive behavioral therapy (CBT) or coordinated delivery of other treatment options and were not supervised by additional mental health specialists. Modest but statistically significant improvements in depression outcomes and patient satisfaction were observed. Limited evidence exists for integrated behavioral health care for peripartum women (Gjerdingen, Crow, McGovern, Miner, & Center, 2009) and ethnic minorities such as Hispanic and Latino(a) patients (Ell et al., 2009). Other populations that could be targeted include immigrant and refugee populations.

Cost and Sustainability

The sustainability of integrated care models is tenuous at best (Gilbody, Bower, & Whitty, 2006), especially in resource-limited safety net settings (Palinkas, Ell, Hansen, Cabassa, & Wells, 2011). The high cost of these programs, in terms of workforce, information technology, time and space, is an obvious barrier to sustainability. Many of these programs are supported by temporary grant funding and foundation support, or are implemented in resource-rich health maintenance organizations such as the Group Health Cooperative (the origin of the IMPACT model). A significant gap remains in our understanding of how to implement the integrated care interventions in small-to medium-sized, independent primary care practices. There is a need to better understand the circumstances under which integration is cost-effective (what must we pay to yield clinically significant improvements in health at the population level?) and yields cost-offset (does increased investment in care in the short term yield lower costs in the long term?). Many evaluations of financial outcomes have followed reports of clinical outcomes for a range of study designs, from randomized trials to program evaluation, in the context of providing behavioral health services in medical settings (c.f., Blount et al., 2007). Generally speaking, integrated behavioral health care is more acutely expensive than usual care, but yields better outcomes and may offset costs in the long run (Gilbody, Bower, & Whitty, 2006). Business models that enable billing and payment for integrated behavioral health services are needed (Blount et al., 2007). Emerging models of pay for performance and accountable care organizations (ACOs) are dramatically restructuring the incentives for chronic disease care delivery, and may serve as a boon for attempts to implement sustainable integrated behavioral health care programs.

Implementation and Dissemination

The Veteran Health Administration (VHA) Quality Enhancement Research Initiative (QUERI) is a methodology for quality improvement and evaluation of implementation and dissemination of evidence-based practices (Rubenstein, Mittman, Yano, & Mulrow, 2000). It draws upon both quantitative and qualitative methods. The VHA is applying this methodology to the evaluation of their national implementation and dissemination of collaborative care in their Translating Initiatives for Depression into Effective Solutions (TIDES) model of collaborative care for depression

(Luck et al., 2009; Stetler et al., 2006). In this model, the importance of the national leadership, sustainable business models, and clinical feasibility and effectiveness is explicit. There is an emphasis on determining elements of integrated behavioral health care that should be standardized versus customized across the different sites (e.g., the extent to which there should fidelity vs. flexibility in the model). Results of a large-scale evaluation have not been published, although there is evidence that translation of the TIDES model into practice leads to better depression outcomes; they have also seen increased support for the TIDES model at the national policy level (Rubenstein et al., 2010). This and other research on implementation and dissemination of integrated behavioral health care models is a growing area of focus (c.f., Katon, Unutzer, Wells, & Jones, 2010).

Complementary Research Methodologies: Filling the Evidence Gaps

The nature of research on integrated behavioral health care has generally commanded "effectiveness" rather than "efficacy" trials. For instance, there are challenges with respect to randomization and adherence to protocol in "real world" settings, and ethical concerns regarding. Thus, this body of research often reflects the characteristics of pragmatic trials, in which the comparison group is "usual care" or even "enhanced usual care," by which patients and providers are allowed or even encouraged to use any of the standard resources for managing mental illness in their system (e.g., provider or self-referral to specialty mental health).

The traditional bias towards randomized controlled trials (with randomization at the individual patient level) as the gold standard for testing the efficacy of integrated care interventions continues to exist, but may be considered tempered by increased perceptions of value of more pragmatic designs for testing effectiveness in more naturalistic settings. More commonly, we see cluster randomization (randomization at the level of providers or sites, to reduce contamination effects) and stratified or permuted block randomization (randomization within groups of patients with common characteristics). Also, there has been increasing opportunity for the use of quasi-experimental designs, such as interrupted time series or regression discontinuity designs, to evaluate the effects of integrated care interventions that are implemented at a particular point in time or targeted to at-risk populations in a given setting. With an increased emphasis on translational and dissemination research, these rigorous-but-not-randomized designs will be especially useful to consider.

Quasi-experimental Designs

The use of quasi-experimental designs in evaluations of quality improvement or other implementation or dissemination projects can provide strong evidence of the impact of integrated care. Expert opinion, funding streams, and the realities of today's health care industry dictate designs that deviate from traditional randomized trials (pragmatic trials, quasi-experimental designs, and research otherwise focused on translation) are needed (Kessler & Glasgow, 2011). The DIAMOND project described above represents a quasi-experimental design. These trials are uniquely suited to evaluate packages of care interventions where the individual elements of the package are not being evaluated, rather the overall effectiveness of the package and potential influence of context are of interest (Macpherson, 2004). Pragmatic trials are especially suited to evaluation of complex interventions such as integrated care. The strengths of these designs must be balanced against the need for larger sample sizes and the inability to tease apart components of the intervention. For example, the Robert Wood Johnson-supported Michigan Depression in Primary Care project was run as a pragmatic trial, in that there were both intervention and control practices, but no true randomization protocol. Individual practices had some freedom in how they implemented the process of referring to care managers, and care managers, while they had a general protocol to follow, this was not scripted in the traditional sense of a treatment manual.

Although it is the weakest of the quasi-experimental designs, the pre-post, single group design can still provide some information about changes occurring within an organization following the implementation of an integrated care model. For instance, evaluation of the St. Louis Initiative for Integrated Care Excellence (SLI²CE) (Brawer, Martielli, Pye, Manwaring, & Tierney, 2010) involved such a design. The primary problem with this design is its susceptibility to threats to internal validity, especially history, maturation, and testing threats. Even when no adequate comparison group is available, though, design elements (e.g., multiple baselines and follow-ups) can be incorporated to strengthen the study. An interrupted time series design can yield stronger conclusions—when an abrupt, persistent, and significant change in the trajectory of the outcome occurs at the same moment in time as when the intervention was imposed, it is unlikely that any other factor caused that change.

Qualitative Research

Qualitative methods (semi-structured interviews and focus groups, primarily) have been used to explore a variety of subjective, experiential aspects of integrated behavioral health care, and are often embedded to assist with interpretation of quantitative outcome measures. Most commonly, qualitative designs are used to explore barriers and facilitators to the adoption of integrated behavioral health care models (Gask, 2005; Kilbourne et al., 2008; Nutting et al., 2008; Palinkas, Ell, et al., 2011). Gask (2005) interviewed 45 mental health workers, primary care physicians, and other personnel involved in the interface between mental health and primary care in a group-model HMO, to examine perceived barriers to integration. In her analysis, grounded in Activity Theory, there were both "overt" and "covert" barriers. Overt barriers included cost, structural barriers to interdisciplinary communication related to patient self-referrals in a carve-out mental health system, and lack of colocation, which prevents easy, informal interaction between primary care and mental health providers. Covert barriers included differences in attitudes and conceptual perspectives on the provision of mental health care. For instance, mental health workers were frustrated by the apparent "learned helplessness" of primary care providers faced with patients with complex mental health issues, while primary care providers were put off by some mental health specialists' tendency to eschew on-the-spot consultation and open access (e.g., the tradition of the "50-minute hour"). There were also concerns about the perceived value of the breadth of the generalist PCP expertise versus the depth of the specialist mental health provider expertise, and differences in perspectives on whose responsibility it is to ensure that patients with mental health needs are seen (the patient's or the health care system's).

A qualitative study involving semi-structured interviews led to the identification of several benefits, barriers, and best practices in the implementation and dissemination of the RESPECT-D care management intervention (Nutting et al., 2008). Thematic analysis (applying a coding scheme to interview transcripts using qualitative analysis software, e.g., ATLAS.ti) was conducted across four waves of interviews with primary care clinicians, care managers, and mental health professionals (varying in their involvement with and enthusiasm for the care management program). Noting widespread endorsement of the value of the care manager for the treatment of depression, tempered by the expected financial and organizational change process barriers, the investigators concluded that "the major barriers to more widespread use of care management in depression are largely economic and related less to attitudes and preferences of primary care clinicians" (p. 35). Additional themes concerned the identification of patients most likely to benefit from care manager contact (e.g., patients undergoing a change in a care plan), the importance of a mental health specialist (e.g., psychiatrist) supervising the care manager, the importance of on-site care management (vs. centralized or located otherwise off-site), and the essential foundation of a good relationship between the primary care clinician and the care manager.

A notable gap in the qualitative literature is consideration of patient and family perspectives (patient satisfaction surveys notwithstanding), including issues pertaining to patient engagement, patient experience, patient preference, and the role of the patient in integrated behavioral health care teams. Qualitative designs also lend themselves well to studying values, principles, and attitudes towards integrated behavioral health care practices and the experiences of interdisciplinary collaboration. For instance, what is the process by which behavioral health providers and medical providers learn to communicate, develop mutual respect for and understanding of each other's skills and conceptual models, and negotiate the balance of power and shared decision making (in concert with the patient/family) on a case-by-case basis? What are the perceived barriers to effective collaboration, and how do these influence the effective implementation and dissemination of integrated behavioral health care systems? Using semi-structured interviews and a grounded theory approach to analysis, Henke, Chou, Chanin, Zides, and Scholle (2008) evaluated physician perceptions of barriers to depression care, and perceived utility of chronic care model-based interventions for depression in primary care. The providers in this study endorsed care management, mental health integration, and education, but felt that mental health consultation models were less helpful. It was subsequently suggested that attempts to implement models endorsed by providers would be more successful. Such qualitative research may therefore aid in hypothesis generation for future implementation research.

Mixed Method Designs

Mixed method designs interweave quantitative and qualitative design elements, often in an iterative fashion such that the richness of the analysis deepens as the study progresses (Palinkas, Aarons, et al., 2011). Mixed methods can be used in both experimental and observational research and evaluation. A prime example is the CADET project. CADET is a large pragmatic cluster randomized controlled trial of collaborative care for depression in the United Kingdom as part of the National Health Service (Richards et al., 2009). It is a phase III trial following the purportedly successful implementation of phase I and II demonstrations (Richards et al., 2008). The model consists of case management, with a patient management plan and education. To address potential threats to validity stemming from contamination effects, randomization occurred at the practice level. Providers belonging to usual care practices receive no recommendations for altering their typical depression care (e.g., prescriptions of antidepressants and referring to specialty care), except when suicide risk is identified. Both quantitative and qualitative methods are being used to assess a variety of outcomes. Clinical and cost outcome data are primarily quantitative, relying upon validated tools such as the PHQ-9 for depression severity, the SF-36 for quality of life, and the CSQ8 for patient satisfaction, as well as objective administrative data on utilization and costs. Process outcome data are primarily qualitative and are based on interviews concerning mechanisms of change and processes of implementation of the intervention. Results are not yet available.

Observational (Correlational) Designs

The apparent variability in the ways in which different organizations have chosen to implement integrated behavioral health care presents the opportunity to conduct observational comparative effectiveness research (OCER) on integrated behavioral health care in real-world settings. Community-based participatory research approaches, described in Chap. 6, are another way to build on the principles and objectives of integrated behavioral health care. However, a major barrier to conducting this type of research is the lack of well-validated measurement tools or even agreement on the discrete domains or elements of integration that should be measured. Work on integrated behavioral health care metrics has only just begun (Kessler & Miller, 2011).

Analytic Strategies

Under what circumstances is integrated behavioral health care effective? For whom is it effective? In what contexts and settings is it effective? Questions such as these are appropriately answered by testing for effect modification, or moderation, of the relationship between condition (intervention vs. control) and the study outcomes. For instance, in the PROSPECT study, the presence or absence of a series of comorbid medical conditions was tested as a moderator of the intervention effect on remission rates for depression (Bogner et al., 2005). While two of 16 conditions (atrial fibrillation and chronic pulmonary disease) significantly predicted odds of remission in the usual care condition, no conditions were associated with remission in the intervention condition, and there were no significant interactions after adjusting for multiple comparisons. In another study, although not a moderation analysis, higher scores on measures of anxiety and bipolar disorder at baseline were positively associated with odds of being a nonresponder to a collaborative care program for depression (Angstman, Dejesus, & Rohrer, 2010). It is a well-known phenomenon that detecting significant interaction effects is underpowered, however. Large-scale comparative effectiveness research presents the opportunity to plan for subgroup analysis and testing moderation.

Summary and Conclusions

The state of the evidence for integrated behavioral health care is strong in certain domains (e.g., protocol-driven, depression-focused randomized trials), but still emerging or weak in others (e.g., real-world implementation of non-disease-specific models). Questions of essential elements, effective dissemination and implementation strategies, and the impact of interventions in the context of primary care multimorbidity remain. Meta-analyses show that integrated behavioral health care can lead to better outcomes (e.g., improved rates of remission, reduced symptomology, improved functioning). We now need to focus research efforts on exploring the settings and organizational contexts in which they can be effectively and efficiently implemented, and expanding integrated behavioral health care models to offer care beyond particular mental health conditions.

Furthermore, consensus is needed in order to develop general principles about what constitutes an integrated behavioral health care model, so that the evidence can provide adequate guidance to those organizations seeking to implement such a model. Peek's lexicon (Peek, 2011) is a promising attempt to bring robust organizing principles to the integrated behavioral health care research domain, and highlights the lack of evidence for what he describes as a paradigm case. More recent research on Strosahl's primary mental health care model and the Depression in Primary Care demonstration projects more closely approximate the paradigm case for collaborative care. As potentially more sustainable healthcare delivery system approaches, these contemporary models are richer and more complex, and address more of the structural features and processes of integrated behavioral health care than did the classic models. The trade-off has been that these models are less amenable to classic randomized trial designs, and the evidence relies upon less rigorous evaluation methods. Indeed, conducting a randomized trial for every possible permutation of integrated behavioral health care would be cost prohibitive. New and innovative methods such as mixed methods (Palinkas, Aarons, et al., 2011), pragmatic trials (Zwarenstein et al., 2008), quality improvement evaluations (Rubenstein et al., 2000), and other emerging research and evaluation methods (Damschroder et al., 2009; Katon et al., 2010; Proctor et al., 2009) appropriate for translation, dissemination, and implementation research—beyond the traditional randomized trial—are needed to fill these evidence gaps.

Acknowledgments The authors wish to acknowledge the expertise of our many esteemed colleagues and collaborators who practice, study, and promote integrated behavioral health care in the "real world" every day. Their experiences and expertise informed the direction and content of this chapter.

References

Alexopoulos, G. S., Katz, I. R., Bruce, M. L., Heo, M., Ten Have, T., Raue, P., et al. (2005). Remission in depressed geriatric primary care patients: A report from the PROSPECT study. *The American Journal of Psychiatry, 162*(4), 718–724. doi:162/4/718 [pii] 10.1176/appi.ajp. 162.4.718.

Alexopoulos, G. S., Reynolds, C. F., Bruce, M. L., Katz, I. R., Raue, P. J., Mulsant, B. H., et al. (2009). Reducing suicidal ideation and depression in older primary care patients: 24-month outcomes of the PROSPECT study. *The American Journal of Psychiatry, 166*(8), 882–890. doi:appi.ajp. 2009.08121779 [pii] 10.1176/appi.ajp.2009.08121779.

Alford, D. P., LaBelle, C. T., Kretsch, N., Bergeron, A., Winter, M., Botticelli, M., et al. (2011). Collaborative care of opioid-addicted patients in primary care using buprenorphine: Five-year experience. *Archives of Internal Medicine, 171*(5), 425–431. doi:171/5/425 [pii] 10.1001/archinternmed.2010.541.

Angstman, K. B., Dejesus, R. S., & Rohrer, J. E. (2010). Correlation between mental health co-morbidity screening scores and clinical response in collaborative care treatment for depression. *Mental Health in Family Medicine, 7*(3), 129–133.

Ansseau, M., Dierick, M., Buntinkx, F., Cnockaert, P., De Smedt, J., Van Den Haute, M., et al. (2004). High prevalence of mental disorders in primary care. *Journal of Affective Disorders, 78*(1), 49–55. doi:S0165032702002197 [pii].

Areán, P. A., Ayalon, L., Jin, C., McCulloch, C. E., Linkins, K., Chen, H., et al. (2008). Integrated specialty mental health care among older minorities improves access but not outcomes: Results of the PRISMe study. *International Journal of Geriatric Psychiatry, 23*(10), 1086–1092.

Asarnow, J. R., & Albright, A. (2010). Care management increases the use of primary and medical care services by people with severe mental illness in community mental health settings. *Evidence-Based Nursing, 13*(4), 128–129. doi:13/4/128 [pii] 10.1136/ebn.13.4.128.

Asarnow, J. R., Jaycox, L. H., Duan, N., LaBorde, A. P., Rea, M. M., Murray, P., et al. (2005). Effectiveness of a quality improvement intervention for adolescent depression in primary care clinics: A randomized controlled trial. *Journal of the American Medical Association, 293*(3), 311–319. doi:293/3/311 [pii] 10.1001/Journal of the American Medical Association.293.3.311.

Babor, T. F., McRee, B. G., Kassebaum, P. A., Grimaldi, P. L., Ahmed, K., & Bray, J. (2007). Screening, brief intervention, and referral to treatment (SBIRT): Toward a public health approach to the management of substance abuse. *Substance Abuse, 28*(3), 7–30.

Bartels, S. J., Coakley, E. H., Zubritsky, C., Ware, J. H., Miles, K. M., Arean, P. A., et al. (2004). Improving access to geriatric mental health services: A randomized trial comparing treatment engagement with integrated versus enhanced referral care for depression, anxiety, and at-risk alcohol use. *The American Journal of Psychiatry, 161*(8), 1455–1462.

Beck, B. J., & Gordon, C. (2010). An approach to collaborative care and consultation: Interviewing, cultural competence, and enhancing rapport and adherence. *Medical Clinics of North America, 94*(6), 1075–1088. doi:S0025-7125(10)00135-5 [pii] 10.1016/j.mcna.2010.08.001.

Berwick, D. M., Nolan, T. W., & Whittington, J. (2008). The triple aim: Care, health, and cost. *Health Affairs, 27*(3), 759–769. doi:10.1377/hlthaff.27.3.759.

Blount, A. (2003). Integrated primary care: Organizing the evidence. *Families, Systems & Health, 21*(2), 121–133.

Blount, A., Kathol, R., Thomas, M., Schoenbaum, M., Rollman, B. L., O'Donohue, W., et al. (2007). The economics of behavioral health services in medical settings: A summary of the evidence. *Professional Psychology-Research and Practice, 38*(3), 290–297. doi:10.1037/0735-7028.38.3.290.

Bogner, H. R., Cary, M. S., Bruce, M. L., Reynolds, C. F., 3rd, Mulsant, B., Ten Have, T., et al. (2005). The role of medical comorbidity in outcome of major depression in primary care: The PROSPECT study. *The American Journal of Geriatric Psychiatry, 13*(10), 861–868. doi:13/10/861 [pii] 10.1176/appi.ajgp. 13.10.861.

Bogner, H. R., & de Vries, H. F. (2008). Integration of depression and hypertension treatment: A pilot, randomized controlled trial. *Annals of Family Medicine, 6*(4), 295–301. doi:6/4/295 [pii] 10.1370/afm.843.

Bower, P., Gilbody, S., Richards, D., Fletcher, J., & Sutton, A. (2006). Collaborative care for depression in primary care. Making sense of a complex intervention: Systematic review and meta-regression. *The British Journal of Psychiatry, 189*, 484–493. doi:189/6/484 [pii] 10.1192/bjp.bp. 106.023655.

Brawer, P. A., Martielli, R., Pye, P. L., Manwaring, J., & Tierney, A. (2010). St. Louis initiative for integrated care excellence (SLI(2)CE): Integrated-collaborative care on a large scale model. *Families, Systems & Health, 28*(2), 175–187. doi:2010-15711-009 [pii] 10.1037/a0020342.

Bruce, M. L., Ten Have, T. R., Reynolds, C. F., Katz, I. I., Schulberg, H. C., Mulsant, B. H., et al. (2004). Reducing suicidal ideation and depressive symptoms in depressed older primary care patients: A randomized controlled trial. *Journal of the American Medical Association, 291*(9), 1081–1091. doi:10.1001/Journal of the American Medical Association.291.9.1081 291/9/1081 [pii].

Butler, M., Kane, R. L., McAlpin, D., Kathol, R. G., Fu, S. S., Hagedorn, H., et al. (2008). *Integration of Mental Health/Substance Abuse and Primary Care No. 173*. Prepared by the Minnesota Evidence-Based Practice Center under Contract No. 290-02-0009. (AHRQ Publication No. 09-E003). Rockville, MD: Agency for Healthcare Research and Quality.

Butler, M., Kane, R. L., McAlpine, D., Kathol, R., Fu, S. S., Hagedorn, H., et al. (2011). Does integrated care improve treatment for depression? A systematic review. *The Journal of Ambulatory Care Management, 34*(2), 113–125. doi:10.1097/JAC.0b013e31820ef605 00004479-201104000-00004 [pii].

Collins, C., Hewson, D. L., Munger, R., & Wade, T. (2010). *Evolving models of behavioral health integration in primary care*. New York: Milbank Memorial Fund.

Craven, M., & Bland, R. (2006). Better practices in collaborative mental health care: An analysis of the evidence base. *Canadian Journal of Psychiatry, 51* (Suppl 1), 7S–72S.

Damschroder, L. J., Aron, D. C., Keith, R. E., Kirsh, S. R., Alexander, J. A., & Lowery, J. C. (2009). Fostering implementation of health services research findings into practice: A consolidated framework for advancing implementation science. *Implementation Science, 4*, 50. doi:1748-5908-4-50 [pii] 10.1186/1748-5908-4-50.

Depression Guideline Panel. (1993). *Depression in primary care*. Rockville, MD: U.S. Dept. of Health and Human Services, Public Health Service, Agency for Health Care Policy and Research.

Dietrich, A. J., Oxman, T. E., Williams, J. W., Jr., Schulberg, H. C., Bruce, M. L., Lee, P. W., et al. (2004). Re-engineering systems for the treatment of depression in primary care: Cluster randomised controlled trial. *British Medical Journal, 329*(7466), 602. doi:10.1136/bmj.38219.481250.55 bmj.38219.481250.55 [pii].

Doherty, W. J., McDaniel, S. H., & Baird, M. A. (1996). Five levels of primary care/behavioral healthcare collaboration. *Behavioral Healthcare Tomorrow, 5*(5), 25–27.

Donabedian, A. (1988). The quality of care. How can it be assessed? *Journal of the American Medical Association, 260*(12), 1743–1748.

Druss, B. G., Rohrbaugh, R. M., Levinson, C. M., & Rosenheck, R. A. (2001). Integrated medical care for patients with serious psychiatric illness: A randomized trial. *Archives of General Psychiatry, 58*(9), 861–868. doi:yoa20292 [pii].

Druss, B. G., von Esenwein, S. A., Compton, M. T., Rask, K. J., Zhao, L., & Parker, R. M. (2010). A randomized trial of medical care management for community mental health settings: The Primary Care Access, Referral, and Evaluation (PCARE) study. *The American Journal of Psychiatry, 167*(2), 151–159. doi:appi.ajp. 2009.09050691 [pii] 10.1176/appi.ajp.2009.09050691.

Ell, K., Katon, W., Cabassa, L. J., Xie, B., Lee, P. J., Kapetanovic, S., et al. (2009). Depression and diabetes among low-income Hispanics: Design elements of a socioculturally adapted collaborative care model randomized controlled trial. *International Journal of Psychiatry in Medicine, 39*(2), 113–132.

Ell, K., Katon, W., Xie, B., Lee, P. J., Kapetanovic, S., Guterman, J., et al. (2010). Collaborative care management of major depression among low-income, predominantly Hispanic subjects with diabetes: A randomized controlled trial. *Diabetes Care, 33*(4), 706–713. doi:dc09-1711 [pii] 10.2337/dc09-1711.

Engel, C. C., Oxman, T., Yamamoto, C., Gould, D., Barry, S., Stewart, P., et al. (2008). RESPECT-Mil: Feasibility of a systems-level collaborative care approach to depression and post-traumatic stress disorder in military primary care. *Military Medicine, 173*(10), 935–940.

Etz, R. S., Cohen, D. J., Woolf, S. H., Holtrop, J. S., Donahue, K. E., Isaacson, N. F., et al. (2008). Bridging primary care practices and communities to promote healthy behaviors. *American Journal of Preventive Medicine, 35*(Suppl. 5), S390–S397. doi:S0749-3797(08)00673-9 [pii] 10.1016/j.amepre.2008.08.008.

Felker, B. L., Chaney, E., Rubenstein, L. V., Bonner, L. M., Yano, E. M., Parker, L. E., et al. (2006). Developing effective collaboration between primary care and mental health providers. *Primary Care Companion to the Journal of Clinical Psychiatry, 8*(1), 12–16.

Fortney, J. C., Pyne, J. M., Edlund, M. J., Robinson, D. E., Mittal, D., & Henderson, K. L. (2006). Design and implementation of the telemedicine-enhanced antidepressant management study. *General Hospital Psychiatry, 28*(1), 18–26. doi:S0163-8343(05)00115-5 [pii] 10.1016/j.genhosppsych.2005.07.001.

Fortney, J. C., Pyne, J. M., Edlund, M. J., Williams, D. K., Robinson, D. E., Mittal, D., et al. (2007). A randomized trial of telemedicine-based collaborative care for depression. *Journal of General Internal Medicine, 22*(8), 1086–1093. doi:10.1007/s11606-007-0201-9.

Foy, R., Hempel, S., Rubenstein, L., Suttorp, M., Seelig, M., Shanman, R., et al. (2010). Meta-analysis: Effect of interactive communication between collaborating primary care physicians and specialists. *Annals of Internal Medicine, 152*(4), 247–258. doi:152/4/247 [pii] 10.1059/0003-4819-152-4-201002160-00010.

Gask, L. (2005). Overt and covert barriers to the integration of primary and specialist mental health care. *Social Science & Medicine, 61*(8), 1785–1794. doi:S0277-9536(05)00155-3 [pii] 10.1016/j.socscimed.2005.03.038.

Gilbody, S., Bower, P., Fletcher, J., Richards, D., & Sutton, A. J. (2006). Collaborative care for depression: A cumulative meta-analysis and review of longer-term outcomes. *Archives of Internal Medicine, 166*(21), 2314–2321. doi:10.1001/archinte.166.21.2314.

Gilbody, S., Bower, P., & Whitty, P. (2006). Costs and consequences of enhanced primary care for depression: Systematic review of randomised economic evaluations. *The British Journal of Psychiatry, 189*, 297–308. doi:189/4/297 [pii] 10.1192/bjp.bp. 105.016006.

Gjerdingen, D., Crow, S., McGovern, P., Miner, M., & Center, B. (2009). Stepped care treatment of postpartum depression: Impact on treatment, health, and work outcomes. *Journal of the American Board of Family Medicine, 22*(5), 473–482. doi:22/5/473 [pii] 10.3122/jabfm.2009.05.080192.

Henke, R. M., Chou, A. F., Chanin, J. C., Zides, A. B., & Scholle, S. H. (2008). Physician attitude toward depression care interventions: Implications for implementation of quality improvement initiatives. *Implementation Science, 3*, 40. doi:1748-5908-3-40 [pii] 10.1186/1748-5908-3-40.

Katon, W., & Schulberg, H. C. (1992). Epidemiology of depression in primary care. *General Hospital Psychiatry, 14*(4), 237–247.

Katon, W. J., & Seelig, M. (2008). Population-based care of depression: Team care approaches to improving outcomes. *Journal of Occupational and Environmental Medicine, 50*(4), 459–467. doi:10.1097/JOM.0b013e318168efb7 00043764-200804000-00011 [pii].

Katon, W., Unutzer, J., Wells, K., & Jones, L. (2010). Collaborative depression care: History, evolution and ways to enhance dissemination and sustainability. *General Hospital Psychiatry, 32*(5), 456–464. doi:S0163-8343(10)00062-9 [pii] 10.1016/j.genhosppsych.2010.04.001.

Katon, W. J., Von Korff, M., Lin, E. H., Simon, G., Ludman, E., Russo, J., et al. (2004). The pathways study: A randomized trial of collaborative care in patients with diabetes and depression. *Archives of General Psychiatry, 61*(10), 1042–1049. doi:61/10/1042 [pii] 10.1001/archpsyc.61.10.1042.

Kessler, R., & Glasgow, R. E. (2011). A proposal to speed translation of healthcare research into practice dramatic change is needed. *American Journal of Preventive Medicine, 40*(6), 637–644. doi:S0749-3797(11)00162-0 [pii] 10.1016/j.amepre.2011.02.023.

Kessler, R., & Miller, B. F. (2011). A framework for collaborative care metrics. In C. Mullican (Ed.), *AHRQ Publication No. 11-0067* (pp. 17–23). Rockville, MD: Agency for Healthcare Research and Quality.

Kilbourne, A. M., Biswas, K., Pirraglia, P. A., Sajatovic, M., Williford, W. O., & Bauer, M. S. (2009). Is the collaborative chronic care model effective for patients with bipolar disorder and co-occurring conditions? *Journal of Affective Disorders, 112*(1–3), 256–261. doi:S0165-0327(08)00174-2 [pii] 10.1016/j.jad.2008.04.010.

Kilbourne, A. M., Irmiter, C., Capobianco, J., Reynolds, K., Milner, K., Barry, K., et al. (2008). Improving integrated general medical and mental health services in community-based practices. *Administration and Policy in Mental Health, 35*(5), 337–345. doi:10.1007/s10488-008-0177-8.

Klinkman, M. S., Bauroth, S., Fedewa, S., Kerber, K., Kuebler, J., Adman, T., et al. (2010). Long-term clinical outcomes of care management for chronically depressed primary care patients: A report from the depression in primary care project. *Annals of Family Medicine, 8*(5), 387–396. doi:8/5/387 [pii] 10.1370/afm.1168.

Krahn, D. D., Bartels, S. J., Coakley, E., Oslin, D. W., Chen, H., McIntyre, J., et al. (2006). PRISM-E: Comparison of integrated care and enhanced specialty referral models in depression outcomes. *Psychiatric Services, 57*(7), 946–953. doi:57/7/946 [pii] 10.1176/appi.ps.57.7.946.

Kroenke, K., Bair, M. J., Damush, T. M., Wu, J., Hoke, S., Sutherland, J., et al. (2009). Optimized antidepressant therapy and pain self-management in primary care patients with depression and musculoskeletal pain: A randomized controlled trial. *Journal of the American Medical Association, 301*(20), 2099–2110. doi:301/20/2099 [pii] 10.1001/Journal of the American Medical Association. 2009.723.

Lee, P. W., Dietrich, A. J., Oxman, T. E., Williams, J. W., Jr., & Barry, S. L. (2007). Sustainable impact of a primary care depression intervention. *Journal of the American Board of Family Medicine, 20*(5), 427–433. doi:20/5/427 [pii] 10.3122/jabfm.2007.05.070045.

Lessing, K., & Blignault, I. (2001). Mental health telemedicine programmes in Australia. *Journal of Telemedicine and Telecare, 7*(6), 317–323.

Levkoff, S. E., Chen, H., Coakley, E., Herr, E. C., Oslin, D. W., Katz, I., et al. (2004). Design and sample characteristics of the PRISM-E multisite randomized trial to improve behavioral health care for the elderly. *Journal of Aging and Health, 16*(1), 3–27.

Lin, E. H., Von Korff, M., Ciechanowski, P., Peterson, D., Ludman, E. J., Rutter, C. M., et al. (2012). Treatment adjustment and medication adherence for complex patients with diabetes, heart disease, and depression: A randomized controlled trial. *Annals of Family Medicine, 10*(1), 6–14. doi:10/1/6 [pii] 10.1370/afm.1343.

Luck, J., Hagigi, F., Parker, L. E., Yano, E. M., Rubenstein, L. V., & Kirchner, J. E. (2009). A social marketing approach to implementing evidence-based practice in VHA QUERI: The TIDES depression collaborative care model. *Implementation Science, 4*, 64. doi:1748-5908-4-64 [pii] 10.1186/1748-5908-4-64.

Ludman, E. J., Simon, G. E., Tutty, S., & Von Korff, M. (2007). A randomized trial of telephone psychotherapy and pharmacotherapy for depression: Continuation and durability of effects. *Journal of Consulting and Clinical Psychology, 75*(2), 257–266. doi:2007-04141-006 [pii] 10.1037/0022-006X.75.2.257.

Macpherson, H. (2004). Pragmatic clinical trials. *Complementary Therapies in Medicine, 12*(2–3), 136–140. doi:S0965-2299(04)00080-9 [pii] 10.1016/j.ctim.2004.07.043.

Martin, M. (2012). Real behavior change in primary care. *Families, Systems & Health, 30*(1), 81–81. doi:Doi 10.1037/A0027295.

McGregor, M., Lin, E. H., & Katon, W. J. (2011). TEAMcare: An integrated multicondition collaborative care program for chronic illnesses and depression. *The Journal of Ambulatory Care Management, 34*(2), 152–162. doi:10.1097/JAC.0b013e31820ef6a4 00004479-201104000-00007 [pii].

Miller, B. F., Kessler, R., Peek, C. J., & Kallenberg, G. A. (2011). A national agenda for research in collaborative care. *Papers from the Collaborative Care Research Network Research Development Conference*. (AHRQ Publication No. 11–0067). Rockville, MD: Agency for Healthcare Research and Quality.

Miller, B. F., Mendenhall, T. J., & Malik, A. D. (2009). Integrated primary care: An inclusive three-world view through process metrics and empirical discrimination. *Journal of Clinical Psychology in Medical Settings, 16*, 21–30.

Mokdad, A. H., Marks, J. S., Stroup, D. F., & Gerberding, J. L. (2004). Actual causes of death in the United States, 2000. *Journal of the American Medical Association, 291*(10), 1238–1245. doi:10.1001/Journal of the American Medical Association.291.10.1238 291/10/1238 [pii].

Mokdad, A. H., Marks, J. S., Stroup, D. F., & Gerberding, J. L. (2005). Correction: Actual causes of death in the United States, 2000. *Journal of the American Medical Association, 293*(3), 293–294. doi:293/3/293 [pii] 10.1001/Journal of the American Medical Association.293.3.293.

Muntingh, A. D., van der Feltz-Cornelis, C. M., van Marwijk, H. W., Spinhoven, P., Assendelft, W. J., de Waal, M. W., et al. (2009). Collaborative stepped care for anxiety disorders in primary care: Aims and design of a randomized controlled trial. *BMC Health Services Research, 9*, 159. doi:1472-6963-9-159 [pii] 10.1186/1472-6963-9-159.

Nelson, L. (2012). *Lessons from Medicare's demonstration projects on disease management, care coordination, and value-based payment 1–8*. Retrieved from http://cbo.gov/publication/42860

Nutting, P. A., Gallagher, K., Riley, K., White, S., Dickinson, W. P., Korsen, N., et al. (2008). Care management for depression in primary care practice: Findings from the RESPECT-Depression trial. *Annals of Family Medicine, 6*(1), 30–37. doi:10.1370/afm.742.

Oslin, D. W., Ross, J., Sayers, S., Murphy, J., Kane, V., & Katz, I. R. (2006). Screening, assessment, and management of depression in VA primary care clinics. The Behavioral Health Laboratory. *Journal of General Internal Medicine, 21*(1), 46–50. doi:JGI267 [pii] 10.1111/j.1525-1497.2005.0267.x.

Oxman, T. E., Dietrich, A. J., & Schulberg, H. C. (2005). Evidence-based models of integrated management of depression in primary care. *Psychiatric Clinics of North America, 28*(4), 1061–1077. doi:S0193-953X(05)00078-X [pii] 10.1016/j.psc.2005.09.007.

Oxman, T. E., Dietrich, A. J., Williams, J. W., Jr., & Kroenke, K. (2002). A three-component model for reengineering systems for the treatment of depression in primary care. *Psychosomatics, 43*(6), 441–450.

Palinkas, L. A., Aarons, G. A., Horwitz, S., Chamberlain, P., Hurlburt, M., & Landsverk, J. (2011). Mixed method designs in implementation research. *Administration and Policy in Mental Health, 38*(1), 44–53. doi:10.1007/s10488-010-0314-z.

Palinkas, L. A., Ell, K., Hansen, M., Cabassa, L., & Wells, A. (2011). Sustainability of collaborative care interventions in primary care settings. *Journal of Social Work, 11*(1), 99–117. doi:Doi 10.1177/1468017310381310.

Peek, C. J. (2011). A collaborative care lexicon for asking practice and research development questions. In C. Mullican (Ed.), *AHRQ Publication No. 11-0067* (pp. 25–44). Rockville, MD: Agency for Healthcare Research and Quality.

Pincus, H. A., Pechura, C., Keyser, D., Bachman, J., & Houtsinger, J. K. (2006). Depression in primary care: Learning lessons in a national quality improvement program. *Administration and Policy in Mental Health and Mental Health Services Research, 33*, 2–15.

Pomerantz, A., Cole, B. H., Watts, B. V., & Weeks, W. B. (2008). Improving efficiency and access to mental health care: Combining integrated care and advanced access. *General Hospital Psychiatry, 30*(6), 546–551. doi:S0163-8343(08)00165-5 [pii] 10.1016/j.genhosppsych.2008.09.004.

Pomerantz, A. S., Shiner, B., Watts, B. V., Detzer, M. J., Kutter, C., Street, B., et al. (2010). The White River model of colocated collaborative care: A platform for mental and behavioral health care in the medical home. *Families, Systems & Health, 28*(2), 114–129. doi:2010-15711-005 [pii] 10.1037/a0020261.

Proctor, E. K., Landsverk, J., Aarons, G., Chambers, D., Glisson, C., & Mittman, B. (2009). Implementation research in mental health services: An emerging science with conceptual, methodological, and training challenges. *Administration and Policy in Mental Health, 36*(1), 24–34. doi:10.1007/s10488-008-0197-4.

Pronk, N. P., Peek, C. J., & Goldstein, M. G. (2004). Addressing multiple behavioral risk factors in primary care. A synthesis of current knowledge and stakeholder dialogue sessions. *American Journal of Preventive Medicine, 27*(Suppl. 2), 4–17. doi:10.1016/j.amepre.2004.04.024 S0749379704001047 [pii].

Pyne, J. M., Fortney, J. C., Tripathi, S. P., Maciejewski, M. L., Edlund, M. J., & Williams, D. K. (2010). Cost-effectiveness analysis of a rural telemedicine collaborative care intervention for depression. *Archives of General Psychiatry, 67*(8), 812–821. doi:67/8/812 [pii] 10.1001/archgenpsychiatry.2010.82.

Ray-Sannerud, B. N., Dolan, D. C., Morrow, C. E., Corso, K. A., Kanzler, K. E., Corso, M. L., et al. (2012). Longitudinal outcomes after brief behavioral health intervention in an integrated primary care clinic. *Families, Systems & Health, 30*(1), 60–71. doi:2012-02452-001 [pii] 10.1037/a0027029.

Regier, D. A., Goldberg, I. D., & Taube, C. A. (1978). The de facto US mental health services system: A public health perspective. *Archives of General Psychiatry, 35*(6), 685–693.

Reiss-Brennan, B. (2006). Can mental health integration in a primary care setting improve quality and lower costs? A case study. *Journal of Managed Care Pharmacy, 12*(Suppl. 2), 14–20. doi:2006(12)2: 14-20 [pii].

Reiss-Brennan, B., Briot, P., Daumit, G., & Ford, D. (2006). Evaluation of "depression in primary care" innovations. *Administration and Policy in Mental Health, 33*(1), 86–91. doi:10.1007/s10488-005-4239-x.

Reiss-Brennan, B., Briot, P. C., Savitz, L. A., Cannon, W., & Staheli, R. (2010). Cost and quality impact of Intermountain's mental health integration program. *Journal of Healthcare Management, 55*(2), 97–113. discussion 113–114.

Richards, D. A., Hughes-Morley, A., Hayes, R. A., Araya, R., Barkham, M., Bland, J. M., et al. (2009). Collaborative depression trial (CADET): Multi-centre randomised controlled trial of collaborative care for depression–study protocol. *BMC Health Services Research, 9*, 188. doi:1472-6963-9-188 [pii] 10.1186/1472-6963-9-188.

Richards, D. A., Lovell, K., Gilbody, S., Gask, L., Torgerson, D., Barkham, M., et al. (2008). Collaborative care for depression in UK primary care: A randomized controlled trial. *Psychological Medicine, 38*(2), 279–287. doi:S0033291707001365 [pii] 10.1017/S0033291707001365.

Rollman, B. L., Belnap, B. H., LeMenager, M. S., Mazumdar, S., Houck, P. R., Counihan, P. J., et al. (2009). Telephone-delivered collaborative care for treating post-CABG depression: A randomized controlled trial. *Journal of the American Medical Association, 302*(19), 2095–2103. doi:2009.1670 [pii] 10.1001/Journal of the American Medical Association. 2009.1670.

Roy-Byrne, P. P., Katon, W., Cowley, D. S., & Russo, J. (2001). A randomized effectiveness trial of collaborative care for patients with panic disorder in primary care. *Archives of General Psychiatry, 58*(9), 869–876. doi:yoa20378 [pii].

Rubenstein, L. V., Chaney, E. F., Ober, S., Felker, B., Sherman, S. E., Lanto, A., et al. (2010). Using evidence-based quality improvement methods for translating depression collaborative care research into practice. *Families, Systems & Health, 28*(2), 91–113. doi:2010-15711-004 [pii] 10.1037/a0020302.

Rubenstein, L. V., Mittman, B. S., Yano, E. M., & Mulrow, C. D. (2000). From understanding health care provider behavior to improving health care: The QUERI framework for quality improvement. Quality Enhancement Research Initiative. *Medical Care, 38*(6 Suppl. 1), I129–I141.

Rustad, J. K., Musselman, D. L., & Nemeroff, C. B. (2011). The relationship of depression and diabetes: Pathophysiological and treatment implications. *Psychoneuroendocrinology.* doi:S0306-4530(11)00094-1 [pii] 10.1016/j.psyneuen.2011.03.005.

Saxon, A. J., Malte, C. A., Sloan, K. L., Baer, J. S., Calsyn, D. A., Nichol, P., et al. (2006). Randomized trial of onsite versus referral primary medical care for veterans in addictions treatment. *Medical Care, 44*(4), 334–342. doi:0.1097/01.mlr.0000204052.95507.5c 00005650-200604000-00007 [pii].

Schulberg, H. C. (1991). Mental disorders in the primary care setting. Research priorities for the 1990s. *General Hospital Psychiatry, 13*(3), 156–164.

Simon, G. E., Ludman, E. J., & Rutter, C. M. (2009). Incremental benefit and cost of telephone care management and telephone psychotherapy for depression in primary care. *Archives of General Psychiatry, 66*(10), 1081–1089. doi:66/10/1081 [pii] 10.1001/archgenpsychiatry.2009.123.

Simon, G. E., Ludman, E. J., Tutty, S., Operskalski, B., & Von Korff, M. (2004). Telephone psychotherapy and telephone care management for primary care patients starting antidepressant treatment: A randomized controlled trial. *Journal of the American Medical Association, 292*(8), 935–942. doi:10.1001/Journal of the American Medical Association.292.8.935 292/8/935 [pii].

Solberg, L. I., Glasgow, R. E., Unutzer, J., Jaeckels, N., Oftedahl, G., Beck, A., et al. (2010). Partnership research: A practical trial design for evaluation of a natural experiment to improve depression care. *Medical Care, 48*(7), 576–582. doi:10.1097/MLR.0b013e3181dbea62.

Stetler, C. B., Legro, M. W., Wallace, C. M., Bowman, C., Guihan, M., Hagedorn, H., et al. (2006). The role of formative evaluation in implementation research and the QUERI experience. *Journal of General Internal Medicine, 21*(Suppl. 2), S1–S8. doi:JGI355 [pii] 10.1111/j.1525-1497.2006.00355.x.

Strosahl, K. (1998). Integrating behavioral health and primary care services: The primary mental health care model. In A. Blount (Ed.), *Integrated primary care: The future of medical and mental health collaboration.* New York: W. W. Norton.

Trangle M, Dieperink B, Gabert T, Haight B, Lindvall B, Mitchell J, Novak H, Rich D, Rossmiller D, Setter-lund L, Somers K. Institute for Clinical Systems Improvement. Major Depression in Adults in Primary Care. http://bit.ly/Depr0512. Updated May 2012.

Unutzer, J., Katon, W., Callahan, C. M., Williams, J. W., Hunkeler, E., Harpole, L., et al. (2002). Collaborative care management of late-life depression in the primary care setting. *Journal of the American Medical Association, 288*, 2836–2845.

Unutzer, J., Katon, W. J., Fan, M. Y., Schoenbaum, M. C., Lin, E. H. B., & Della Penna, R. D. (2008). Long-term cost effects of collaborative care for late-life depression. *The American Journal of Managed Care, 14*(2), 95–100.

Unutzer, J., Katon, W., Williams, J. W., Jr., Callahan, C. M., Harpole, L., Hunkeler, E. M., et al. (2001). Improving primary care for depression in late life: The design of a multicenter randomized trial. *Medical Care, 39*(8), 785–799.

Watts, B. V., Shiner, B., Pomerantz, A., Stender, P., & Weeks, W. B. (2007). Outcomes of a quality improvement project integrating mental health into primary care. *Quality & Safety in Health Care, 16*(5), 378–381. doi:16/5/378 [pii] 10.1136/qshc.2007.022418.

Williams, J. W., Jr., Gerrity, M., Holsinger, T., Dobscha, S., Gaynes, B., & Dietrich, A. (2007). Systematic review of multifaceted interventions to improve depression care. *General Hospital Psychiatry, 29*(2), 91–116. doi:S0163-8343(06)00223-4 [pii] 10.1016/j.genhosppsych.2006.12.003.

Williams, J. W., Jr., Katon, W., Lin, E. H., Noel, P. H., Worchel, J., Cornell, J., et al. (2004). The effectiveness of depression care management on diabetes-related outcomes in older patients. *Annals of Internal Medicine, 140*(12), 1015–1024. doi:140/12/1015 [pii].

Zivin, K., Pfeiffer, P. N., Szymanski, B. R., Valenstein, M., Post, E. P., Miller, E. M., et al. (2010). Initiation of Primary Care-Mental Health Integration programs in the VA Health System: Associations with psychiatric diagnoses in primary care. *Medical Care, 48*(9), 843–851. doi:10.1097/MLR.0b013e3181e5792b.

Zwarenstein, M., Treweek, S., Gagnier, J. J., Altman, D. G., Tunis, S., Haynes, B., Moher, D. (2008). Improving the reporting of pragmatic trials: an extension of the CONSORT statement. BMJ, 337, a2390. doi:10.1136/bmj.a2390.

Chapter 6
Community-Based Participatory Research: Advancing Integrated Behavioral Health Care Through Novel Partnerships

Tai J. Mendenhall, William J. Doherty, Jerica M. Berge, James M. Fauth, and George C. Tremblay

Abstract The call for interdisciplinary collaboration in health care is longstanding, and our collective efforts to answer this across mental health and biomedical care and training sites are evolving faster today than ever before. As we do this, it is important to recognize the lived experience, wisdom, and energy of the patients, families, and communities that we serve—and that we, as professionals, advance our effort(s) in a manner that honors this insight. In this chapter, we describe community-based participatory research (CBPR) as a way of partnering professionals with lay communities to work together to create health initiatives that neither group, respectively, could create by itself. We highlight core tenets that guide CBPR and, drawing from our own and others' work, share important lessons learned. We discuss data collection and analysis (qualitative, quantitative, and mixed-methods designs), and offer suggestions and guidance regarding education and training for those interested in learning more about partnering and working with communities in CBPR.

T.J. Mendenhall, Ph.D., LMFT, CFT (✉) • W.J. Doherty, Ph.D., LMFT, LP
Department of Family Social Science, University of Minnesota, 290 McNeal Hall;
1985 Buford Ave, Saint Paul, MN 55108, USA
e-mail: mend0009@umn.edu; bdoherty@umn.edu

J.M. Berge, Ph.D., MPH, LMFT, CFLE
Department of Family Medicine and Community Health,
University of Minnesota Medical School, 516 Delaware Street SE, Minneapolis,
MN 55455, USA
e-mail: mohl0009@umn.edu

J.M. Fauth, Ph.D. • G.C. Tremblay, Ph.D.
Department of Clinical Psychology, Antioch University New England,
40 Avon Street Keene, NH 03431, USA
e-mail: jfauth@antioch.edu; George_tremblay@antiochne.edu

M.R. Talen and A. Burke Valeras (eds.), *Integrated Behavioral Health in Primary Care: Evaluating the Evidence, Identifying the Essentials*, DOI 10.1007/978-1-4614-6889-9_6,
© Springer Science+Business Media New York 2013

The call for interdisciplinary collaboration in health care is a longstanding one, and our collective efforts to do this are evolving across medical- and mental health-training programs and care facilities today more than they ever have. Recent advancements in the Patient-Centered Medical Home (PCMH) movement are arguably pushing team-based approaches in continuous and coordinated care toward the middle of the bell-curve, wherein someday soon our integrated models will represent the rule (not the exception) to how health care is done.

A variety of definitions of what "integrated," "collaborative," or "medical home" sequences look like have been put forth, and efforts by the Agency for Healthcare Research and Quality (AHRQ), Collaborative Care Research Network (CCRN), Collaborative Family Healthcare Association (CFHA), Substance Abuse and Mental Health Services Administration (SAMHSA), and others to standardize and clarify these characterizations are presently underway (AHRQ, 2011; Peek, 2011). Common themes within our increasingly shared lexicon of core concepts within integrated behavioral health care relate to working relationships between components of the larger health care system that represent different care types (e.g., behavioral health care with primary care), providers who represent different disciplines (e.g., a family physician with a family therapist), and/or providers (broadly defined) with the very patients and families that they serve (Peek, 2010).

Our efforts, however, often miss two things that are important to consider: (1) attention to the active role(s) that our patients and their families can play in co-creating their own health, and (2) attention to the potential collective power of broader patient communities in advancing health. Instead, most health care ("collaborative" or otherwise) still frames professionals as the carriers of knowledge/wisdom and providers of services vis-à-vis patients/families who are relatively passive. Further, most care that is provided to said patients/families is delivered to one patient/family at a time, with no mechanism of connecting patients with each other along the way (Doherty, Mendenhall, & Berge, 2010; Mendenhall & Doherty, 2005b; Berge, Mendenhall, & Doherty, 2009).

This is problematic because arguably the greatest untapped resource for improving health is the knowledge, wisdom, and energy of individuals, families, and communities who face challenging health issues in their everyday lives (Doherty et al., 2010; Doherty, Mendenhall, & Berge, 2012). Consider, for example, the following questions: How does somebody recently diagnosed with diabetes really overhaul his/her lifestyle (and stick with it) across diet, physical activity, and disease management arenas? Where is "the line" between supportively reminding someone to check blood sugars and being a "nag"? How can a partner avoid burning out from supporting a mate whose pain is chronic and progressive and whose complaints are never-ending? How does a partner attend to his/her own health and needs as his/her partner continues to decline? How do couples handle the sometimes intrusive roles of health professionals, social services, and/or insurance companies?

As large national and international organizations focused on health (e.g., AHRQ, NIH, WHO) have systematically called for—and advanced funding to support—community-driven and collaborative efforts to address complex health and social problems that are ill-suited for conventional top-down service delivery and/or research endeavors, community-based participatory research (CBPR) has been put forth as a way to partner with our patient communities (AHRQ, 2011; National Center on Minority Health and Health Disparities, 2011). This is an especially timely call within the arenas of integrated behavioral health care, insofar as our strong emphases on relationships and partnerships (between providers themselves and/or providers with patients/families) are well underway. Many are now working to extend these emphases to patient/family communities, and they are creating and implementing supportive care systems that neither providers/researchers nor patients/families could create on their own.

Community-Based Participatory Research

Since its early coining as "Action Research" by Kurt Lewin in the 1940s, many have contributed to advancing an investigative orientation in which academic and professional researchers partner and collaborate with communities who are directly affected by an issue to generate knowledge and solve local problems (AHRQ, 2004; Berge et al., 2009; Mendenhall & Doherty, 2005b). Approaches within this larger frame vary in and across the degrees to which professionals and community members are involved in facilitating group processes, engaged in decision-making and change sequences, and undertaken roles or experiences as (co)learners (Bell et al., 2004; Cornwall & Jewkes, 1995; Wallerstein & Duran, 2006). These approaches have been recognized by unique and overlapping terminologies and labels like "participative research" (Bell et al., 2004) or "participatory research" (PR) (Classen et al., 2008; Torre & Fine, 2005), "participatory action research" (PAR) (Baum, MacDougall, & Smith, 2006; Bell et al., 2004; Braithwaite, Coghlan, O'Neill, & Rebane, 2007; Cammarota & Fine, 2008; Kemmis & McTaggart, 2000; Pyrch, 2007; Pyrch & Castillo, 2001; Rahman & Fals-Borda, 1991), "development leadership teams in action" (DELTA) (Haaland & Vlassoff, 2011), "critical action research" (DePoy, Hartman, & Haslett, 1999), "collaborative inquiry" (Kelly, Mock, & Tandon, 2001), "co-operative inquiry" (Heron & Reason, 2001), and "appreciative inquiry" (Ludema, Cooperrider, & Barrett, 2001). Some have framed their efforts around medical practices (versus specific diseases) in partnership with patient communities, e.g., "practice-based participatory research (PBPR)" (Fauth & Tremblay, 2011), and still others have purposively excluded the word "research" altogether so as to emphasize co-learning and change processes per se (e.g., "participatory action learning" (Wilson, Ho, & Walsh, 2007), "participatory action development" (Lammerink, Bury, & Bolt, 1999)). As aforementioned national and international organizations focused on health have encouraged such community-driven and collaborative efforts, the term "community-based participatory research" (CBPR) has been put forth as an inclusive and characterizing umbrella to connect these like-minded efforts (AHRQ, 2004; Edwards, Lund, Mitchell, & Anderson, 2008; Pan American Health Organization, 2004).

In CBPR, the "community" (however defined) is recognized and honored as a principal unit of identity, with lay members and professionals (e.g., service providers, academic researchers) serving as co-creators of each stage of the process. This

1. Recognition of the community as the principal unit of identity

2. Democratic and equitable partnership between all project members (e.g., community stakeholders, researchers) as collaborators through every stage of knowledge and intervention development

3. Building on the strengths and resources within the community

4. Promoting co-learning and capacity-building between and among partners

5. Deep investment in change that carries with it an element of challenging the status quo and improving the lives of members in a community or practice

6. Cyclical process in which problems are identified, solutions to address problems are developed within the context(s) of the community's existing resources, interventions are implemented, outcomes are evaluated according to what is essential in the eyes of participants, and interventions are modified in accord with new information as necessary

7. Project members' humility and flexibility to accommodate changes as necessary across any part of a project

8. Disseminating findings and new knowledge to and by all partners and constituents in the investigative process

9. Recognition that CBPR can be a slow and messy process, especially during initial phases of development

10. Long-term engagement and commitment to the work

Fig. 6.1 Core assumptions of community-based participatory research

stands in contrast to top-down, hierarchical methods of research that have traditionally been imposed upon communities of interest. Core assumptions guiding CBPR (see Fig. 6.1) advance these partnerships among stakeholders throughout the entire research process, from identifying the problem to implementing (and evaluating) interventions, to disseminating new knowledge and refining interventions in accord to said knowledge. Throughout this work, everyone works together in the context of flattened hierarchies (Bradbury & Reason, 2003; Doherty et al., 2010; Mendenhall & Doherty, 2005b; Scharff & Mathews, 2008; Strickland, 2006).

Key Factors Guiding Professional/Community Partnerships

From the core assumptions outlined above, those most relevant to the relationships maintained by professional and community participants in CBPR are as follows:

Building on strengths and resources. Whereas conventional approaches in health care begin with a deficit-based "needs assessment" so as to inform what reparative professional knowledge or resources to bring into a community from the outside, CBPR partnerships emphasize the identification and advancement of local wisdom, strengths, and energies to solve problems. This then sets the foundation for the equal valuing of professional and lay contributions to the work (Mendenhall & Doherty, 2005a; Reason & Bradbury, 2001, 2006, 2008).

Democratic and equitable partnership. In contrast to conventional top-down, provider-led care, research and public health initiatives, CBPR projects are advanced with a flattened professional hierarchy that honors the unique wisdom and expertise of everyone involved. While health care professionals and aca-demic researchers bring with them a knowledge- and skill-set regarding a chronic illness or investigatory design, for example, patients bring with them a knowledge base regarding what it is like to live with a chronic illness. Patients' family members bring with them wisdom about how to be supportive without being a nag, best strategies for affording indicated foods and medicines, and/or self-care so as to not burn out in the role of an involved caregiver and loved one. Community leaders bring with them knowledge and understanding about the local "pulse" and impact(s) that an illness or health-related issue is having on their people (however defined). By recognizing and honoring all project mem-bers' respective contributions to a larger whole, patients, community stakehold-ers, health care providers, and academic researchers are able to collaborate through every stage of knowledge and intervention development—from early steps in trust-building and defining what is most important to focus on to later steps of project evaluation and establishing long-term sustainability (Christopher, Watts, McCormick, & Young, 2008; Horowitz, Robinson, & Seifer, 2009; Israel, 2005; Wallerstein & Duran, 2010).

Co-learning and capacity building. By focusing on each other's unique strengths and wisdom and working collaboratively together, professionals and lay commu-nity members learn from each other. For example, as patients and families learn about important disease-management sequences and information from providers (e.g., the components of a good diet, indicated amounts of exercise), they are also learning from other patients and families about where to find the most affordable foods or participate in physical activities safely. As providers learn from patients about local value-systems regarding food and health, they are able to advance more sensitive and culturally tailored care, suggestions, and dialogue (Bradbury & Reason, 2003; Doherty et al., 2010; Mendenhall et al., 2010; Minkler & Wallerstein, 2008).

Humility and flexibility. As with any healthy relationship, project members in CBPR maintain a consistent humility regarding the extent of their knowledge, and along with this, a receptivity to others' knowledge. They are responsive to new information that suggests change is necessary across individual (e.g., a patient learning that s/he must alter a dietary or health-related routine) and project/community (e.g., modifying an intervention component in response to evaluation data that show it is or is not working). This can be especially difficult for professional members of the team, as much of their training in medical or graduate school socialized them to function as infallible experts (Hayes, 1996; Mendenhall, 2002; Mendenhall & Doherty, 2003; Minkler, 2000; Minkler & Wallerstein, 2008).

Long-term engagement and commitment to the work. CBPR projects can be very slow and messy to advance, especially during early phases of development, as providers/researchers and patients/families/community members learn to work together in a very different way than they may be accustomed to and/or until a new initiative is firmly grounded in a professional or community organization. Our experience across several projects suggests that one to two years is a reasonable amount of time to expect between first meetings and the launching of action steps and new interventions. It is important that participants understand this from the outset, and that they are invested in the long haul (Doherty et al., 2010; Jones & Wells, 2007; Wallerstein & Duran, 2006; Wallerstein & Duran, 2010).

Data Collection and Analyses in CBPR

An essential element throughout CBPR relates to the clarity of its "R," (e.g., advancing a clear effort in the arenas that project members and others on the outside would call "research"). Because participants (providers, administrators, researchers, patients, families, etc.) are often dealing with novel problems within the unique contexts of local communities, they must be methodologically flexible and eclectic in order to best match data collection efforts with what is going on in the CBPR process (McNicoll, 1999; Mendenhall & Doherty, 2005b). In order to be sensitive to the perspectives and needs of multiple participants, careful use of methods and measures that have high face validity and practical (and immediate) utility are indicated. For this reason, CBPR researchers often gravitate toward qualitative methods of data collection and analysis during early phases of the work. Exploring, for example, participants' subjective experiences can engage communities in identifying concerns that run deep within them, monitor inter-member and inter-group processes as problems are identified, solutions are democratically and collaboratively developed, and/or as action is taken, and assessing satisfaction with the results of new interventions. While objective (read: quantitative) measures of "success" can be created to assess a program's impact on a particular dependent variable (e.g., metabolic control in a local ethnic community), most CBPR studies do not do this until after a project is comparatively underway.

To this end, a myriad of qualitative data in CBPR have been described in the literature, including in-depth interviews (Lindsey & McGuinness, 1998; Mendenhall & Doherty, 2003; Mendenhall, Harper, Stephenson, & Haas, 2011; Razum, Gorgen, & Diesfeld, 1997); naturalistic case studies (Casswell, 2000); reflective journaling and meeting minutes (Hampshire, Blair, Crown, Avery, & Williams, 1999; Nichols, 1995); thematic and content analysis of group process notes and publicly available documents (Nichols, 1995; Razum et al., 1997); focus groups (Small, 1995); participant observation (Lindsey & McGuinness, 1998; Maxwell, 1993); social network mapping (Bradbury & Reason, 2003); and oral histories and open-ended stories (Small, 1995). Access to many of these types of data is generally easy for investigators in CBPR, because the very nature of the work requires that they be active participators in the research that is being evaluated (Mendenhall & Doherty, 2005b).

Whereas qualitative analyses are especially useful in helping researchers to understand participants' contexts, cultures, beliefs, attitudes, community practices, and subjective experiences related to CBPR processes, quantitative measures are most usually and most usefully employed to evaluate an intervention's efficacy (Mendenhall & Doherty, 2005b; Reese, Ahern, Nair, O'Faire, & Warren, 1999). These efforts are also important on "political" grounds, insofar as formally testing for objective change in tangible measures (whatever measures these may be) helps to advance regard by the broader scientific community that the work that is being conducted is rigorous and credible (Minkler & Wallerstein, 2008; National Institutes of Health, 2009).

Consistent with the basic tenets of CBPR, however, it is important to involve participants in selecting what to quantitatively evaluate, test, or measure. For example, in a CBPR initiative designed to reduce smoking on a school campus, participants (researchers and community members) discussed how students' smoking prevalence was—and was not—an important measure of "success." Indeed, student participants saw the number of available after-school activities (which were advanced by the project to target the very stress and boredom that students commonly attributed to smoking) was a more important quantitative measure of success. Put simply, students saw this initial step as a stage-setter for the improved subjective sense of self-efficacy and social support that will eventually help students to quit smoking (Mendenhall, Whipple, Harper, & Haas, 2008b; Mendenhall et al., 2011). In another project, providers involved in a diabetes CBPR initiative for adolescents saw metabolic control as the most important dependent variable of success, whereas adolescent patients' wanted to track school-policies regarding whether students with diabetes were allowed to go on fieldtrips with their peers (Mendenhall & Doherty, 2007b). In these and other CBPR projects, what is tested quantitatively is up to the whole group to decide. It is important to note, too, that quantitative analyses of CBPR projects tend to remain "local"—e.g., for, by, and within the community in which a project is positioned (Mendenhall & Doherty, 2005b). Efforts to test widespread generalizability (e.g., a randomized control trial) are less indicated than efforts to test local effectiveness (e.g., a single-group repeated-measures trial) because CBPR projects are designed purposefully to tap and reflect the unique resources and challenges of their local contexts.

Ultimately, participants in CBPR tend to combine both qualitative and quantitative methods. Using multiple methods over the course of a project enables researchers to triangulate different sources of data, and this increases confidence in conclusions that are drawn (Hagey, 1997; Lindsey & McGuinness, 1998; McKibbin & Castle, 1996; Nichols, 1995). Throughout this and the cyclical processes of CBPR, all data that are collected and analyzed are presented back to the initiative's participants (Hambridge, 2000; Mendenhall & Doherty, 2005b; Meyer, 2000; Nichols, 1995). This facilitates an active and purposeful dialogue between providers, researchers, and community participants about the meanings and usefulness of data, which then informs the generation of ensuing action steps en route to collaboratively identified and mutually shared goals.

Disseminating CBPR

Disseminating research findings is another important aspect of community-based participatory research. This allows for important findings to be distributed to academic researchers, providers, administrators, and the patients/families/communities that are involved in the work. Results communicate success of the project, changes brought about by its labors, and the ongoing efforts that researchers/families/community members are doing to sustain the initiative. CBPR teams, then, collaborate fully in writing and disseminating study findings to professional/scientific communities, community-specific organizations, and the general public. To share knowledge with the scientific community, they target refereed journals and local, national, and international conferences and forums. To share knowledge with community-specific organizations, the local community itself, and the general public, team members connect with community service-providing sites and resources, e.g., targeting local and state-wide public print and electronic media and community events/celebrations (Berge et al., 2009; Minkler & Wallerstein, 2008).

CBPR and Integrated Behavioral Health Care: Advancing the Research Agenda

More and more health care providers and researchers are engaging in CBPR projects and, with this, rigorous expert-driven investigatory methods aimed at widespread generalizability are losing ground to comparatively small but locally relevant and meaningful efforts that are co-created by patient and provider communities working collaboratively together. What was once broadly viewed by academic and research institutions as flimsy or unscientific is now establishing a niche in the world(s) of valued health care research and service-provision (Mendenhall & Doherty, 2005b; Minkler & Wallerstein, 2008). This evolution is advancing in synchrony with our increased emphases on patient/

CBPR, PBPR, and the Integrated Care Evaluation Project

James Fauth and George Tremblay

We illustrate here some of the principles articulated in this chapter through a project designed to explore and improve integrated care as practiced by four primary care clinics in New Hampshire. The Integrated Care Evaluation (ICE) project utilized a close cousin of CBPR, called practice-based participatory research (PBPR) (Fauth & Tremblay, 2011). While similar in many ways, the models diverge in a few respects that we will return to toward the end of the chapter.

What Is Practice-Based Participatory Research (PBPR)?

We developed PBPR as an antidote to failed "dissemination" and "translation" practice change strategies, both of which have foundered repeatedly on the assumption that practitioners should and would absorb and enact the findings from clinical trials. In our view, both of these strategies fall short in over-relying on evidence that is neither credible nor compelling in the eyes of the practice community, and in offering practitioners a one-down position in the science-practice relationship. What distinguishes PBPR is our focus on (1) cultivating a learning orientation in routine clinical settings; (2) taking an open and curious (rather than pejorative) stance toward practice-based departures from evidence-based models (Litaker, Tomolo, Liberatore, Stange, & Aron, 2006); and (3) adopting an incremental, recursive practice change strategy that is informed by key stakeholder learning priorities, local evidence, and systems thinking.

PBPR involves four phases: (1) Planning, (2) Pilot, (3) Discovery, and (4) Quality Improvement planning. Chart I outlines the goals of each phase.

Chart I: Four phases of practice-based participatory research. (Fauth & Tremblay, 2011; Imm et al., 2007; United States Department of Veterans Affairs, 2011).

Phase	Description
I. Planning	Locate practice contexts (settings, focal issues)
	Engage key stakeholders in diagnostic analysis
	Reveal "high leverage" information gaps that inform the design of a formative evaluation plan
II. Pilot Phase	Evaluation plan is implemented, feasibility assessed, power of the findings to inform quality improvement explored, and the plan is improved
III. Discovery Phase	Implementation of the evaluation plan and data collection
IV. Quality Improvement	Data-informed, stakeholder-driven quality improvement (QI) planning framework and feedback process

(continued)

(continued)

Application of PBPR to the Integrated Care Evaluation project

The initial planning phase has been designed around common integrated care components and the assumptions that integrated care depends more on the systematic identification of patients most likely to profit from behavioral health intervention than on the specific intervention model chosen (Gilbody, Bower, & Whitty, 2006) and that patients with non-chronic, mild to moderate distress may most likely benefit from integrated care interventions, whereas more distressed patients need specialty care (Krahn et al., 2006).

Our clinic partners vary widely in size, geography, and behavioral health resources. All four are pioneers in colocated integrated primary care, but none of their practices have been improved or substantiated through an evaluation. During the planning phase, we asked our practice partners to identify a segment of their patient population that placed heavy burdens on their clinic and providers and for whom they imagined that behavioral health expertise would be particularly relevant. Two of the clinics focused on diabetic patients, a third chose chronic pain patients, and the fourth and smallest practice aggregated diabetic, asthmatic, and chronic obstructive pulmonary disease patients.

"Information gaps" were identified with a qualitative method known as diagnostic evaluation (Curran, Mukherjee, Allee, & Owen, 2008), which helps practice stakeholders to make explicit their clinical practice and compares it to evidence-based models of care. This process involved translating the research-tested models into an evidence-based task diagram of integrated care and juxtaposing it to the practice-based task model through task analysis interviews (Annett & Stanton, 2000) with key stakeholders. The diagnostic analysis revealed some similarities between the evidence- and practice-based models (e.g., delivery of brief intervention by colocated behavioral health specialists). A main point of divergence, however, was the reliance on ad hoc clinical judgment for providers to referring to behavioral health versus the evidence-based use of standardized measures and systematic cut-off scores to identify patients.

Pilot study: We then set about designing a quantitative pilot study that would help the clinic staff track how they were allocating behavioral health resources, and would serve to estimate the feasibility of a larger-scale discovery and quality improvement phases of PBPR. Our goal was for the pilot phase to yield a profile of how behavioral health services were allocated based on the level of the patient's emotional distress. We used a standardized measure of emotional distress comprised of the PHQ-9 (Kroenke & Spitzer, 2002) and GAD-7 (Spitzer, Kroenke, Williams, & Lowe, 2011) scales, a functional impairment item from the PHQ (Spitzer, Kroenke, & Williams, 1999), and a

(continued)

(continued)

chronicity item created for this study. We also tracked billing codes for three care types from existing clinic databases: primary care only (PCP), PCPs administering psychotropic medication (MED), and colocated behavioral health intervention (BH).

From these data, we calculated the probability of receiving each care type within the 30-day window following every administration of the EDM. (It is important to note that we did not have EDM data from the patients' first presentation to the clinic, so the resulting probabilities do not indicate a response to initial diagnosis—they represent rolling, 30-day snapshots of care). The results indicated that integrated care at all four clinics was primarily allocated to the most severely distressed and functionally impaired patients. Patients with severe emotional distress were about five times more likely than mildly distressed patients to receive colocated behavioral health. These results, of course, were at odds not only with the theoretical literature and research evidence, which indicate that integrated care is most appropriate and helpful for patients at lower levels of acuity.

In the discovery and QI phases, we facilitated an initial QI process with the pilot findings. We held two meetings at each site, the first of which focused on sharing basic results with as many staff and providers at each site as possible, and the second on utilizing the pilot findings with the "implementation team" at each clinic. There is an investment in new action at two clinics: formation of a QI planning committee at one clinic, and a decision at a second clinic to hire a care manager focused on support and stabilization of severely distressed patients so as to free up the rest of the behavioral health staff to work with less severely afflicted patients (as originally intended).

Convergence and Divergence with CBPR

Consistent with CBPR, we habitually invite stakeholder input, yet we suspect that we are more willing than CBPR to assume an expert role around matters such as research design and the necessary ingredients of practice change. We also take pains to frame our requests for input in a way that respects our stakeholders' autonomy and honors—but does not romanticize or exaggerate—their particular vantage point(s) and expertise.

Allowing the research process to unfold in response to emergent needs and iterative learning cycles, which demands considerable time and flexibility, is typical of both CBPR and PBPR. The planning and pilot phases of the ICE project took nearly three years to complete, with numerous self-corrections and adjustments. Time and flexibility were also critical to developing evaluation

(continued)

(continued)

capacity among our clinic partners. For example, while two sites were quick to initiate data collection, their capture rates soon tapered off, alerting us to logistical barriers that were readily resolved once critical players (e.g., front line staff) were recruited into problem-solving mode. The methodological dynamic of both approaches moves from qualitative to quantitative data and back again. For instance, we used a qualitative method—diagnostic analysis—to inform our quantitative evaluation design. This approach builds on the assumption that baseline data are also necessary to test the extent to which QI efforts actually improve effectiveness.

family-centered medical homes, wherein comprehensive approaches for children, youth, and adults are attended to within settings that facilitate partnerships between individuals/families and respective (and collaborating) members of multidisciplinary care teams (Minkler & Wallerstein; Peek, 2011; Wallerstein & Duran, 2010). Through CBPR methods, the patient/family community partnerships with providers are held up as an essential foundation to create care that is of high quality, culturally competent, strength based, and effective (Chavez, Duran, Baker, Avila & Wallerstein, 2003; Doherty et al., 2010; Tobin, 2000; Ward & Trigler, 2001). Over the last decade, projects driven by this approach have gained credibility through their ability to inform understanding of patients' experiences, improve or generate services, facilitate community outreach and engagement, enhance education, and augment cultural awareness (Chavez et al., 2003; Tobin, 2000; Ward & Trigler, 2001). Projects have advanced improvements in asthma (Brugge, Rivera-Carrasco, Zotter, & Leung, 2010), diabetes (Mendenhall & Doherty, 2003, 2007a), dental and mouth-care practices (Watson, Horowitz, Garcia, & Canto, 2001), smoking cessation (Mendenhall et al., 2011), patient and practitioner satisfaction (e.g., through improved communication and problem-solving skills) (Hampshire et al., 1999; Lewis, Sallee, Trumbo, & Janousek, 2010; Lindsey & McGuinness, 1998; Meyer, 2000; Schulz et al., 2003), and a number of other significant health care foci (Doherty et al., 2012; Mendenhall & Doherty, 2005b).

From this foundation, efforts in CBPR are now underway to further advance the research agenda for collaborative care by extending our attention beyond disease-specific arenas and narrowly defined clinical outcomes (like many CBPR and related research studies regarding collaborative care practices have done to-date) (AHRQ, 2011; Doherty et al., 2012; Fauth & Tremblay, 2011). Understanding(s) about the effects of specific strategies and care processes, levels of integration per se, and financial models of clinical outcomes are sorely needed, alongside regard for broader clinic and health system(s) level functioning (Miller, Kessler, Peek, & Kallenberg, 2010). In order to do this, we must first establish a common language and lexicon of terms and definitions to consistently guide researchers, systems (re) designers, experts in quality improvement and performance measurement, policy-makers, and patients/citizens (Peek, 2010). This aligns well with CBPR's emphasis on involving all stakeholders collectively and throughout the aforementioned iterative process(es) of research and intervention development and improvement (Mendenhall & Doherty, 2005b; Minkler & Wallerstein, 2008). Indeed, to do less would be to fall back on conventional provider-led, expert-driven methods of defining care parameters, and to leave behind the voices of the very people that our efforts are oriented to helping.

Following recommendations put forth by the Agency for Healthcare Research and Quality (AHRQ) and Miller, Kessler, Peek, and Kennenberg (AHRQ, 2011; Miller et al., 2010), we must then begin asking descriptive questions to create systematically articulated pictures of how collaborative practices are carried out, followed by evaluative questions that assess outcomes across clinical, operational, and financial foci. CBPR is, again, well equipped to answer these calls. By engaging all stakeholders in care processes, comprehensive descriptions of clinical practices can be gleaned (e.g., providers can describe who they see in their practices and in what care settings; administrators can describe processes by which patients are identified and how care is coordinated and paid for; patients and family members can describe their experiences in working with clinic providers and staff throughout care sequences). To evaluate outcomes connected to a practice's care, engaged stakeholders' voices will similarly inform what is discovered (e.g., providers and patients can describe clinical outcomes related to health; providers and administrators can describe health system processes related to clinic flow and interdisciplinary collaboration; administrators and patients can describe the financial costs related to care initiation and maintenance). Efforts to engage in collaborative efforts such as these (e.g., that involve all stakeholders versus researchers (only) or administrative personnel (only)) are now emerging, as leaders in the field are working to advance CBPR methods into larger health systems. See Fauth and Tremblay's example, using "practice-based participatory research" (Fauth & Tremblay, 2011), in Box 1, above.

Leading Organizations in Health-Related CBPR

In addition to its increasing visibility in health-related foci, community-based participatory research has extended into the overlapping arenas of business, public policy, food-distribution practices, education, housing, and family time (Bogart & Uyeda, 2009; Bradbury-Huang, 2010; Jacobs, 2010; Kwok & Ku, 2011; Weaver-Hightower, 2010). It is thereby challenging to single out single organizations in this movement, because to do so in one area is to neglect pioneering groups in other areas. Having prefaced the following with this caveat, examples of leading organizations in CBPR partnerships around health include the following.

Citizen Professional Center

The University of Minnesota's (UMN) Citizen Professional Center (Doherty et al., 2012) advances a mission to prepare professionals for effective democratic engagement with communities and in generating community-based research that advances knowledge and solves local problems. This work has encompassed more than a dozen projects to-date that have collectively bridged medical and mental health providers and researchers with a broad range of organizations representing a myriad of ethnic minority groups, health and social concerns, and socioeconomic strata. For example, the *Family Education Diabetes Series* (FEDS) is a health promotion initiative that works actively with urban-dwelling American Indians (AIs) to achieve and maintain healthy lifestyles through culturally relevant dietary and physical activity sequences (Department of Indian Work, 2010). The *Students Against Nicotine and Tobacco Addiction* (SANTA) project is a smoking cessation project for teenagers and young adults created in partnership with the Hubert H. Humphrey Job Corps Center, and works through a combination of student-led activities designed to combat stress and boredom (Hubert H.Humprey Job Corps Center, 2011). The *Hmong Women United Against Depression* (HWUAD) initiative represents a partnership between a primary care clinic's staff and local elders/leaders positioned within the Twin Cities' immigrant community (Doherty et al., 2010). The *Citizen Father Project* works to support, educate, and develop healthy, active fathers and to rebuild family and community values (Goodwill/EasterSeals Minnesota, 2011). For a complete list and description of these projects, their partnering organizations, and related literature/publications, go to: www.citizenprofessional.com.

Center for Participatory Research

The University to New Mexico's (UNM) Center for Participatory Research (UNM, 2011) advances a mission to support a collaborative environment between university and community partners to improve health and life quality. This work has encompassed a variety of initiatives, which have endeavored to create and apply new knowledge. For example, the *Research for Improved Health* study represents an in-depth effort to investigate promoters and barriers to CBPR in American Indian/Alaska Native (AI/AN) communities to reduce health disparities (Hicks, 2011; Hicks & Wallerstein, 2011). The *Stop Smoking, Enjoy Pregnancy Project* (STEP) is a smoking cessation initiative designed purposively for women who are expecting, and aims to create a means to adapt its efforts across both private and public institutions (Center for Participatory Research, 2011c). The *Depression Among Off-Reservation American Indian Women* project is working to create an AI community and academic research infrastructure to identify culturally specific and personal explanations for depression, alongside effective solutions and strategies to allay it (Center for Participatory Research, 2011a). Additionally, the Center for Participatory Research is working in the arenas of tobacco use and cessation among lesbian, gay, bisexual, and transgender persons, and will use knowledge gained to advance culturally appropriate and effective interventions across a variety of care sites (Center for Participatory Research, 2011b). For a complete list and description of these projects, their partnering organizations, and related literature/publications, go to: http://hsc.unm.edu/som/fcm/cpr.

Detroit Community-Academic Urban Research Center

Partnered with the University of Michigan's Schools of Public Health, Nursing, Social Work, and several other community organizations, the Detroit Community-Academic Urban Research Center (Detroit Community-Academic Urban Research, 2011a) advances a mission to identify problems affecting the health of urban residents and conduct interdisciplinary CBPR to recognize and build upon resources and strengths already within their communities. This organization involves multiple research and intervention projects targeting health disparities across a broad range of foci. For example, the *Neighborhoods Working in Partnership: Building Capacity for Policy Change* project is working to extend community voices into the policy-making arenas to impact local, state, regional, and national policies oriented to the creation of safe and healthy neighborhoods for urban-dwelling children and families (Detroit Community-Academic Urban Research, 2011d). The *Healthy Environments Partnership—Lean and Green in Motown Project* (LGM) endeavors to better understand the impact(s) of interventions that include environmental change efforts on increasing physical activity and promoting healthy diets (Detroit Community-Academic Urban Research, 2011b). The *Healthy Mothers on the Move/ Madres Saludables En Movimiento* (Healthy MOMS) is working to advance and evaluate the effectiveness of a social support healthy lifestyle intervention that targets behavioral and clinical risk factors for type 2 diabetes among pregnant and postpartum women (Detroit Community-Academic Urban Research, 2011c). For a complete list and description of these projects, their partnering organizations, and related literature/publications, go to: http://www.detroiturc.org.

Leadership Strategies

Figure 6.2 presents a summary of key leadership and action strategies that we have learned for the initiation and conduct of CBPR (Doherty & Mendenhall, 2006; Doherty et al., 2010; Mendenhall et al., 2010). In the early phases of a project's evolution, we have found that it is best to request little or no financial support from key professionals and/or administrative leaders because this helps to facilitate their buy-in while at the same time allowing the project to evolve sans external pressures in terms of time or outcomes/deliverables. This enables professionals and community members to extend considerable attention to "going deep" in identifying health-related issues that are of great concern to all involved. Before inviting a large group of community leaders to begin generating solutions and/or interventions, it is important for a small group of community members with personal experience (but not with institutional priorities or constraints) to establish consensus in its focus and desire to proceed. As the project's membership is then thoughtfully expanded and its momentum increases, community and citizen dimensions of the issue are perused, which then informs the development and implementation of action initiatives.

Throughout this journey, key processes and guiding principles of CBPR are advanced and maintained. Democratic planning and decision-making are carried out through each step of the work. Professionals and community members continue to learn from each other, and project results continue to inform intervention designs and revisions (if/as indicated). Attention is consistently paid to identifying and developing new leaders, who then carry forward the project's efforts over time and en route to its larger mission(s) of effecting widespread and beneficent change.

1. *Get buy-in from key professional leaders and administrators*

    These are the gatekeepers who must support the initiation of a project based on its potential to meet one of the goals of the health care setting. However, we have found it best to request little or no budget, aside from a small amount of staff time, in order to allow the project enough incubation time before being expected to justify its outcomes

2. *Identify a health issue that is of great concern to both professionals and members of a specific community (clinic, neighborhood, cultural group in a geographical location)*

    Stated differently, the issue must be one that a community of citizens actually cares about—not just something that we think they should care about. And the professionals initiating the project must have enough passion for the issue to sustain their efforts over time

3. *Identify potential community leaders who have personal experience with the health issue and who have relationships with the professional team*

    These leaders should generally be ordinary members of the community who in some way have mastered the health issue in their own lives and who have a desire to give back to their community. "Positional" leaders who head community agencies are generally not the best group to engage at this stage, because they bring institutional priorities and constraints

4. *Invite a small group of community leaders (3-4 people) to meet several times with the professional team to explore the issue and see if there is a consensus to proceed with a larger community project*

Fig. 6.2 Action strategies for CBPR and Citizen Health Care

These are preliminary discussions to see if a project is feasible and

to begin creating a professional/citizen leadership group

5. *This group decides on how to invite a larger group of community leaders (10-15) to begin the process of generatinvg the project*

One invitational strategy we have used is for providvers to nominate patients and family

members who have lived expertise with a health issue and who appear to have leadership

potential

6. *Over the next six months of biweekly meetings, implement the following steps of community organizing:*

   i.   *Exploring the community and citizen dimensions of the issue in depth*

   ii. *Creating a name and mission*

   iii. *Doing one-to-one interviews with a range of stakeholders*

   iv. *Generating potential action initiatives, processing them in terms of the citizen health care model and their feasibility with existing community resources*

   v.   *Deciding on a specific action initiative and implementing it*

7. *Employ the following key Citizen Health Care processes:*

   i.   *Democratic planning and decision making at every step.*As mentioned before, this

        requires training of the professionals who bring a disciplined process model and a

        vision of collective action that does not lapse back into the conventional

        provider/consumer model, but who do not control the outcome or action steps the

        group decides to take

   ii. *Mutual teaching and learning among community members.*Action initiatives

        consistent with the model first call upon the lived experience of community

        members, with the support of professionals, rather than recruiting community

        members to support a professionally created initiative

Fig. 6.2 (continued)

iii. *Creating ways to fold new learnings back into the community.* All learnings can become "community property" if there is a way for them to be passed on. Currently, we have vehicles for professionals to become "learning communities," but few vehicles outside of Internet chat rooms for patients and families to become learning communities

iv. *Identifying and developing leaders.* The heart of community organizing is finding and nurturing people who have leadership ability but who are not necessarily heads of organizations with turfs to protect

v. *Using professional expertise selectively —"on tap," not "on top."* In this way of working, all knowledge is public knowledge, democratically held and shared when it can be useful. Professionals bring a unique font of knowledge and experience— and access to current research —to Citizen Health Care initiatives. But everyone else around the table also brings unique knowledge and expertise. Because of the powerful draw of the provider/consumer way of operating, professionals must learn to share their unique expertise when it fits the moment, and to be quiet when someone else can just as readily speak to the issue. A community organizing axiom applies here: Never say what someone in the community could say, and never do what someone else in the community could do

vi. *Forging a sense of larger purpose beyond helping immediate participants.* Keep the Big, Hairy, Audacious Goal (BHAG) in mind as you act in a local community. This work is not just about people helping people; it is about social change towards more activated citizens in the health care system and larger culture. This understanding inspires members about the larger significance of their efforts. It also attracts media and other prominent community members to seek to understand, publicize, and disseminate Citizen Health Care projects

Fig. 6.2 (continued)

1. This work is about identity transformation as a citizen professional, not just about

   learning a new set of skills

2. It is about identifying and developing leaders in the community more than about a specific

   issue or action

3. It is about sustained initiatives, not one-time events

4. Citizen initiatives are often slow and messy, especially during the gestation period

5. You need a champion with influence in the institution

6. Until grounded in an institution's culture and practices, these initiatives are quite vulnerable

   to shifts in the organizational context

7. A professional who is putting too much time into a project is over-functioning and not using

   the model. We have found that the average time commitment to be on the order of 6-8 hours

   per month, but over a number of years

8. External funding at the outset can be a trap because of timelines and deliverables, but

   funding can be useful for capacity building to learn the model, and for expanding the

   scope of citizen projects once they are developed

9. The pull of the traditional provider/consumer model is very strong on all sides; democratic

   decision-making requires eternal vigilance

10. You cannot learn this approach without mentoring, and it takes upto two years to get good at it

Fig. 6.3 Lessons learned in CBPR and citizen health care

Lessons Learned

Figure 6.3 presents a summary of key lessons that we have learned in our CBPR efforts (Doherty & Mendenhall, 2006; Doherty et al., 2010; Mendenhall et al., 2010). Two lessons relate to time. First, doing this work does not require a large amount of professionals' time (six to eight hours per month, on average), but it does require a long-term commitment (several years or more). Second, learning how to do this kind of work requires mentorship. Simply reading about CBPR (or listening to a presentation about it at a professional conference) and then directly proceeding with a project can be likened to reading a book about how to ride a bicycle and then expecting to embark upon a trip without falling. There are no quick ways to teach professionals the public skills of engaging other citizens in CBPR or related community organizing projects with flattened hierarchies; direct mentorship (with frequent stops and starts, trials and errors, and discussion/pro-cessing) is necessary.

CBPR projects tend to be very vulnerable to dissolution without strong buy-in from an administrative leader and champion within the provider/researcher side of the professional/community partnership. This person does not have to be an active member of the project itself, but s/he tends to play a strong role in backing and supporting early efforts in getting something started in a variety of ways, e.g., permitting involved professionals to devote work time to the project, advocating for the project, and/or defending it against efforts by other organization personnel who do not support it. Relatedly, CBPR projects can be vulnerable to shifts in organizational contexts if they are not well grounded into an organization's culture before said shifts occur. For example, an early project called *Partners in Diabetes* (Mendenhall, 2002; Mendenhall & Doherty, 2007a) was disbanded when its partnering residency clinic transitioned to a private practice, whereas the aforementioned Family Education Diabetes Series project has survived several years of organizational, funding, and administrative changes since its establishment as a foundational part of its hosting organization's wares within its local American Indian community (Doherty et al., 2010; Mendenhall et al., 2010).

It is also important to highlight how strong the pull of the traditional doctor-patient model is, and that maintaining collaborative and democratic efforts in CBPR requires eternal vigilance. This pull comes from both sides. For example, it can feel very natural for a provider to prematurely take over or offer solutions to a group (because his/her socialization through graduate or medical school was such that this is what s/he is "supposed" to do in his/her "day job"). It can feel equally natural for community members to defer to providers for guidance, because most of us have been socialized to be passive recipients of care when we see the doctor and/or to follow authority figures' directions.

Finally, CBPR must meet the needs of professionals for satisfying work. We have found that if this public practice fits within one's values and vision, providers and researchers can experience an expanded sense of professional contribution, as well as a closer relationship to local communities. If health care is to be redesigned in the United States (and most argue that it must be), doing so will require that we adopt new forms of partnership between professionals and the patient and family citizens that seek our care. The driving mission behind this work is to create a democratic model of health care that unleashes the capacity and energy of ordinary citizens as producers of health for themselves and their communities.

Sustainability of Care

History is full of shining examples of "community projects" that fizzled or stopped altogether as soon as external funding ran out or their charismatic leader(s) left. A key tenet of CBPR is that this not happen, for the reason that extant community resources and energies are tapped and project ownership is shared collectively by a group of citizens that inhabit a project or are somehow connected to it (Doherty & Mendenhall, 2006; Mendenhall & Doherty, 2005b; Wallerstein & Duran, 2003). Through the collaborative processes outlined in this chapter, consecutive generations of lay and clinical leaders work together to challenge the notion (frequently espoused by academic- and/or health-related fields and literature) that "care" or "research" can only be carried out if/when it is first funded by monies secured by professionals—and/or that programs/interventions can only be sustained if funded by monies that are secured in such a manner. Consider specific projects, already highlighted above, as examples of this sustainability:

The *Family Education Diabetes Series* (FEDS) is a CBPR project created through the collaborative efforts of providers at the University of Minnesota and local leaders in the Saint Paul/Minneapolis American Indian (AI) community (Mendenhall et al., 2010; Mendenhall, Seal, GreenCrow, LittleWalker, & BrownOwl, 2012). Initiated in 2001 without any external funding, participants worked to engage low-income, urban-dwelling AIs and their families in an active forum of education, fellowship, and support through its mission to improve the health and well-being of American Indian people in manners that embrace their heritage, values, and culture(s). This work has functioned, and continues to function, with and without external funding. For example, intervention resources (such as food) have at times been provided through the collective contributions of participants, themselves, and at other times through local State and foundation grants. Professionals' involvement has sometimes been funded by grant monies; other times, it has been advanced through voluntary means and/or viewed as part of "outreach" or "community-oriented" components within existing professional job descriptions. The overall project's sustainability has thereby been enhanced because it is not dependent on external funding or the charisma and leadership of a single person (e.g., one community elder/leader, one University "PI").

The *Students Against Nicotine & Tobacco Addiction* (SANTA) initiative began in 2006. This work engages local providers in partnership with students, teachers, and administrators at the Hubert H. Humphrey Job Corps Center in St. Paul, MN, to address on-campus smoking (and the concomitant reduction of students' stressors and the adoption of healthier lifestyles). Its mission is to improve the health and well-being of students at Job Corps through smoking cessation, education, stress reduction, and support. As project members have worked together to answer the question, "How do we keep SANTA going as an initiative that is owned-and-operated by the community in which it is positioned?" They have come to believe its sustainability as a realistic and expected outcome because (1) participating members are highly invested in the project surviving long after they have graduated, retired, or otherwise revised the foci of their current work, and (2) no independent student-based group or organization in the history of Job Corps has ever lasted as long as the SANTA initiative already has. The initiative continues to function with and without external funding, advancing a variety of lively on-campus activities, health and wellness education series, and group and 1:1 supportive forums (Mendenhall et al., 2011, 2008b).

The *Hmong Women United Against Depression* (HWUAD) project began in 2005. This work engages local providers and residents of the Hmong community in a collaborative partnership oriented to investigating, understanding, and improving the lives of patients and refugees who are struggling with a myriad of stressors related to depression, chronic physical pain, and psychosocial difficulties associated with immigration (Doherty et al., 2010; Mendenhall, Kelleher, Baird, & Doherty, 2008a). Its mission is to tap the resources and wisdom of the Saint Paul Hmong community to empower, support, encourage, and offer hope to Hmong women and their families who live with depression. Over time the initiative has partnered with local ethnic food markets, public social and meeting places, community events, schools, and health care sites—and it continues to evolve with the needs and interests of its members and the larger community in which its work is positioned.

While most existing literature reflects the investigatory efforts of providers or professional researchers who conducted projects that they secured funding for to create, advance, and/or evaluate, CBPR does not function this way. This work supports the notion that both research and intervention/practice efforts can be advanced without depending on (or being delayed by) external funding. Indeed, waiting for external funding is conceptually inconsistent with CBPR tenets because to do so would be to rely on professionals' efforts in grant-writing while simultaneously prioritizing their needs for work-related status or laudation (which aligns with top-down, provider-driven sequences that are incompatible with genuine participatory approaches). To advance a project in such a way would be to place principal responsibility for an initiative's livelihood on said professionals (Doherty et al., 2010; Mendenhall et al., 2010). In CBPR, professional expertise should be "on tap," not "on top."

Quality of Evaluation and Strength of Research Evidence

While most agree that the guiding principles of CBPR are sensible in the design and implementation of interventions targeting complex social and medical presentations, it is important to evaluate the effectiveness of this type of approach. Put simply: Does CBPR work? To answer this question, efforts to move past qualitative accounts (only) that capture this research process(es) and/or the understandings/resources it taps along the way are advancing now more than ever before. And the short answer is that, yes, CBPR appears to work.

Exhaustively reviewing or presenting all outcome studies in CBPR is beyond the scope of this chapter, insofar as the approach has been employed across hundreds of professional fields targeting innumerable topics and challenges. Echoing this widespread visibility and scope, CBPR within the medical professions has been similarly advanced and evaluated across a range of health foci, including (as noted earlier): obesity, diabetes, healthy diet, smoking cessation, asthma, dental and mouth-care practices, management of preoperative fasting, accident reduction, safe sexual practices, midwifery, living with disabilities, and overall physical well-being (Barrett, 2011; Brugge et al., 2010; Davis & Reid, 1999; Doherty et al., 2010; Garwick & Auger, 2003; Gallagher & Scott, 1997; Hampshire et al., 1999; Kondrat

& Julia, 1998; Lewis et al., 2010; Lindsey & McGuinness, 1998; Mendenhall & Doherty, 2005b; Meyer, 2000; Schulz et al., 2003; Stevens & Hall, 1998). The following is a brief, but more detailed, review of two of these topics.

CBPR Targeting Diabetes in the American Indian Community

Many providers and patient communities are beginning to engage in novel and collaborative partnerships that honor and tap resources across professional and lay groups where diabetes is of high concern, and CBPR is a leading methodology guiding this work (Lewin, 1946; Mendenhall & Doherty, 2003, 2005b). Principal reasons justifying this approach in American Indian communities rest in its contrast to AIs' earlier experiences with conventional research (e.g., work conducted by outsiders through top-down, expert-driven methods) that has tended to benefit researchers more than Native people (e.g., advancing professionals' prestige and/or tenure), pathologized American Indians as dysfunctional, and not directly informed or advanced the communities they were supposed to help (e.g., study results not shared or integrated/advanced into new services and outreach) (Burhansstipanov, Christopher, & Schumacher, 2005; Davis & Reid, 1999; Gone, 2009). Emerging projects support the utility of CBPR in co-creating medically sound programs that are sensitive to local customs and cultural traditions. For example, Castro, O'Toole, Brownson, Plessel, and Schauben (2009) found that integrating culturally relevant sequences like talking circles and community forums in standard education and exercise led to improvements in disease knowledge and management. Garwick and Auger (2003) partnered with AI teenagers to increase awareness of asthma and inform providers about how to offer more culturally sensitive and appropriate care. Potvin and colleagues (2003) partnered with AIs and local education systems to create sustainable school-based health programs that combine culturally relevant activities and health education. Steckler and colleagues (2002) collaborated with American Indian and non-AI researchers and staff to incorporate cultural information into curricula for elementary school-aged children, alongside recognizing and emphasizing the importance of family and community involvement. Mendenhall and colleagues (2010, 2012), in the *Family Education Diabetes Series* project presented above, have worked through University/Clinic/Community partnerships in CBPR to improve health in the American Indian community through significant reductions in weight, metabolic control (A1c), and blood pressure.

CBPR Targeting Smoking Cessation in Adolescents and Young Adults

As the health care field(s) has begun to more aggressively address smoking cessation in adolescents and young adults (e.g., most work to-date has focused on adult samples), it has become increasingly clear that the unique challenges, resources, indicated interventions, and processes of implementing interventions for young people are not well understood by researchers positioned in academia who tackle smoking from an adult-centric, top-down service-delivery foundation and approach. Consistent with the notion that oftentimes the best person to talk with a teenager is another teenager, researchers are aligning with the CBPR principle that recognizes that the greatest untapped resource in our efforts is the lived experience and wisdom of the very individuals and groups that we seek to influence. Through the employment of CPBR methods involving both professional and community participants, Tsark and colleagues (2001) addressed the need for culturally/ethnically appropriate and relevant approaches to address tobacco use among Native Hawaiians. The collaborative process was effective in the construction of a user-friendly survey tool to gather data from a broad range of community groups and constituencies, community-specific findings with direct application to ongoing intervention design(s), and expanded local capacity for health promotion on a larger scale. Powers and colleagues (1989) employed similar methods with a very different group. Engaging young mothers as active participators in CBPR to reduce smoking behaviors, the Nottingham Mother's Stop Smoking Project was designed and implemented successfully in a small New Zealand community. Burton and colleagues (2004) are currently working in partnership with the Chinese American community in New York City, and have developed a multimodal intervention to reduce smoking behaviors in young adults that encompasses awareness campaigns, telephone support and services, print materials and neighborhood groups (outcome data are being collected now, and should be available soon). In Pennsylvania and New Jersey, Ma and colleagues (2004) are similarly working to engage members of the local Asian community to address tobacco and cancer control. Mendenhall and colleagues (2008b, 2011), in the *Students Against Nicotine and Tobacco Addiction* project outlined above, have worked through University/Clinic/Community partnerships to improve health in HHH Job Corps community through increased activities to reduce stress and concomitant reductions in smoking frequency and status.

CBPR Outcome Studies: What Do They Really Tell Us?

The common thread that runs through these and related projects is that CBPR methodology serves to engage community members as active participators in research and care that is oriented to something that they are invested in and care deeply about. Unlike conventional investigatory approaches evaluating outcomes—e.g., those that seek to design a single intervention that can be transported across different communities (with positive quantitative results that are replicated time-and-again to prove its merit)—CBPR researchers seek to develop interventions that are immediately relevant to the specific communities in which they are positioned. By addressing local and unique challenges in-context, and tapping local wisdom and unique resources in-context, participants in CBPR are increasingly (and repeatedly) showing the world that their efforts work. And while widespread generalizability of any single CBPR intervention is not realistic (or sought), the immediate relevance and positive outcomes for local communities is seen as worth the trade-off (Hambridge, 2000; McGarvey, 1993; Morrison & Lilford, 2001). What CBPR outcome studies tell us, then, is that engaging in such efforts where they have not heretofore been advanced is worth the risk. Others have done it; why not us?

Education and Training

A variety of opportunities for education and training in professional/community partnerships and CBPR are available across local university and community sites, for example, University of California-Berkley (2010), University of Michigan (2011), and University of Minnesota (2011); open national and international forums, like American Public Health Association (2009) and American Sociological Association (2009); and competitive/by-invitation-only workshops/seminars, like National Institutes of Health (2007, 2009). Common themes across these venues include attention to key tenets that guide and define participatory approaches (as outlined above); how professionals and community members work to redefine their roles within care and investigatory sequences; and practical and methodological challenges and strategies within the conduct of CBPR, such as trust-building processes, meeting-facilitation skills, working with IRBs, and disseminating findings (Community-Campus Partnerships for Health, 2010; Dalal, Skeete, Yeo, Lucas, & Rosenthal, 2009; United States Department of Health & Human Services, 2011; Wilson et al., 2006).

Parallel to processes common in the field, education and training sequences in CBPR tend to be interdisciplinary in nature insofar as professionals and community members from a variety of backgrounds tend to learn together. As they are exposed to each other's respective disciplines and disciplinary cultures, they are also made familiar with investigations across a wide range of presenting issues (not just health-related ones). This educational journey serves to facilitate an erosion of turf-battles and professional-socialization regarding "experts'" roles, and sets the stage for working within the contexts of collaborative and flattened hierarchies that permeate effective and successful professional/community partnerships (National Institutes of Health, 2007, 2009; University of Michigan, 2011; University of Minnesota, 2011).

Closing Thoughts

At the outset of this chapter, we maintained that the call for interdisciplinary collaboration in health care is something that most practicing providers have heard about, and that our early and collective efforts to answer this call are evolving across training programs and care facilities, alike. As we do this, however, it is essential that we not forget to include the patients and families that we serve. Indeed, the greatest untapped resource for improving health is the knowledge, wisdom, and energy that they have acquired through facing and living with challenging issues in their everyday lives.

Through the use of CBPR methods, we (all) are able to contribute professional and personal pieces to a larger mosaic of care that neither providers nor community members could, respectively, do by themselves. Ultimately what we create can advance a broader scope than any (interdisciplinary, collaborative, or otherwise) top-down, provider-led, one-patient-at-a-time model could reach. Projects are sustainable, too, by nature of their being owned-and-operated by the communities that they are positioned in (vs. relying wholly on professional leadership or grant-funding for support). Participants in CBPR believe in what they are doing, and are energized by the collective energy they share to promote broad and meaningful change.

References

Agency for Healthcare Research and Quality. (2004). *Community-based participatory research: Assessing the evidence*. Rockville: Author.

Agency for Healthcare Research and Quality. (2011). A national agenda for research in collaborative care: Papers from the Collaborative Care Research Network research development conference. *Agency for Healthcare Research and Quality*. Available at: http://www.ahrq.gov/research/collaborativecare/

American Public Health Association. (2009). *Applying community-based participatory research at the National Institutes of Health*. In Special session at the 137th annual meeting of the American Public Health Association Philadelphia, PA.

American Sociological Association. (2009). *Community-based participatory research (CBPR): When academic/research institutions meet the real world*. Special session at the 104th annual meeting of the American Sociological Association San Francisco, CA.

Annett, J., & Stanton, N. (2000). *Task analysis*. Boca Raton: CRC Press.

Baum, F., MacDougall, C., & Smith, D. (2006). Participatory action research. *Journal of Epidemiology and Community Health, 60*, 854–857.

Bell, J., Cheney, G., Hoots, C., Kohrman, E., Schubert, J., Stidham, L., et al. (2004). *Comparative similarities and differences between action research, participative research, and participatory action research*. Seattle, WA: Antioch University Seattle.

Berge, J., Mendenhall, T., & Doherty, W. (2009). Using Community-Based Participatory Research (CBPR) to target health disparities in families. *Family Relations, 58*, 475–488.

Bogart, L., & Uyeda, K. (2009). Community-based participatory research: Partnering with communities for effective and sustainable behavioral health interventions. *Health Psychology, 28*, 391–393.

Bradbury, H., & Reason, P. (2003). Action research: An opportunity for revitalizing research purpose and practices. *Qualitative Social Work, 2*, 155–175.

Bradbury-Huang, H. (2010). The action research contribution to education. *Action Research, 8*, 115–116.

Braithwaite, R., Coghlan, S., O'Neill, M., & Rebane, D. (2007). Insider participatory action research in disadvantaged post-industrial areas: The experiences of community members as they become community based action researchers. *Action Research, 5*, 61–74.

Brugge, D., Rivera-Carrasco, E., Zotter, J., & Leung, A. (2010). Community-based participatory research in Boston's neighborhoods: A review of asthma case examples. *Archives of Environmental & Occupational Health, 12*, 70–76.

Burhansstipanov, L., Christopher, S., & Schumacher, S. (2005). Lessons learned from community-based participatory research in Indian country. *Cancer, Cancer, Culture and Literacy Supplement, 12*(Suppl 2), 70–76.

Burton, D., Fahs, M., Chang, J., Qu, J., Chan, F., Yen, F., et al. (2004). Community-based participatory research on smoking cessation among Chinese Americans in Flushing, Queens, New York City. *Journal of Interprofessional Care, 18*, 443–445.

Cammarota, J., & Fine, M. (2008). *Revolutionizing education: Youth participation action research in motion.* New York: Routledge.

Casswell, S. (2000). A decade of community action research. *Substance Use and Abuse, 35*, 55–74.

Castro, S., O'Toole, M., Brownson, C., Plessel, K., & Schauben, L. (2009). A diabetes self-management program designed for urban American Indians. *Public Health Research, Practice, and Policy, 6*, 1–8.

Center for Participatory Research. (2011a). *Depression among off-reservation American Indian women.* University of New Mexico. Available at: http://hsc.unm.edu/SOM/fcm/cpr/mini-Grants.shtml

Center for Participatory Research. (2011b). *Exploring factors that influence tobacco use and cessation among lesbian, gay, bisexual, transgender and queer people in New Mexico.* University of New Mexico. Available at: http://hsc.unm.edu/SOM/fcm/cpr/miniGrants.shtml

Center for Participatory Research. (2011c). *Stop Smoking, Enjoy Pregnancy Project* (STEP). University of New Mexico. Available at: http://hsc.unm.edu/SOM/fcm/cpr/miniGrants.shtml

Chavez, V., Duran, B., Baker, Q. E., Avila, M. M., & Wallerstein, N. (2003). The dance of race and privilege in community-based participatory research. In M. Minkler & N. Wallerstein (Eds.), *Community based participatory research for health* (pp. 81–97). San Francisco: Jossey-Bass.

Christopher, S., Watts, V., McCormick, A., & Young, S. (2008). Building and maintaining trust in a community-base participatory research partnership. *American Journal of Public Health, 98*, 1398–1406.

Classen, L., Humphries, S., Fitzsimons, J., Kaaria, S., Jimenez, J., Sierra, F., et al. (2008). Opening participatory spaces for the most marginal: Learning from collective action in Honduran hillsides. *World Development, 36*, 2402–2420.

Community-Campus Partnerships for Health. (2010). An introduction to community-based participatory research at the National Institutes of Health: A road map to funding. *Proceedings at the Community-Campus Partnerships for Health Conference*, Portland, OR.

Cornwall, A., & Jewkes, R. (1995). What is participatory research? *Social Science & Medicine, 41*, 1667–1676.

Curran, G., Mukherjee, S., Allee, E., & Owen, R. (2008). A process for developing an implementation intervention: QUERI series. *Implementation Science*. Available at: http://www.ncbi.nlm.nih.gov/pubmed/18353186

Dalal, M., Skeete, R., Yeo, H., Lucas, G., & Rosenthal, M. (2009). A physician team's experiences in community-based participatory research: Insights into effective group collaborations. *American Journal of Preventive Medicine, 37*, S288–S291.

Davis, S. M., & Reid, R. (1999). Practicing participatory research in American Indian communities. *American Journal of Clinical Nutrition, 69*, 755S–759S.

Department of Indian Work. (2010). Family Education Diabetes Series (FEDS). St.Paul Area Council of Churches. Available at: http://www.spacc.org/index.asp?Type=B_BASIC&SEC=%7BBC584B39-8D75-4718-ADF2-3657E5DE125D%7D&DE=.

DePoy, E., Hartman, A., & Haslett, D. (1999). Critical action research: A model for social work knowing. *Social Work, 44*, 560–569.

Detroit Community-Academic Urban Research Center. (2011a). *About URC.* Detroit Community-Academic Urban Research Center. Available at: http://www.detroiturc.org/index.php?option=com_content&view=frontpage&Itemid=17

Detroit Community-Academic Urban Research Center. (2011b). *Healthy Environments Partnership – Lean and Green in Motown Project (LGM)*. Detroit Community-Academic Urban Research Center. Available at: http://www.detroiturc.org/index.php?option=com_content&view=article&id=18#19

Detroit Community-Academic Urban Research Center. (2011c). *Healthy Mothers on the Move/ Madres Saludables En Movimiento (Healthy MOMS)*. Detroit Community-Academic Urban Research Center. Available at: http://www.detroiturc.org/index.php?option=com_content&view=article&id=18#21

Detroit Community-Academic Urban Research Center. (2011d). *Neighborhoods working in partnership: Building capacity for policy change*. Detroit Community-Academic Urban Research Center. Available at: http://www.detroiturc.org/index.php?option=com_content&view=article&id=18#16

Doherty, W., & Mendenhall, T. (2006). Citizen health care: A model for engaging patients, families, and communities as co-producers of health. *Families, Systems & Health, 24*, 357–362.

Doherty, W., Mendenhall, T., & Berge, J. (2010). The families & democracy and citizen health care project. *Journal of Marital and Family Therapy, 36*, 389–402.

Doherty, W., Mendenhall, T., & Berge, J. (2012). Citizen Professional Center. University of Minnesota. Available at: http://www.cehd.umn.edu/cpc/projects.html

Edwards, K., Lund, C., Mitchell, S., & Anderson, N. (2008). Trust the process: Community-based research partnerships. *Journal of Aboriginal and Indigenous Community Health, 6*, 187–199.

Fauth, J., & Tremblay, G. (2011). Beyond dissemination and translation: Practice based participatory research. *Psychotherapy Bulletin*. Available at: http://www.divisionofpsychotherapy.org/wp-content/uploads/2011/03/Bulletin46-1.pdf

Gallagher, E., & Scott, V. (1997). The STEPS project: Participatory action research to reduce falls in public places among seniors and persons with disabilities. *Canadian Journal of Public Health, 88*, 129–133.

Garwick, A. W., & Auger, S. (2003). Participatory action research: The Indian family stories project. *Nursing Outlook, 51*, 261–266.

Gilbody, S., Bower, P., & Whitty, P. (2006). Costs and consequences of enhanced primary care for depression: Systematic review of randomised economic evaluations. *The British Journal of Psychiatry, 189*, 297–308.

Gone, J. P. (2009). A community-based treatment for Native American historical trauma: Prospects for evidence-based practice. *Journal of Consulting and Clinical Psychology, 77*, 751–762.

Goodwill/EasterSeals Minnesota. (2011). *Citizen Father Project*. Goodwill/EasterSeals Minnesota. Available at: http://www.opnff.net/Files/Admin/Citizen%20Father%20Project%20brochure.v6.pdf

Haaland, A., & Vlassoff, C. (2011). Introducing health workers for change: From transformation theory to health systems in developing countries. *Health Policy and Planning, 16*(Suppl 1), 1–6.

Hagey, R. S. (1997). The use and abuse of participatory action research. *Chronic Disease & Cancer, 18*, 1–4.

Hambridge, K. (2000). Action research. *Professional Nurse, 15*, 598–601.

Hampshire, A., Blair, M., Crown, N., Avery, A., & Williams, I. (1999). Action research: A useful method of promoting change in primary care? *Family Practice, 16*, 305–311.

Hayes, P. (1996). Is there a place for action research? *Clinical Nursing Research, 5*, 3–5.

Heron, J., & Reason, P. (2001). The practice of co-operative inquiry: Research "with" rather than "on" people. In P. Reason & H. Bradbury (Eds.), *Handbook of action research: Participative inquiry and practice* (pp. 179–188). London: Sage.

Hicks, S. (2011). *What predicts outcomes in CBPR?* Presentation at the American Academy of Health Behavior Hilton Head, SC.

Hicks, S., & Wallerstein, N. (2011). Research for improved health: A national study of community-academic partnerships. National Congress of American Indian Policy Research Center (NCAIPRC). Available at: http://narch.ncaiprc.org/documentlibrary/2011/08/NARCH5CBPR-Flyer2-090911.pdf

Horowitz, C., Robinson, M., & Seifer, S. (2009). Community-based participatory research from margin to mainstream: A researchers prepared? *Circulation, 119*, 2633–2642.

Hubert H.Humprey Job Corps Center. (2011). *Hubert H. Humphrey Job Corps Center.* United States Department of Labor. Available at: http://huberthhumphrey.jobcorps.gov/home.aspx

Imm, P., Chinman, M., Wandersman, A., Rosenbloom, D., Guckenburg, S., & Leis, R. (2007). *Preventing underage drinking: Using getting to outcomes with the SAMHSA Strategic Prevention Framework to achieve results.* National Organizations for Youth Safety. Available at: http://www.rand.org/pubs/technical_reports/TR403.html

Israel, B. (2005). Introduction to methods in community-based participatory research for health. In B. Israel, E. Eng, A. Schulz, & E. Parker (Eds.), *Methods in community based participatory research for health* (pp. 3–29). San Francisco: Jossey-Bass.

Jacobs, G. (2010). Conflicting demands and the power of defensive routines in participatory action research. *Action Research, 8*, 367–386.

Jones, L., & Wells, K. (2007). Strategies for academic and clinician engagement in community-participatory partnered research. *Journal of the American Medical Association, 296*, 407–410.

Kelly, J., Mock, L., & Tandon, D. (2001). Collaborative inquiry with African American community leaders: Comments on a participatory action research process. In P. Reason & H. Bradbury (Eds.), *Handbook of action research: Participatory inquiry and practice* (pp. 348–355). London: Sage.

Kemmis, S., & McTaggart, R. (2000). Participatory action research. In N. Denzin & Y. Lincoln (Eds.), *Handbook of qualitative research* (pp. 567–605). Thousand Oaks, CA: Sage.

Kondrat, M., & Julia, M. (1998). Democratizing knowledge for human social development: Case studies in the use of participatory action research to enhance people's choice and well-being. *Social Development Issues, 20*, 1–20.

Krahn, D., Battels, S., Coakley, E., Chen, H., Chung, H., Ware, J., et al. (2006). PRISM-E: Comparison of integrated care and enhanced specialty referral models in depression outcomes. *Psychiatric Services, 57*, 946–953.

Kroenke, K., & Spitzer, R. (2002). The PHQ-9: A new depression diagnostic and severity measure. *Psychiatric Annals, 32*, 509–515.

Kwok, J., & Ku, H. (2011). Making habitable space together with female Chinese immigrants to Hong Kong: An interdisciplinary participatory action research project. *Action Research, 6*, 261–283.

Lammerink, M., Bury, P., & Bolt, E. (1999). An introduction to participatory action development. *Participatory Learning and Action, 35*, 29–33.

Lewin, K. (1946). Action research and minority problems. *Journal of Social Issues, 2*, 34–46.

Lewis, K., Sallee, D., Trumbo, J., & Janousek, K. (2010). Use of community-based participatory research methods in adults' health assessment. *Journal of Applied Psychiatry, 40*, 195–211.

Lindsey, E., & McGuinness, L. (1998). Significant elements of community involvement in participatory action research: Evidence from a community project. *Journal of Advanced Nursing, 28*, 1106–1114.

Litaker, D., Tomolo, A., Liberatore, V., Stange, K., & Aron, D. (2006). Using complexity theory to build interventions that improve health care delivery in primary care. *Journal of General Internal Medicine, 21*, 30–34.

Ludema, J., Cooperrider, D., & Barrett, F. (2001). Appreciative inquiry: The power of the unconditional positive question. In P. Reason & H. Bradbury (Eds.), *Handbook of action research: Participative inquiry and practice* (pp. 189–199). London: Sage.

Ma, G., Toubbeh, J., Su, X., & Edwards, R. (2004). ATECAR: An Asian American community-based participatory research model on tobacco and cancer control. *Health Promotion Practice, 5*, 382–394.

Maxwell, L. (1993). Action research: A useful strategy for combining action and research in nursing? *Canadian Journal of Clinical Nursing, 4*, 19–20.

McGarvey, H. E. (1993). Participation in the research process. Action research in nursing. *Professional Nurse, 8*, 372–376.

McKibbin, E., & Castle, P. (1996). Nurses in action: An introduction to action research in training. *Curationis, 19*, 35–39.

McNicoll, P. (1999). Issues in teaching participatory action research. *Journal of Social Work Education, 35*, 51–62.

Mendenhall, T. (2002). *Partners in diabetes: The process and evolution of a democratic citizenship initiative in a medical context* [dissertation]. University of Minnesota.

Mendenhall, T., Berge, J., Harper, P., GreenCrow, B., LittleWalker, N., WhiteEagle, S., et al. (2010). The Family Education Diabetes Series (FEDS): Community-based participatory research with a Midwestern American Indian community. *Nursing Inquiry, 17*, 359–372.

Mendenhall, T., & Doherty, W. J. (2003). Partners in diabetes: A collaborative, democratic initiative in primary care. *Families, Systems & Health, 21*, 329–335.

Mendenhall, T., & Doherty, W. (2005a). Partners in diabetes: A new initiative in primary care. In R. Kane, R. Priester, & A. Totten (Eds.), *Meeting the challenge of chronic illness* (pp. 121–122). Baltimore: John Hopkins University Press.

Mendenhall, T., & Doherty, W. J. (2005b). Action research methods in family therapy. In F. Piercy & D. Sprenkle (Eds.), *Research methods in family therapy* (2nd ed., pp. 100–117). New York: Guilford Publications.

Mendenhall, T., & Doherty, W. (2007a). Partners in diabetes: Action research in a primary care setting. *Action Research, 5*, 378–406.

Mendenhall, T., & Doherty, W. (2007b). The ANGELS (A Neighbor Giving Encouragement, Love and Support): A collaborative project for teens with diabetes. In D. Linville & K. Hertlein (Eds.), *The therapist's notebook for family healthcare*. New York: Hayworth Press.

Mendenhall, T., Harper, P., Stephenson, H., & Haas, S. (2011). The SANTA Project (Students Against Nicotine and Tobacco Addiction): Using community-based participatory research to improve health in a high-risk young adult population. *Action Research, 9*, 199–213.

Mendenhall, T., Kelleher, M., Baird, M., & Doherty, W. (2008a). Overcoming depression in a strange land: A Hmong woman's journey through the world of Western Medicine. In R. Kessler (Ed.), *Collaborative medicine case studies* (pp. 327–340). New York: Springer.

Mendenhall, T., Whipple, H., Harper, P., & Haas, S. (2008b). Students Against Nicotine and Tobacco Addiction (S.A.N.T.A.): Community-based participatory research in a high-risk young adult population. *Families, Systems & Health, 26*, 225–231.

Mendenhall, T., Seal, K., GreenCrow, B., LittleWalker, K., & BrownOwl, S. (2012). Family Education Diabetes Series (FEDS): Improving health in an urban-dwelling American Indian community. *Qualitative Health Research, 22*, 1524–1534.

Meyer, J. (2000). Using qualitative methods in health related action research. *British Medical Journal, 320*, 178–181.

Miller, B., Kessler, R., Peek, C., & Kallenberg, G. (2010). *Establishing the research agenda for collaborative care*. Agency for Healthcare Research and Quality. Available at: http://www.ahrq.gov/research/collaborativecare/collab1.htm

Minkler, M. (2000). Using participatory action research to build healthy communities. *Public Health Reports, 115*, 191–197.

Minkler, M., & Wallerstein, N. (2008). *Community based participatory research for health* (2nd ed.). San Francisco: Jossey-Bass.

Morrison, B., & Lilford, R. (2001). How can action research apply to health services? *Qualitative Health Research, 11*, 436–449.

National Center on Minority Health and Health Disparities. (2011). NCMHD Community Based Participatory Research Initiative. National Institutes of Health. Available at: http://www.nimhd.nih.gov/our_programs/communityParticipationResearchasp.

National Institutes of Health. (2007). *Summer institute: Design and development of community-based participatory research in health*. National Institutes of Health. Available at: http://obssr.od.nih.gov/summerinstitute2007/about.html

National Institutes of Health. (2009). *Summer institute: Community-based participatory research targeting the medically underserved*. National Institutes of Health. Available at: http://conferences.thehillgroup.com/si2009/about.html

Nichols, B. (1995). Action research: A method for practitioners. *Nursing Connections, 8*, 5–11.

Pan American Health Organization. (2004). *Participatory evaluation of healthy municipalities: A practical resource kit for action.* Washington, DC: Author.

Peek, C. (2010). *A collaborative care lexicon for asking practice and research development questions.* Agency for Healthcare Research and Quality. Available at: http://www.ahrq.gov/research/collaborativecare/collab3.htm

Peek, C. (2011). *A collaborative care lexicon for asking practice and research development questions.* Agency for Healthcare Research and Quality. Available at: http://www.ahrq.gov/research/collaborativecare/collab3.htm

Potvin, L., Cargo, M., McComber, A. M., Delormier, T., & Macaulay, A. C. (2003). Implementing participatory intervention and research in communities: Lessons from the Kahnawake Schools Diabetes Prevention Project in Canada. *Social Science & Medicine, 56,* 1295–1305.

Powers, F., Gillies, P., Madeley, R., & Abbot, M. (1989). Research in an antenatal clinic: The experience of the Nottingham Mothers' Stop Smoking Project. *Midwifery, 5,* 106–112.

Pyrch, T. (2007). Participatory action research and the culture of fear: Resistance, community, hope and courage. *Action Research, 5,* 199–216.

Pyrch, T., & Castillo, M. (2001). The sights and sounds of Indigenous knowledge. In P. Reason & H. Bradbury (Eds.), *Handbook of action research: Participative inquiry and practice* (pp. 379–385). London: Sage.

Rahman, A., & Fals-Borda, O. (1991). *A self-review of PAR in action and knowledge: Breaking the monopoly with participatory action research.* London: Intermediate Technology Publications.

Razum, O., Gorgen, R., & Diesfeld, H. J. (1997). Action research in health programmes. *World Health Forum, 18,* 54–55.

Reason, P., & Bradbury, H. (2001). *Handbook of action research: Participative inquiry and practice.* London: Sage.

Reason, P., & Bradbury, H. (2006). *Handbook of action research: Concise* (Paperbackth ed.). London: Sage.

Reason, P., & Bradbury, H. (2008). *The SAGE handbook of action research* (2nd ed.). Los Angeles: Sage.

Reese, D., Ahern, R., Nair, S., O'Faire, J., & Warren, C. (1999). Hospice access and use by African Americans: Addressing cultural and institutional barriers through participatory action research. *Social Work, 44,* 549–559.

Scharff, D., & Mathews, K. (2008). Working with communities to translate research into practice. *Journal of Public Health Management and Practice, 14,* 94–98.

Schulz, A., Israel, B., Parker, E., Lockett, M., Hill, Y., & Wills, R. (2003). Engaging women in community-based participatory research for health: The east side village health worker partnership. In M. Minkler & N. Wallerstein (Eds.), *Community-based participatory research for health* (pp. 293–315). San Francisco: Jossey-Bass.

Small, S. (1995). Action-oriented research: Models and methods. *Journal of Marriage and the Family, 57,* 941–955.

Spitzer, R., Kroenke, K., & Williams, J. (1999). *Validation and utility of a self-report version of PRIME-MD: The PHQ primary care study* (Vol. 282). Chicago: American Medical Association.

Spitzer, R., Kroenke, K., Williams, J., & Lowe, B. (2011). A brief measure for assessing generalized anxiety disorder: The GAD-7. *Archives of Internal Medicine, 166,* 1092–1097.

Steckler, A., Ethelbah, B., Martin, C., Stewart, D., Pardilla, M., Gittelsohn, J., et al. (2002). Lessons learned from pathways process evaluation. In A. Steckler & L. Linnan (Eds.), *Process evaluation for public health interventions and research* (pp. 268–287). San Francisco: Jossey-Bass.

Stevens, P., & Hall, J. (1998). Participatory action research for sustaining individual and community change: A model of HIV prevention education. *AIDS Education and Prevention, 10,* 387–402.

Strickland, C. (2006). Challenges in community-based participatory research implementation: Experiences in cancer prevention with Pacific Northwest American Indian tribes. *Cancer Control, 13,* 230–236.

Tobin, M. (2000). Developing mental health rehabilitation services in a culturally appropriate context: An action research project involving Arabic-speaking clients. *Australian Health Review, 23,* 177–184.

Torre, M., & Fine, M. (2005). Don't die with your work balled up in your fists: Contesting social injustice through participatory research. In B. Leadbeater & N. Way (Eds.), *Urban girls revisited: Building strengths* (pp. 221–240). New York: New York University Press.

Tsark, J. A. (2001). A participatory research approach to address data needs in tobacco use among Native Hawaiians. *Asian American and Pacific Islander Journal of Health, 9*, 40–48.

United States Department of Health & Human Services. (2011). *Community-based participatory research.* Available at: http://obssr.od.nih.gov/scientific_areas/methodology/community_based_participatory_research/index.aspx

United States Department of Veterans Affairs. (2011). *QUERI implementation guide.* Available at: http://www.queri.research.va.gov/implementation/section_1/

University of California-Berkley. (2010). *Community-based participatory research courses.* Available at: http://campuslife.berkeley.edu/sites/campuslife. berkeley.edu/files/UCB_CBPR_Courses.pdf

University of Michigan. (2011). *School of public health academic courses: HBEHED733 community-based participatory research.* Available at: http://www.sph.umich.edu/iscr/caid/display_course.cfm?CourseID=HBEHED733

University of Minnesota. (2011). *Community based participatory research and social work.* Available at: http://blog.lib.umn.edu/cehd/insideout/2011/04/free_workshop_community_based.html

University of New Mexico. (2011). *Center for participatory research.* Available at: http://hsc.unm.edu/som/fcm/cpr/

Wallerstein, N., & Duran, B. (2003). The conceptual, historical, and practice roots of community-based participatory research and related participatory traditions. In M. Minkler & N. Wallerstein (Eds.), *Community based participatory research for health* (pp. 27–52). San Francisco: Jossey-Bass.

Wallerstein, N., & Duran, B. (2006). Using community-based participatory research to address health disparities. *Health Promotion Practice, 7*, 312–323.

Wallerstein, N., & Duran, B. (2010). Community-based participatory research contributions to intervention research: The intersection of science and practice to improve health equity. *American Journal of Public Health, 100*, S40–S46.

Ward, K., & Trigler, J. S. (2001). Reflections on participatory action research with people who have developmental disabilities. *Mental Retardation, 39*, 57–59.

Watson, M., Horowitz, A., Garcia, I., & Canto, M. (2001). A community participatory oral health promotion program in an inner-city Latino community. *Journal of Public Health Dentistry, 61*, 34–41.

Weaver-Hightower, M. (2010). Using action research to challenge stereotypes: A case study of boys' education work in Australia. *Action Research, 8*, 333–356.

Wilson, V., Ho, A., & Walsh, R. (2007). Participatory action research and action learning: Changing clinical practice in nursing handover and communication. *Journal of Children's and Young People's Nursing, 1*, 85–92.

Wilson, N., Minkler, M., Dasho, S., Carrillo, R., Wallerstein, N., & Garcia, D. (2006). Training students as facilitators in the Youth Empowerment Strategies (YES!) Project. *Journal of Community Practice, 14*, 201–217.

Chapter 7
Integrated Behavioral Health in Public Health Care Contexts: Community Health and Mental Health Safety Net Systems

Danna Mauch and John Bartlett

Abstract With growing research-based evidence of clinical and cost improvements, the integration of behavioral health and primary care in the safety net public health care system is moving from the realm of early adopters and program innovators to the mainstream. This chapter is designed to provide readers with useable information on behavioral health care integration in the safety net health care system, the characteristics of people who depend upon that system, and the elements of workable integrated care models that can be brought to scale. The chapter reviews the clinical, delivery system, and cost outcomes associated with fragmented, siloed care versus integrated care. The chapter outlines the history of safety net care systems and the divergent legislative, financing and regulatory factors that established and preserved separation between community health centers and community behavioral health organizations. Recent public policy initiatives that promote care integration and adoption of integrated behavioral health care models in public health settings are discussed. Five case examples were drawn from the ranks of federally qualified community health centers and community behavioral health organizations to illustrate the opportunities and challenges in adoption of integrated care in the safety net. Essential components of sustainable integrated care initiatives are analyzed and include: organization and governance, organizational and staff culture, clinical systems and protocols, practice management and financial systems, and practice-based quality improvement and evaluation.

D. Mauch, Ph.D. (✉)
Abt Associates, 55 Wheeler Street, 02138 Cambridge, MA, USA
e-mail: Danna_mauch@abtassoc.com

J. Bartlett, M.D., MPH
Mental Health Program, The Carter Center One Copenhill,
453 Freedom Parkway, 30307 Atlanta, GA, USA
e-mail: John.Bartlett@emory.edu

M.R. Talen and A. Burke Valeras (eds.), *Integrated Behavioral Health in Primary Care: Evaluating the Evidence, Identifying the Essentials*, DOI 10.1007/978-1-4614-6889-9_7, © Springer Science+Business Media New York 2013

Introduction

With growing research-based evidence of clinical and cost improvements, the integration of behavioral and primary care in the safety net public health care system is moving from the realm of early adopters and program innovators to the mainstream. As research reveals that integration yields gains in health care outcomes for patients and reductions in care costs for payers, policymakers and insurers are promoting larger scale implementation. HRSA and SAMHSA now fund demonstrations at 64 organizations through their Primary and Behavioral Health Care Integration (PBHCI) Program (Substance Abuse and Mental Health Services Administration [SAMHSA], 2012). In addition, provisions of the Affordable Care Act will drive integration as health homes and Accountable Care Organizations (ACOs) are established in response to new performance incentives in the Medicaid and Medicare insurance programs that are the largest sources of reimbursement to the safety net system. However, while there are a number of demonstrations in play with evaluations pending, there is a shortage of guidance on best approaches to achieving integration that produces positive results for both providers and administrators, as well as for systems.

This chapter is designed to provide readers with useable information on behavioral health care integration in the safety net health care system, the characteristics of people who depend upon that system, and the elements of workable integrated care models that can be brought to scale. We anticipate demand for this knowledge will grow as integrated behavioral health care efforts expand in response to the considerable increases in funding—an estimated $11 billion for health centers alone—provided to the safety net through the Affordable Care Act (Rosenbaum et al., 2011).

Value of Integrated Behavioral Health Care in Public Health

Scope of the problem: Incidence, prevalence, and treatment rates. More than 72 million people (15 million children and 57 million adults), representing an estimated 23 % of the US population, are affected by mental health and/or substance use disorders (MH/SUD) each year (SAMHSA, 2011). These conditions often begin in childhood and adolescence, and can co-occur with another behavioral health condition and/or other medical conditions.

Long delays persist between onset of behavioral health conditions and diagnosis and treatment, which cause unnecessary morbidity and disability. The delay between diagnosis and treatment typically ranges from 6 to 8 years for individuals who eventually received treatment for mood disorders and between 9 and 23 years for those who sought treatment for anxiety disorders (Wang et al., 2005). In general, rates of treatment are low compared to the reported rates of prevalence. Many (about 90 %) receive behavioral treatment in the primary or general medical setting, while 68 % get no treatment or get under-treatment for their behavioral health conditions

(Kessler et al., 2005). While 29 % of individuals with chronic health conditions have mental health problems, most receive little treatment for their behavioral health conditions and therefore have poorer outcomes, for both the behavioral and the chronic medical conditions (Butler et al., 2008; Kessler et al., 2005).

The Affordable Care Act of 2012 aims to expand insurance coverage to some 32 million previously un- or underinsured individuals, 7.6 million of whom will need mental health services in a given year (Garret, Holahan, Cook, Headen, & Lucas, 2009). This newly insured population is relatively older, less educated, more racially diverse, and has a lower income than current privately insured populations. Sixty-five percent of individuals who will purchase coverage will have been previously uninsured and thus have significant unmet health care needs, 25 % of which will may require MH/SUD services (Garret et al.). Therefore, the expansion of health insurance coverage through ACA will result in a tremendous increase in the demand for behavioral health care services, including SUD treatment, and most of this demand must be met through the safety net system.

Societal costs associated with untreated mental health and substance use conditions include lost wages, reduced productivity, education, social welfare, criminal justice, and overall medical costs (Kessler et al., 2008; Miller & Hendrie, 2008). When health care and social program costs are added, the total estimated economic burden of serious mental illness reaches $317 billion per year, an estimate that does not include certain costs of comorbid conditions, incarceration, homelessness, and early mortality (Insel, 2008; O'Connell, Boat, & Warner, 2009). General health care costs are higher for persons with mental health conditions, as these conditions are associated with increased rates of morbidity and mortality, decreased adherence to treatment recommendations, and more frequent use of high cost care settings. The large disease burden associated with untreated mental health conditions is an important consideration in integrating behavioral health in primary care settings to capitalize on the cost-effectiveness of timely and appropriate prevention and treatment.

Safety net care systems play a large role in serving individuals who are at higher risk for behavioral, mental, and other health conditions and for those who develop chronic conditions. Integrating care effectively in safety net systems, therefore, has the potential to positively impact the health status and life course of individuals and the social and economic burden.

Parallel and Divergent Histories: Background of FQHCs and CMHCs

Despite common population characteristics and common values about addressing health care disparities, early efforts to bring behavioral health and primary care together were ultimately unsuccessful, as separate legislative and grant initiatives separated the safety net system into different silos for medical and behavioral health care. These silos were respectively administered by the Health Resources and

Services Administration (HRSA) for Federally Qualified Health Centers (FQHCs) and Rural Health Centers (RHCs) and by (initially) the Alcohol, Drug Abuse, and Mental Health Administration (ADAMHA) of the National Institute of Mental Health (NIMH), and later by the Substance Abuse and Mental Health Services Administration (SAMHSA) for Community Mental Health Centers (CMHCs), and Community Behavioral Health Organizations (CBHOs). This separation of over-sight, regulation, and funding has historically greatly complicated efforts to drive closer collaboration between the two systems.

Safety net health care systems were established to serve individuals who tradition-ally lacked access to private hospitals and medical practices, due to social, economic, insurance, and geographic and/or health status reasons. Although models vary across urban, rural, and other communities, safety net systems traditionally include public hospitals, community health and mental health centers, specialty and school-based clinics, physician practices, and local health departments. Safety net providers and systems typically operate in communities with high prevalence of identified social determinants of health risk factors, including poverty and its association with racial, cultural, and linguistic minorities. Half of all uninsured persons and 58 % of low-income uninsured persons are minorities (Chapa, 2011; Urban Institute, 2010) and disparities in access to care experienced by cultural and linguistic minorities occur at nearly twice the rate as persons in poverty of all races (Chapa, 2011). Safety net pro-viders were first focused on uninsured and underinsured individuals, such as migrant workers and homeless persons. However, because many private providers refused to accept Medicaid due to the low reimbursement rates, many Medicaid recipients also depend on the safety net providers. Since a steep rise in the cost of health care benefits and the economic downturn in 2008, a growing number of previously insured persons are using the safety net for their health care needs (Jones & Sajid, 2009).

According to Health Resources and Services Administration (HRSA, 2010), nearly 20 million individuals were served in FQHCs, 35 % of whom were under 20 years old and 7 % over age 65. Approximately half (51 %) of patients reported that they were white, 20.6 % reported that they were black or African-American, and another 10 % included Native American, Asian, Native Hawaiian, and other Pacific Islanders (20 % of patients refused to report their race). Two thirds of FQHC patients have incomes at or below 150 % of the federal poverty level (FPL). In 2010, 37.5 % of FQHC patients were uninsured, 38.5 % were covered by Medicaid, 7.5 % were covered by Medicare, and 2.5 % were covered by other public insurance, with fewer than 14 % privately insured (HRSA).

Unfortunately, comparative figures for CMHCs and CBHOs are not uniformly reported. Of the estimated 10.5 million low income individuals served in a given year, about half were treated in CBHOs, with the balance of those individuals seen in pri-mary care and other settings (National Council for Community Behavioral Health care, 2009). The majority of individuals served in CBHOs have moderate to high impairment, usually associated with serious emotional disturbance or serious mental illness, with more than 70 % among them Medicaid recipients and 21 % uninsured. Among children aged 4–17, 5.3 % had experienced definite or severe emotional or behavioral difficulties and 13.7 % experienced minor difficulties (SAMHSA, 2012).

As part of the health care safety net, community mental health centers (CMHCs) and community health centers (CHCs) were initially established to serve individuals regardless of ability to pay. CMHCs have long provided care for free or on a sliding fee scale basis to individuals who may have been insured for other health conditions, but were effectively uninsured or underinsured for prevention and treatment of mental health conditions due to persistent discrimination in insurance coverage for mental health conditions, even in public insurance programs. Until now, state budget appropriations and federal block grant funds have filled some of the gaps in insurance reimbursement.

As noted above, safety net systems play a major role in the delivery of behavioral health treatment for several reasons: (1) gaps in coverage for these services under private insurance, (2) negative impact of mental health and substance use on patient functioning, and (3) barriers for patients in accessing public disability and Medicaid benefits. Approximately 77 % of all funding for all substance abuse treatment and 58 % of all funding for mental health treatment come from public sector dollars (Levit et al., 2008; Mark et al., 2007).

Historical Perspective on Divergent Funding, Policies, and Regulations

As was noted above, community health centers (CHCs) and community behavioral health organizations (CBHOs) share common ground in their missions to target underserved and disadvantaged populations with high health risk and medical need. However, different policy, legislative, regulatory, and reimbursement strategies have evolved into separate service delivery and funding systems that impact the capacity for integration of behavioral health and primary care on many levels.

Community Mental Health Centers (CMHCs) were first established under the Retardation Facilities and Community Mental Health Centers Construction Act of 1963 (Public Law 88-164, 1963). The Act envisioned the creation of 3,000 centers throughout the USA to provide universal access to care in home communities as an alternative to institutional care (Foley & Sharfstein, 1983). The initial program was targeted as a mental health safety net to all members of the community, regardless of ability to pay, and covered five core services, including outpatient, inpatient, consultation/education, partial hospitalization, and emergency/crisis intervention. While CMHCs did not typically provide primary care services on site, they sometimes provided support or onsite services at CHC locations, under their consultation/liaison services.

CMHC funding rose and fell throughout the next several decades. Starting in 1966, funding for community mental health centers decreased as dollars were consolidated into Block Grants provided directly to the states (Finegold, Wherry, & Schardin, 2004). CMHCs came to depend increasingly on state contracts, seeking reimbursement through Medicaid, and pursuing federal grants for community support and child and adolescent systems of care. The early focus on preventive care, consultation and liaison, and frontline mental health services was replaced by mental health care for children and adults with serious mental illness. This shift moved CMHC into specialty care centers rather than mental health promotion and prevention centers. Consequently, aligning the mission of prevention and health promotion with CHCs was lost. Recently, however, there has been a renewed vision of integrating medical and mental health and a realignment of the mission of CBHOs within primary health care. They have regained a principal function of coordinating and integrating aspects of mental health treatment, addiction treatment, with primary care (Sharfestein, 2000).

Community Health Centers (CHCs) were first funded under the Economic Opportunity Act (EOA) of 1964, and like the CMHC Act, were provided grants for both construction and operations. Many of the early CHCs either had mental health practitioners on staff or, as noted above, worked collaboratively with local CMHCs through consultation/liaison services. Later, Federally Qualified Health Centers (FQHCs) were funded, pursuant to Section 330 of the Public Health Service Act, initially passed in 1975 (42 USCS § 254b). FQHCs receive grants under Section 330 to address the health prevention, treatment, and rehabilitation needs of medically underserved groups. While these groups include those who are uninsured, underinsured, or have poor access due to social, racial, and cultural disparities, there are also four specific provisions of the FQHC grant programs targeted to certain groups, including:

- Community Health Center Program—Section 330(e) providing primary care to medically underserved, uninsured, and underinsured, including services delivered in school-based health
- Migrant Health Center Program—Section 330(g)
- Health Care for the Homeless Program—Section 330(h) and
- Public Housing Primary Care Program—Section 330(i)

Enabling legislation and regulations governing CHCs and FQHCs require the entities to be either not-for-profit/charitable organizations or public/governmental organizations located in a medically underserved area (MUA) and are dedicated to serving a medically underserved population (MUP). Regulations further require FQHCs to provide a core set of clinical services delivered by a multidisciplinary, culturally and linguistically competent, licensed health care professionals working in the clinic or through partnership agreements.

In recent years, HRSA has made some strategic investments in the capabilities of FQHCs, including the requirement that FQHC grantees to adopt electronic health records and report to the Uniform Data System (UDS), and participate in national quality assurance efforts, such as the Health Disparities Collaboratives. HRSA has played a significant role in leading the development of FQHCs and RHCs and is instrumental in sustaining the current strength of community health centers.

In striking contrast, the CMHC Act is no longer operative and CMHCs, now often referred to as CBHOs, no longer have standard federal grant support or associated requirements. Those that receive SAMHSA Block Grant funds have certain reporting requirements, but typically, requirements for staffing, facility, clinical operations, reporting, and quality improvement are tied to state licensure requirements, or payer demands, from Medicaid or state agency funding, with some block grant funding to certain entities. CMHCs rarely enjoy the advantages of cost-based reimbursement, construction loans, or favorable drug pricing, unless the states in which they operate elect to provide some of these benefits. CMHCs are staffed differently, according to reimbursement and licensure standards, and frequently use persons with lived experience or who are in recovery as peer educators, support staff, or program staff. Moreover, there has been little to no strategic investment in the development of CBHO capabilities, in contrast to that of HRSA in the FQHCs.

Divergent Funding and Reimbursement Between FQHCs and CBHOs

Financing and reimbursement have long posed barriers to the integration of behavioral health and primary care. While FQHCs and CBHOs share payer mix profiles that are similar in their heavy concentration of persons with public insurance, there are significant differences in the methods and rates of free care, Medicaid and Medicare reimbursement available to these respective safety net entities (see Chap. 8 for more on funding). CBHOs now depend largely on state contracts and Medicaid reimbursement rates are often set at rates well below cost. By contrast, FQHCs have significant financial advantages and cover the costs of uncompensated primary health care, reimbursement under the Prospective Payment System (PPS), and other incentives such as "first dollar" of services rendered to Medicare beneficiaries or co-payment waivers. FQHCs also get support for health care infrastructure such as federal loans for capital and information technology (IT) improvements, costs of developing and operating managed care and practice management networks or health plans, and access to favorable drug pricing from manufacturers.

In summary, the missions of FQHCs and CBHOs are closely aligned in serving disadvantaged groups with lower incomes and higher health risks. While there is overlap in pediatric and adult populations served, FQHCs enjoy considerable reimbursement advantages over those available to CBHOs. FQHCs, because of their experience with primary and specialty care, as well as more universal adoption of EHRs that link practice and financial systems, have advantages as sites for integrated care. However, there is the potential to merge these two care systems. The ACA, health care reform act, and parity laws between medical and mental health care may hold the policy and regulatory reforms for service delivery and payment structures to end the discriminatory coverage practices, and expand health care coverage for the population. These changes create the infrastructure, which can create critical support and an environment for integrated care in safety net systems.

Integrated Health Care Initiatives in Safety Net Systems

Integration of behavioral health and primary care has the opportunity to change the development and course of health for the community in multiple ways. Weaving together systems of care that have historically been separate and not equal will be a challenging task but opportunity to implement evidence-based and promising practices in screening, health promotion, prevention, early intervention, and continuing care are on the rise.

Although safety net primary health care settings have some advantages for integrating mental health, previous attempts have historically fallen far short in terms of quality and sustainability of care (Katon et al., 2001; Wang et al., 2005). Historically, primary care providers and mental health providers function in referral and parallel practice models rather than team-based care. PCPs too often fail to identify patients with behavioral health conditions, and when they do, treatment is too often suboptimal, with limited application of evidence-based practices, overreliance on medication, and limited monitoring and poor follow-up care (Kessler et al., 2005; Wang et al., 2005b; Wang, Demler, & Kessler, 2002). Disparities in quality and appropriateness of treatment are far greater for persons from racial and ethnic minorities and low-income groups (Alegria et al., 2008; González et al., 2008). Patients with serious mental illness who have behavioral health services, on the other hand, have limited access or collaboration with primary care providers.

Effectively provided integrated care can lead to cost savings (Rost, Pyne, Dickinson, & LoSasso, 2005; Wang, Simon, & Kessler, 2003), although other studies cite modest cost increases associated with additional medication, visits, and phone contacts for the treatment of depression (Croghan & Brown, 2010). Evidence on the positive results of integration persuaded the Institute of Medicine (IOM, 2001) to recommend integration of mental health and physical health services as one element of a broader strategy to close the quality gap in health treatment.

Stakeholders in Emerging Initiatives: Federal, State, and Local Levels

SAMHSA and HRSA are in the process of evaluating grant funded demonstrations of integrated behavioral and primary care in safety net health care systems that target publicly insured and uninsured persons, including those with chronic mental health and medical conditions. Demonstration funds are provided for FQHCs that are embedding behavioral health specialists into primary care teams that have potential for promotion, prevention, universal screening and early intervention, as well as treatment of co-occurring conditions. Funds are also directed to embedding on-site primary care practitioners into CBHO settings in which persons with serious and disabling mental health conditions are already established in care. Sites under study include mature initiatives such as Cherokee Health Systems, as well as more recent integration and collaborative care efforts developed in local communities through the California Integrated Behavioral Health Project and Maine Health's Mental Health Integration Program. Intermountain Health Systems recently reported evidence on the effectiveness of their integration efforts in a cross section of their system's primary care clinics serving publicly insured persons, producing increased outpatient use and reduced emergency department use, inpatient use and cost of care

(Reiss-Brennan, Briot, Savitz, Cannon, & Staheli, 2010). Integrated programs have demonstrated outcomes such as decreased emergency department visits and decreased hospital admissions (Begley et al., 2008; Frequent Users of Health Services Initiative, 2008; Green, Singh, & O'Byrne, 2010; Katon et al., 2010; Marr, Pillow, & Brown, 2008).

The current approaches to integrated care in the safety net system reflect the same conceptual frameworks and practice models of behavioral/primary care integration as are found in the private sector, adjusted for the characteristics of the safety net population. These conceptual frameworks reflect the evolution in thinking and evidence about integrated behavioral and primary care, including debates about the role of the generalist (primary care practitioner) versus specialist (behavioral health practitioner) that surround the integration of mental health into primary care. They also reflect different paths that the evolution of mental health treatment in primary care has taken. Some of these models have grown from community practice and others emerged from tightly regulated clinical trials.

For example, some safety net community health centers (including FQHCs and RHCs) have, with HRSA support, adopted the Strosahl model, a population-based approach driven by the concept that behavioral health conditions and care are primary drivers of medical utilization, requiring a primary mental health care model in which the behavioral health provider operates as an integral member of the primary care team, assessing risk, screening for emerging behavioral conditions, and providing brief interventions while providing consultation to the primary care physician. While providers and administrators are becoming familiar with these aspects of care, there are often unsystematic processes for incorporating these elements into the new culture of integrated care. This model of care may have conceptual viability but lacks sufficient data for advancing evidence-based practices. Consequently, the translational evidence for evaluation of the outcomes when behavioral health is incorporated into primary health care settings in the safety net is limited.

Drivers of Integrated Behavioral Health Care on Federal/State/Regional Levels

Integrated behavioral health care is a natural direction for safety net providers for a variety of reasons. In an era when there are clear conflicts between supporters of ACA's proposed expansion of access to comprehensive and affordable health insurance for millions of formerly uninsured and underinsured individuals and the needs of payers, such as Medicaid, to reduce costs during the current state budget crises, any intervention which holds promise to address both sides of the conflict is of obvious interest. Currently, however, state and federal payers are recognizing that they supply most of the health care resources for the safety net population through siloed and uncoordinated funding channels, resulting in both higher costs and lower clinical efficacy (J. Unutzer, May 25, 2012, personal communication). These parties have, for example, identified that 5 % of Medicaid beneficiaries drive 50 % of total

Medicaid spending, in part because care is fragmented and poorly coordinated (Kaiser, 2007). Since safety net CHCs and CBHOs serve many of the highest risk and highest cost patients, the integration of these two safety net systems holds promise to bend a significant section of the cost curve.

Implementation science would argue that the adoption of integrated behavioral health and primary care is an example of "the uptake of research findings into routine health care in clinical, organizational, or policy contexts." In practice, however, the adoption of integrated care in safety net systems has emerged in response to other drivers of change. These drivers are (1) the safety net's response to and dependence on funds from a variety of targeted public payer programs and initiatives (an example is the practice of Sutton's Law—go where the money is); (2) the shared mission and values of the medical and mental health safety net provider systems and the overlapping characteristics of the patient population they serve; and (3) the role of visionary leaders in response to patient need, staff demands, and grant incentives, to solve local access and financing challenges for underserved patients.

The Federal Level: Programs and Funds

The Health Resources Services Administration (HRSA) and the Substance Abuse and Mental Health Services Administration (SAMHSA) have been the drivers toward integrated care on the Federal level. They have contributed to the development of both the infrastructure (e.g., health information technology capabilities) and, increasingly, appropriated funds for designing targeted integrated care initiatives.

HRSA and SAMHSA (with its predecessor roots in NIMH) historically have addressed the same public health populations, but promoted different strategies and investments over the years. Over the years, CMHC state block grants were associated with decreases in both funding levels and control over programming and strategic direction for CMHCs and CBHOs. HRSA, on the other hand, was able to preserve direct grants to FQHCs and RHCs, building more consistent practice models and infrastructure investments that leave many CHCs in a stronger position to support systems that integrate behavioral health care. This relatively stronger position is founded on: the ability to capitalize on comprehensive services and add funding to primary care clinics for behavioral health services through the Expanded Services (ES) grant mechanism; established EHRs with embedded practice protocols; and prospective payment revenue streams that more easily cover preventive and care management functions, as well as certain uncompensated care, required for effective integrated care in the safety net. SAMHSA has used demonstration and services innovation grants, for example, System of Care (SOC) grants that establish integrated behaviorally enhanced pediatric medical homes, and the Primary and Behavioral Health Care Integration (PBHCI) Grants, to promote integrated care. However, the PBHCI Grants are more often focused on integrating limited primary care resources into CBHOs.

In 2009, SAMHSA and HRSA jointly funded the Center for Integrated Health Solutions (CIHS) to improve access to comprehensive integrated medical and behavioral services for persons with mental health and substance use conditions through either primary care or behavioral health specialty organizations. CIHS is a national training and technical assistance center in support of partnerships designed to develop or expand primary health care services for persons with serious and persistent mental illness (SPMI) in the safety net. Through the efforts of the CIHS, with PBHCI Grants as the main support, safety net organizations from both the CHC and the CBHO areas are supported in their efforts to move beyond the traditional, siloed model in which all behavioral health prevention, treatment, and recovery support services are delivered in specialty settings, to more integrated approaches. CIHS supports a range of approaches, from colocation through collaboration to full integration, and grant sites are scattered throughout the country. CIHS is now beginning to address the issue of achieving greater scale through its various programs. These programs are in the early stages of evaluation and consequently, we have limited data to evaluate the effectiveness and efficiency of these integrated behavioral health care models.

Impact of State and Drivers in State and Regional Care Integration Initiatives

In a similar fashion, a number of state and regional level initiatives have also supported the safety net provider system toward integrated care initiatives. There are larger scale integration initiatives in safety net systems, using co-location and integrated behavioral health care models on the State and County level. For example, the Harris County Hospital District in Texas, the fourth largest safety net health system in the USA, implemented a pilot Community Behavioral Health Program in 2004, which expanded in 2005. The Harris County program used two strategies to improve access and results of care to an uninsured population: colocating behavioral health staff in 11 community health centers to provide behavioral health services; and expanding the scope of behavioral health screening and intervention provided by PCPs practicing in the centers. Results showed increases in access, timeliness of treatment, and units of service received, clinical functioning, and provider satisfaction for an average cost of $268 per patient served (Begley et al., 2008). In 2005, the Montgomery County Cares initiative was established in Maryland to implement a depression/anxiety integrated behavioral health care project. Using the IMPACT Model's evidence-based depression care approach, multidisciplinary teams were established in a network of three community health center primary care clinics. PCPs screened and referred patients to the teams, targeting to persons with medical conditions who required treatment for comorbid depression, anxiety, and/or risky substance use. Unique characteristics of the patient population, comprised in the majority of immigrants, drove adaptations to the model and produced successful outcomes. In a quasi-experimental design, statistically significant clinical improvements were seen in PHQ-9 and GAD-7 scores for those patients referred to the program, with per patient costs for team services ranging from $455 to $660 (Katman, Pauk, & Alter, 2011).

In a recent initiative to support a unified statewide approach to integration of behavioral health and primary care in safety net systems, the State of Washington implemented the Mental Health Integration Program (MHIP). Using resources assembled at the AIMS Center at the University of Washington, more than 200 CHCs and CMHCs are engaged in delivering integrated care guided by evidence-based practices and protocols based on the IMPACT model. In this approach, primary care provider participants use a population-based approach to screen all adult patients for depression using valid and reliable mental health screening, use medication management and evidence-based behavioral health treatments, and they refer patients to CMHCs to provide more intensive mental health services for individuals. In 2009, government payers introduced a pay-for-performance (P4P) incentive to adopt several quality indicators in the program designed to promote timely follow-up of patients, provide psychiatric consultation to those whose clinical status did not improve, and track psychotropic medications. Performance incentives seemed to further improve results with increases in timely follow-up care (from 53 % to 72 % of patients), psychiatric consults for treatment planning (from 49 % to 60 % of patients), and reduction in time to improvement of depression symptoms measured by the PHQ9. As noted, this work is based on the IMPACT model, which was developed for the treatment of comorbid depression (not all behavioral health conditions) in older adults (not all age groups). This work has since been applied to a broader population of individuals of various ages and diagnoses, served across a range of safety net provider clinics and community health centers (Unutzer et al., 2012).

In Georgia, the state associations for both the safety net primary care (Georgia Association for Primary Care) and behavioral care providers (Georgia Association of Community Service Boards) have started a statewide learning collaborative on integrated care. In collaboration with the Carter Center, a 501c3 not-for-profit organization started by the former president and first lady, Jimmy and Rosalynn Carter, headquartered in Atlanta, over 20 local partnerships between FQHCs and CBHOs are being introduced to the latest evidence-based and best field practices from around the nation through a series of didactic and interactive learning sessions. The training initiative targets both clinical and administrative staff, including physicians; depending on the target audience, topics vary to address respective roles and responsibilities. Both medical and behavioral health safety net providers participate in the training. Champions for the initiative include the Carter Center and Healthcare Georgia Foundation. The Healthcare Georgia Foundation, the legacy foundation from the privatization of Blue Cross Blue Shield of Georgia, provides the main financial support for the collaborative.

On a regional level, The Depression Improvement Across Minnesota, Offering a New Direction (DIAMOND) Project, which links collaborative care functions, such as behavioral health coaches, care managers, patient registries, and data tracking, with primary care practices under a sustainable reimbursement structure that adds a monthly case rates for care management functions to the traditional fee-for-service approach Mental Health Weekly, 2008). DIAMOND is based on the IMPACT model and is carried out through collaboration among nine health plans, 25 medical groups, and more than 80 primary care clinics in Minnesota, many of which serve safety net populations. The evaluation of the program to date has shown clinically significant rates of improvement in depressive symptomatology and functioning two to three times that achieved with more traditional care (e.g., 60–80 % as opposed to 30 %). There have also been significant increases in provider and patient satisfaction with care. In addition, because the regional business community has been involved in the project from its initiation, changes in productivity and absenteeism with collaborative treatment of depression have also been measured; the evaluation has shown a positive relationship between decreased PHQ-9 scores and absenteeism and an inverse relationship between the same PHQ-9 scores and presenteeism. Monthly reports are provided to both the primary care clinics and the affiliated health plans; this practice has served to promote excellent buy-in and cooperation among the various partners. The major limitation identified to date is the focus on the single issue of depression, as opposed to a wider range of behavioral health issues. Plans are currently underway to add screening, brief intervention, and referral to treatment for risky drinking (SBIRT), an evidence-based practice recognized by the National Quality Forum. The project has also recently been awarded a grant from the Innovation center at CMS to add collaborative management of associated chronic medical conditions. Limitations of the DIAMOND Project center on its exclusive focus on Depression; moreover, PCP settings may be challenged to implement multiple, diagnosis-specific behavioral health screening and treatment initiatives (e.g., depression, substance abuse, anxiety, PTSD) (AIMS Center, 2012; Hunkeler et al., 2006; Katon et al., 1996).

Drivers of Integrated Behavioral Health Care in Regional Communities

Organizational success is often touted as dependent on a strongly articulated and shared vision and mission. Successful safety net provider organizations that are practicing integrated care identified such a clear sense of mission as essential to forging agreement about care integration and making necessary operational changes to support the new direction. When these organizations look at missions that target improvements in health status and quality of life for individuals who depend on the safety net, many of whom have multiple health risks and/or chronic conditions, and look at the needs manifesting in their patients, the rationale for and benefits of integrated care are hard to deny.

The Impact of Leadership on the Adoption of Integrated Care by Safety Net Providers

The leaders of safety net provider organizations operate in some of the most difficult terrain within the overall health care delivery landscape. Committed by their mission to serve many of the highest risk and highest cost patients, who often have comorbid chronic medical and behavioral issues, the leaders of safety net organizations face significant clinical challenges on a daily basis. At the same time, these same leaders, especially those from CBHOs, operate in a complex, changing, and perpetually underfunded revenue environment. These challenges cause some organizations to adopt inwardly focused, survival-oriented attitudes while others foster extremely high degrees of innovation and flexibility. It is the latter organizations that have both recognized the need for integrated care in the clients they serve, as well as the determination and creativity to make it possible to provide it. Time and again, early adopters of integrated care within the safety net provider community begin their integrated care initiatives without a solid long-term organizational or financial plan in place, perhaps in response to a specific Federal or state program, and oftentimes with no secure outside revenue stream available. At a conference at the National Center for Primary Care (NCPC) at Morehouse School of Medicine (2008), a group of early adopters of integrated care agreed that they championed their initiatives most often from a patient-centered care frame of reference, because it was clear that many of their clients had comorbid medical and behavioral issues. Ultimately, however, the value of the integrated care provided more than compensated for the effort, from a cost-savings point of view (e.g., reduced rehospitalizations, fewer ER visits), from a provider and patient satisfaction point of view, or because of improved clinical outcomes for both the behavioral and the medical conditions (NCPC).

Introduction to Case Examples

CHCs and CBHOs are main suppliers of care in the safety net, serving populations in high need of comprehensive, integrated care and holding promise for significant health and cost improvements. Increasing numbers of these organizations are attempting integration, without the benefit of substantial outcome evidence or technical guidance derived from evaluations of experience in the safety net. Some are using the technical assistance resources available through the AIMS Center and the Center for Integrated Health Strategies (CIHS) described earlier; others are fashioning their own response to implementing integrated care. Five integrated care initiatives are profiled below. The organizations were selected to represent a mix of experienced, early adopters and more recent implementers of integrated behavioral health and primary care. The five profiles also represent several organizational models, including: one with dual FQHC/CBHO licensure and multiple lines of health and specialty behavioral health business; two with FQHC licensure and a behavioral health business line; and two with CBHO licensure, one of which has a FQHC partner. Several of these profiled organizations have been the beneficiaries of HRSA 330 grants, two received early CMHC grants, and several are drawn from a growing group of SAMHSA/HRSA PBHCI grantees, with some sites receiving support from both sources.

	Pioneers and early adopters	Recent implementers
Organizational origins	10 years or longer	5 years or fewer
Legacy CHC	Chase Brexton	Lone Star
	• Mainstream	• Mainstream
	• Targeted to universal	• Universal
	• Integrated	• Integrated
Legacy CBHO	Cherokee	Cobb and Douglas & Shawnee Pilot
	• Mainstream	
	• Universal	• Targeted
	• Integrated primary care/ care colocated	• Series of pilots, taken hold with current physical colocation of primary care team

Regardless of their origins, these organizations are driven by a shared mission to serve individuals with high social and health risk with comprehensive care responses delivered without regard for the ability to pay. In each case, clinical and executive leaders in the profiled organizations recognized the bidirectionality of behavioral and other health conditions, the poorly addressed complex health needs of their patients, and the value of preserving existing treatment relationships. Moreover, these organizations, like the many other safety net providers they represent, are determined to serve their patients without clearly defined clinical protocols or financial stability, yet. They have a shared vision for team-based service for a target population of complex (medically and psycho-socially) underserved patient population. In sharing their mission and experiences, these organizations are contributing to an emerging knowledge base to support broad implementation of integrated care.

Profiles of Safety Net Organizations Engaged in Providing Integrated Care

Chase Brexton Health Services, Baltimore MD: FQHC with On-Site, Integrated Mental Health and Substance Abuse Services

History and service overview. Chase Brexton Health Services was founded in 1978 as a gay health clinic, and by the early 1980s was largely focused on serving a targeted population of individuals with HIV/AIDS. In 1991, they received a HSRA grant to add mental health and case management services and, by 1995, expanded to offer primary care services to a more universal population of all eligible persons in the communities they serve. Chase Brexton became an FQHC in 1999, soon began to offer dental services, and expanded their mental health and substance use services to all populations. Within a few years, they earned Joint Commission accreditation. Chase Brexton began its exploration of integrated care in 2002 as a result of participation in the Federal Bureau of Primary Care's Health Disparities Collaborative.

Chase Brexton recognized the importance of using their FQHC as a base for colocated services, which were developed into fully integrated care to respond to their own patient's experience and the emerging evidence that most people access health care, including behavioral health care, via primary care.

Chase Brexton is one of the largest FQHCs in Maryland, serving nearly 20,000 children and adults in 2011, with just fewer than 150,000 patient visits (Annual Report, 2011). Chase Brexton has four comprehensive clinic sites serving Baltimore City, Baltimore County, Howard County, and Talbot County providing: primary medical care, dental services, mental health services, substance use services, HIV/AIDS testing and medical care, sub-specialty medicine, women's wellness services, on-site pharmacy, nutritional services, case management including entitlement counseling; nursing services, and chronic disease care management. Care management services, provided by the treatment team, are targeted to three areas: chronic disease management, cancer prevention/screening, and HIV. Behavioral health services provide frontline care, specialty services, and behavioral medicine delivered by health psychologists who have been trained to work with medical patients on psychosocial conditions affecting their treatment (www.chasebrexton.org). They offer intensive case management service and care management, as noted above, for individuals with serious mental illness. Case managers assist patients with entitlement enrollment, health and wellness program linkages, access to transportation, and other required referrals. Staff members work with clients to identify barriers to health care and implement mitigation strategies to overcome them.

HOW: Team-based care/staffing roles and communication. Chase Brexton employs multidisciplinary team-based care, integrated care protocols, cross-training for staff, and shared communication and medical record functions. The integrated behavioral health care team includes nurses, medical assistants, pharmacists, psychologists, psychiatrists, dentists, therapists, and case managers. The intensive case management and care management teams include licensed clinical social workers, peer advocates, and patient navigators. In addition to cross-training their own staff, Chase Brexton has implemented a training program with 16 colleges and universities in their area to develop students interested in their integrated care approach. The EHR contains a number of tools to support the assessment, diagnosis, and treatment of persons with complex health conditions. Treatment planning encompasses both primary care and behavioral health care screening, assessment, diagnosis, and health and wellness services.

Shared patient population/targeted or universal. As detailed in the Overview above, Chase Brexton began serving a targeted patient population of gay persons, began providing more comprehensive and integrated care in response to the complex needs of patients with HIV/AIDS, and then extended their services to the broader, more universal community population.

Systematic clinical protocols and pathways. Systematic clinical approach Communications among clinical staff are facilitated by interdisciplinary team meetings and a shared and integrated electronic health record, Centricity. Chase Brexton is renovating a recently purchased physical plant to reconfigure office and treatment space to support delivery of integrated care, using a "pod" model of care, based on

Fig. 7.1 Chase Brexton patient mix by insurance service

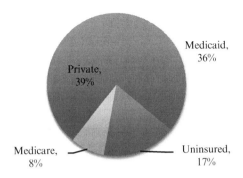

work in a Denver, Colorado FHQC, where the configuration of space, called "colloca-tion," situates the treatment team (medical providers, case/care managers, behavioral health psychologist, nurse, and adjunct specialties) in an open, central room, sur-rounded by exam rooms, thus actually supporting a coordinated team approach to care.

SUPPORTED BY: Office practice, leadership alignment and business model. Chase Brexton's high commercial insurance rate may be attributable to mission to serve the Lesbian, Gay, Bisexual, and Transgender community in Baltimore, many of whom are employed and insured (See Fig. 7.1). Supporting an integrated care model is made difficult by Maryland Medicaid's policy prohibiting same-day billing for medical and behavioral care, even though the health and behavior codes exist to cover integrated care. In order to support integrated care and remain fiscally sound, Chase Brexton relies on reimbursement for its services eligible for fee-for-service payment and on federal and foundation grants to support the remainder of its health care ser-vices, as well as close management of care, expenses, and staff productivity. Patients on integrated teams are more likely to attend appointments, reducing losses associated with "no-show" appointments.

Continuous quality improvement and effectiveness. Chase Brexton employs the PDSA (Plan, Do, Study, Act) model for quality improvement and applies it across their programs. Staff teams meet and discuss needs ranging from modifying the electronic health record and better coordinating scheduling to decreasing no-show rates. Teams develop new approaches, implement them, and evaluate outcomes. They have recently upgraded their electronic health record software, in part to be able to query medical records and produce outcome data, as they currently lack a comprehensive, systematic way of doing so.

Strengths, challenges, and insights. In Chase Brexton's experience, the strength of the initiative is that integrated care programs address the disparities that continue to surround treatment for mental health and substance use conditions for their histori-cal targeted patient population, as well as for the more recently adopted universal community population. The challenge is that true integrated care requires a philo-sophical shift from a more traditional, prescriptive doctor-patient paradigm to one that incorporates more dialog between care providers and their patients. Chase Brexton identified two important insights go to the value of tackling challenges to implement integrated care. The first is that when behavioral health is made a part of medical treatment, it reduces stigma and allows diagnoses to be made earlier, which is key to improving health outcomes. The second is that in their experience, involving patients in their care early in the process is essential to engaging them in decision making, and this increases patient support of the care plan and retention in care.

Cherokee Health Systems, Ease Tennessee: Dual Licensure as a CMHC and a FQHC

History and services overview. Cherokee Health Systems began its operations as a CMHC in the early 1960s, initiating outreach services for primary care in 1969, a role in which the current CEO was first hired for. Implementing its vision to provide universal access to comprehensive care for needy, underserved populations with "intertwined" conditions and needs, the first primary care clinic at Cherokee was established in 1984. In 1987, they adopted a troubled community health clinic at the request of the federal Bureau of Primary Health Care, leading to federal funding in 2000 and an FQHC grant in 2002. Cherokee is one of a handful of organizations in the country to pioneer the use of both CMHC and FQHC licensure to cover health needs for its client population (D. Freeman, June 12, 2012, personal communication).

HOW: Team-based care/Staffing roles and communication. Cherokee provides team-based comprehensive primary care and specialty behavioral health care services and supports, and addresses acute and chronic health conditions with prevention, treatment, rehabilitation, and care management. Cherokee operates clinics, programs, and support services in 23 locations with a staff composition of more than 500 including psychologists, physicians, social workers, nurses, community public health specialists, and administrative support staff.

The integrated primary care team staff serves individuals who are being screened or have been diagnosed with any mental health or substance use conditions as well as those with serious and disabling conditions who prefer to be served by the primary care team. Behavioral health services provided through the primary care team include patient education, behavioral management, and treatment for all behavioral health conditions. Specialty behavioral health clinics and services are also available, focused mainly on persons with serious and disabling behavioral health conditions.

Shared patient population/Targeted or universal. Cherokee's patient population is drawn from 13 counties in Eastern Tennessee and last year Cherokee served approximately 55,000 persons. Cherokee patients have a broad range of medical diagnoses. Of those patients served in the primary care clinics, 17 % meet the State of Tennessee's definition for serious and persistent mental illness (SPMI), yet care is managed in an integrated care setting. In Cherokee's specialty behavioral health programs, 80 % (25,000 persons) fit this SPMI definition.

Systematic clinical approach. Cherokee used team-based integrated care, well-articulated clinical pathways from the point of intake, evidence-based practices, cross-training, case conferencing, a robust electronic health record, routinely recorded measures, and quality improvement reports to support its behavioral health and primary care integration. As an early adopter of the patient-centered medical home (PCMH) concept, Cherokee has created an integrated "health home" with the behavioral health specialist embedded in the primary health care team, providing timely, on-site assessment, brief intervention and consultation to the team's patients, with further consultation to the medical staff on treatment plans and referrals for specialty behavioral care. Every team member has care management responsibilities embedded in the team-based treatment process.

Cherokee providers employ evidence-based practices with fidelity to practice standards, recruiting properly trained professional staff with the credentials prescribed by fidelity standards. This is reinforced with onsite training, shadowing and supervision, and scheduled case conferences. Providers team together to share coverage and provide availability to their patients around the clock for urgent clinical conditions, keeping the locus of care within Cherokee and avoid unnecessary use of emergency department and hospital care.

SUPPORTED BY: Office practice, leadership and business model. The intake and assessment interview is performed by a designated team member and addresses both behavioral health and primary care needs. For challenging cases, the team will schedule one to one and a half hours to convene the full team and review all information available on the patient, with the team leader facilitating input from all staff and formulating an integrated care plan. Routine treatment team meetings review the most critical 15–25 cases in each meeting. Weekly team meetings and grand rounds provide additional opportunities for cross-fertilization. The director of psychiatry holds grand rounds and provides routine telephonic consultation to PCPs and care teams.

Case Managers provide significant field-based services and handle coordination with other systems of care, particularly for individuals with chronic and disabling conditions. Primary care and specialty clinics operate in the same buildings, further supporting staff and care integration.

Medicaid is the largest payer and Tennessee's program supports care integration, permitting same-day billing for primary care and behavioral care delivered to the same patient (See Fig. 7.2). When new health behavior and assessment CPT codes were released, Cherokee approached Tennessee Medicaid to implement the codes, which in turn directed the Medicaid HMOs and MCOs to reimburse for the codes under their respective contracts. Case Managers are funded through managed care contract capitations or billed to Medicaid Rehab option.

Cherokee's financing structure is critical to supporting the integrated care model; global payments are preferred over FFS payments, and align with goals to reduce encounters (See Fig. 7.3).

Continuous quality improvement and effectiveness. The organization uses data to support care team efforts and focus resources; for example, selected clinical and utilization measures are tracked across the patient population and the primary care teams are notified of numbers that exceed established thresholds or benchmarks.

Fig. 7.2 Cherokee patient
mix by insurance service

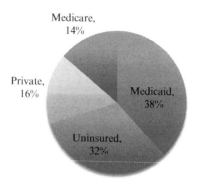

Fig. 7.3 Cherokee revenue
sources

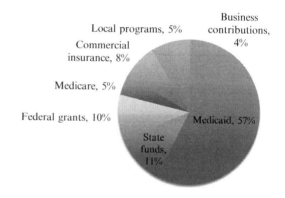

   Quality Improvement (QI) and Monitoring is managed by the Cherokee clinical
leadership team composed of five directors—Primary Care, Psychiatry, Community
Mental Health, Integrated care, and Pharmacy. The HRSA Uniform Data System
(UDS) Report and the FQHC Health Plan report drive feedback on selected clinical
measures of PCMH, meaningful use, and other measures required by payers and
designed by Cherokee staff members. All staff members receive bonuses for hitting
QI measures for efficiency, patient satisfaction, and clinical indicators. Tennessee
Blue cross-examined Cherokee utilization data and, comparing Cherokee to the
mean utilization levels of other regional providers, found that: ER utilization was
lower at 32 % of levels used in other primary care systems; hospital days were lower
at 63 % of others' levels; and specialty visits were also lower at 58 % of the number
of visits provided by other organizations; while overall costs were lower at only
78 % of what was incurred in other Tennessee provider systems (See Fig. 7.4).

Strengths, challenges, and insights. Cherokee has developed and documented integrated care practice protocols and adheres to evidence-based practices, measures
care activities, and reports results that indicate positive impacts on access,

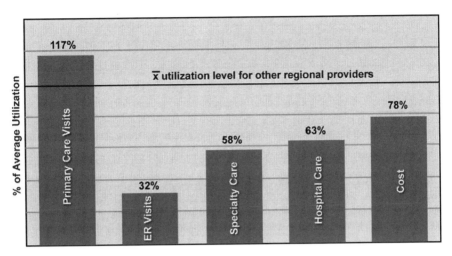

Fig. 7.4 Mean patient health care utilization by Cherokee Health Systems as compared to other regional providers (Source: Blue Cross Blue Shield of Tennessee)

utilization, and costs. However, scheduling extended hours for behavioral health consultants and other staff needs to be flexible to provide same-day access to care as needed; otherwise, patients will go to the emergency department. Establishing clinical and administrative workflows that promote alignment and integration of staff is essential. A multidimensional staff communication infrastructure is crucial for coordinated care.

Cobb and Douglas County Community Service Boards: County Community Services Board Clinic with Embedded FQHC Partner Clinical Team

History and services overview. The Cobb County Community Services Board and the Douglas County Community Services Board (CSB) are public agencies serving Cobb, Douglas, and Cherokee Counties, Georgia. The agency provides support to over 14,000 people annually, including approximately 3,000 patients in the Cobb County Jail. Together, the CSBs employ 400 staff at 20 sites.

HOW: Team-based care/Staffing roles and communication. The integrated care team changed from a physician's assistant, a registered nurse, a nurse care manager, and two care managers (one RN and one social worker) to include an MSW Care Manager, a Wellness Coordinator, a Peer Specialist (20 hours a week, serves as a Health Coach), and an hourly Data Manager, through their partnership contract with West End FQHC. The MSW care manager is actively engaged in the linkage process, as well as in integration and referrals to specialty care.

They are partnered with the West End FQHC, which has a "wing" in the CSB clinic that is supported by a SAMHSA PBHCI grant. Additional alliances have been formed with key health delivery structures in the community to support comprehensive integrated care, complemented by a Medicaid Disease Management Project supported by APS. In 2007, the Cobb and Douglas CSB leaders acted on their concerns about early mortality due to preventable medical conditions among their dual diagnosis and behavioral health clients, and initiated a partnership with Benjamin Druss, MD, at Emory University to apply for and win a NIMH research demonstration grant. The grant allowed them to run a home study demonstration project targeted at bringing FQHC services into the CMHC setting to improve the array of services provided to individuals with SPMI and comorbid cardiometabolic disorders, and funded the services of a doctor, a physician's assistant (PA), and a registered nurse (RN). The NIMH funding was extended to 2010, at which time the CSB was awarded one of SAMHSA's Primary Care Behavioral Health Integration (PCBHI) Grants, which allowed them to extend their partnership with the West End FQHC.

Patient population/Targeted or universal. The CSB primarily serves a population diagnosed with serious and persistent mental illness (SPMI). Their integrated care initiative is targeted to their core clients who also have comorbid cardiometabolic conditions.

Systematic clinical approach. The CSB employs the Four Quadrant model, in which wellness is addressed at all levels of care. They employ evidence-based practices, including peer support services targeted at wellness and recovery, integrated dual disorders treatment (IDDT), and they utilize the Best Practice of Chronic Care Model. Four levels of treatment are provided, including universal PCP screening for physical conditions via self-report and lab tests; a staff appointment for one of the screened-for conditions, during which basic follow-up and wellness is provided; then, more intensive services; and finally, wellness services with a focus on preventive measurement and active self-management.

SUPPORTED BY: Office practice, leadership and business model. The Cobb and Douglas CSB has developed what they term a "Primary Care hallway," which allows them to integrate staff for patient flow. They have made this hallway part of their circle of holistic care to more fully integrate services. Their medical and behavioral staff members shadow each other to learn from one another and become familiar with each approach to care. The Master's-level social worker is engaged with training on site and they have a certification program pending for integrated care. The Cobb and Douglas CSB participates in the Learning Academy run by the CIHS and Mental Health Corporations of America, which focused on cardiometabolic conditions.

The integrated care program receives PBHCI grant funding, as noted above, and Kaiser Permanente grant funds that supports the partnership with the West End FQHC (See Fig. 7.5).

Continuous Quality Improvement (CQI). The Cobb and Douglas CSB collects SAMHSA's required TRAC measures and continues to routinely assess and record

Fig. 7.5 Cobb and Douglas
CSB funding sources

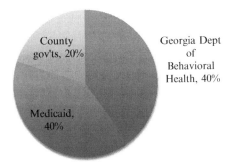

results of various clinical metrics associated with the NIMH study. They have made their intake process a common point, which drives quality data and efficiency. The Cobb and Douglas CSB focuses on medical metrics because their program aims to address chronic health conditions.

Strengths, challenges, and insights. West End is sophisticated and progressive, and has provided a partnership of equals and strong cultural match in taking informed risks to innovate and improve care for their clients. If this relationship with the West End FQHC continues to evolve positively, they will seek to colocate permanently and will bill Medicare and Medicaid once ACA expands eligibility. This will allow both entities to bill according to their licenses to all third party payers. They are also exploring the idea of sending CSB behavioral health staff to the West End FQHC, which would build on a small study involving West End patients with depression. On the other hand, the CSB cannot bill for PCP services provided to indigent, non-Medicaid and Medicaid clients, but the "out of clinic" rate under the Rehab Option can cover behavioral health services provided at West End clinics at a higher rate of reimbursement than when delivering behavioral health care in the CSB clinics.

The CSB has successfully implemented measures-driven integrated care and is producing results and data to guide future implementation efforts. The partnership with West End is spawning interest in other community infrastructure efforts, including partnering with WellStar Health System and the Cobb County Public Health system to develop a process to address health disparities with the CSB serving as the behavioral health provider at any new clinics.

Lone Star Circle of Care, Georgetown TX: FQHC with In-House Behavioral Health Services

History and services overview. Lone Star Circle of Care (LSCC) became a Federally Qualified Health Center (FQHC) in 2002, at which time, like other CHCs, it contracted with community providers, including CMHCs, to deliver mental health services to its primary care clients (G. Jensen & K. Kotrla, May 2, 2012, personal communication; Lone Star, 2012). In 2006, LSCC began providing mental health and substance misuse services in-house to address gaps in the community service network, colocating provider employees of a separate organization in the LSCC clinics. To strengthen its medical home offering, Lone Star then chose to develop behavioral health and psychiatry services into a new business line with services offered in-house by Lone Star staff; this is now its largest business line. Lone Star now provides a network of 27 clinics serving clients in a large geographic area of Central Texas, including pediatric, family practice, OB-GYN, dentistry, vision, geriatric care, and psychiatry and behavioral health, which offers adult, child and adolescent, geriatric and addictions treatment.

HOW: Team-based care/Staffing roles and communication. They employ 36 behavioral health providers including 13 psychiatrists (adult, geriatric, and child/adolescent), and 24 therapists (Psychologists, Licensed Professional Counselors, and Licensed Clinical Social Workers), and they will soon employ Psychiatric Nurse Practitioners. LSCC embeds behavioral health staff in all of its primary care clinics, providing a "behaviorally enhanced health home" to patients.

Shared patient population/Targeted or universal. More than 50 % of LSCC patients are Latino and approximately 20 % of its behavioral health clients are monolingual Spanish. Patients can choose whether to use Lone Star as their medical home for both primary care and behavioral health services, or they can access its psychiatric clinics while maintaining a medical home with another provider. Lone Star provides approximately 360,000 patient encounters per year, with 52,000 of these visits projected in behavioral health.

Systematic clinical approach. Lone Star strives to employ evidence-based practices and national clinical practice guidelines to structure effective care delivery. These include motivational interviewing (MI), CBT and DBT, the Corel Guidelines for patients on second generation antipsychotics, American Psychiatric Association Practice Guidelines and the American Academy of Child and Adolescent Psychiatry Practice Parameters as clinical standards of care for its behavioral health providers. LSCC collects standardized screening data using the Mood Disorder Questionnaire (MDQ), the Patient Health Questionnaire-9 (PHQ-9) for adults, and the Vanderbilt Assessment Scale to monitor children's symptoms. For patients seeking care, whether they are new or established, their first encounter is with the Patient Navigation Center (PNC), a call center that provides patients with a single point of contact for all 27 clinics and seven service lines. The Patient Navigation Center has a variety of staff including eligibility specialists, patient service representatives, and registered nurses who support behavioral health, in addition to other service lines. PNC staff helps the client with care choices, location, and team preferences to determine the best fit for the patient's medical home, and also determine insurance status or Medicaid eligibility, providing enrollment assistance if needed. Uninsured patients are served on sliding fee scale or as an unfunded patient. The PNC has access to nurse referral specialists who handle patient triage and prescription questions, facilitating the work of the integrated medical team.

SUPPORTED BY: Office practice, leadership and business model. The standardized screening data discussed above is slated to be embedded as standard protocols in Lone Star's electronic health record (NextGen). Lone Star also employs an

Fig. 7.6 Lone Star payer mix

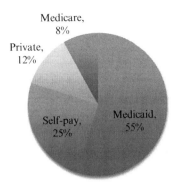

internal governance structure called the Behaviorally Enhanced Health care Integration Council (BEHIC), which meets on monthly basis, involving all service line medical directors and senior managers (finance, quality, PNC). The goal of the BEHIC meetings is to focus attention across all service lines on integrating behavioral health care.

Seventy percent of Lone Star's operating revenue comes from patient revenue and 30 % comes from grant or other partnership resources (see Fig. 7.6). Lone Star requires their providers to be Medicaid certified. Financial sustainability demands focus on three metrics: staff skill mix, balanced payer mix, and high productivity.

Continuous quality improvement and effectiveness. Lone Star places a premium on meeting quality standards, ranging from conformance with meaningful use standards to Joint Commission accreditation and NCQA Level 3 patient-centered medical home certification. Quality Councils operate for each health service line and organization wide. The behavioral health quality council is planning to include patients on the council. Lone Star tracks patient satisfaction and symptom reduction, such as the PHQ and Vanderbilt standardized screening tools, and they are adopting new tools to measure quality of life. LSCC monitors various operational measures, like the wait time between primary care intake and referral to specialists, and shares outcomes data with staff. Patients show positive results of care integration efforts including improvements in physical health status and daily activity performance levels, and decreased in PHQ-9 depression symptom scores, with symptom alleviation within a month after beginning care and sustaining across a 24-month period.

Strengths, challenges, and insights. The single access point through the Patient Navigation Center is a novel and important process for matching patient needs with health care resources at the beginning of care. The inclusion of standard screening tools to assess patient's mental health functioning is also an important part of screening all patients for behavioral-mental health care. The implications of incorporating this data into patient care, standard protocols, or treatment plans are in the early stages of investigation. LSCC's largest challenge is in trying to respond to rising demand for care and to address unmet needs in settings outside of its operations, including schools and nursing facilities, and reaching patient and remote facilities in need of psychiatric care and consultation delivered via telemedicine (Lone Star, 2012).

Insights: LSCC identifies several factors in effective implementation of an integrated behavioral health program including: focus on mission, entrepreneurial leadership, creating a PCMH, employing evidence-based screening and treatment, using technology to support communications and track results, and active partnering with other health care entities in the community to increase access and continuity of care for Lone Star patients.

Shawnee Mental Health Center, Portsmouth OH: CMHC with In-House Primary Care Services

History and services overview. Shawnee Mental Health Center, incorporated as a CMHC in 1973, has four clinics serving three rural counties in Southeast Ohio, all of which are located in federally underserved health areas (D. Thacker, May 2, 2012, personal communication).

HOW: Team-based care/Staffing roles and communication. Moved by evidence that early mortality and morbidity among individuals with serious mental illness was largely attributable to preventable health conditions, Shawnee clinical and administrative leaders explored health home and integrated care models. They were successful in securing planning grant funds from the Health Foundation of Cincinnati and operations grant funding from SAMHSA's PBHCI initiative. Shawnee's integrated care initiative has grown from one primary care practitioner addressing the most serious somatic health needs of people with serious mental illness in its behavioral health clinics to providing integrated primary care to a broader community population in all clinics.

Shawnee's staffing mix consists of: Support staff, nurses, Psychologists, LPNs, Peer Wellness Coaches, and Psychiatric and Family Nurse Practitioners, who have been prescribing privileges. All new Shawnee clients are offered access to integrated PCP services, unless they choose to maintain an established PCP relationship.

Shared patient population/Targeted or universal. Shawnee clients are primarily Appalachian; with 98 % white, 1 % African-American, and 1 % others; 60 % of patients are female and 40 % male. Most clients have high behavioral health needs and moderate to high primary care needs. Top behavioral health diagnostic categories include mood and psychotic disorders, and primary care diagnoses are most frequently dyslipidemia, diabetes, hypertension, respiratory, and tobacco dependence.

Systematic clinical approach. Clients first meet with an integrated team member. Nurse Practitioners, working with a supervising physician, use standard protocols to assess for chronic medical conditions including hypertension, obesity, tobacco, diabetes. Depending on his/her needs, there may be a "warm hand off" from behavioral

Fig. 7.7 Shawnee MHC'
payer mix

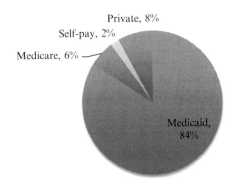

health to primary care staff, or behavioral health clinicians will participate in primary care visits that are coordinated by a Nurse Practitioner. Patient progress is monitored using clinical interviews. Care management services are offered to clients needing assistance with coordinating care, like appointment reminders or follow-up. The case/care managers, LPNs, and peer wellness coaches work to provide both behavioral health and primary care services.

SUPPORTED BY: Office practice, leadership and business model. Shawnee uses a variety of mechanisms to support communications among integrated care staff. All clinics hold daily team meetings and use phone consultations, email, and impromptu conversations to ensure care coordination. They recently revised the layout of clinical space to colocate practitioners and have already seen improved communications and care coordination. Patients have access to a 24-hour hotline and the appropriate care team responds. They expect that their new EHR system will also help to enhance case coordination among practitioners.

While Shawnee bills all payer sources available, the SAMHSA grant is essential to the support for its integrated services (See Fig. 7.7). Grant funds cover gaps as the integrated care patient load grows to a sustainable level and experience is gained with billing third parties for the range of primary and specialty functions provided to patients. Shawnee recognizes that financial sustainability depends on expanding integrated care to the broader population, including children and family members of their current clients. This latter strategy aligns with Shawnee's health home philosophy to work with the entire family to improve outcomes.

Continuous quality improvement and effectiveness. Shawnee employs diagnostic assessment guidelines that meet CARF accreditation standards, adding questions about patients' health history and PCP to their intake interview. Staff use motivational interviewing with clients and provide peer wellness coaching and other peer support. Other evidence-based practices include an organization-wide tobacco cessation program using Tobacco Recovery Across the Continuum (TRAC) program, offering nicotine replacement treatment, monitoring tobacco use with a carbon monoxide monitor. Shawnee contracts with Case Western University to evaluate its integrated care program, looking at outcome measures for morbidity and management of diabetes, hypertension, and emergency room use. They also serve as an experimental group in SAMHSA's PBHCI nationwide study, with results expected after 2013.

Strengths, challenges, and insights. Shawnee identifies problems in billing Medicare, with reimbursement rates reduced by 20–30 % when there is a behavioral health diagnosis associated with primary care claims. They have also struggled to secure adequate psychiatry coverage in rural areas, particularly in the child psychiatry specialty. Shawnee contracts with a child psychiatrist in another state who provides services via telepsychiatry and comes on site one or two days per month. They are exploring collaborative models where psychiatrists provide oversight and consultation and nurse practitioners provide direct services. Another observation is that providing primary care inside a behavioral health clinic requires cross-training and mutual understanding of respective primary care and behavioral health practice cultures and expectations of patients, rules and regulations, which necessitates a redefinition of integrated protocols.

Essentials for Implementing Integrated Behavioral Health Care in Public Health

Because of these differences in use of terms and application of models, the discussion of implementation, across different settings, scanning different models, is focused on "organizational factors" and "integrated care functions," elements that are comparable at an operational level. Mission, values, and leadership are, as discussed earlier, important drivers of integrated care for persons who have or are at risk for comorbid health conditions. As outlined for the integrated care sites profiled above, a range of clinical and system functions are similarly essential to deliver effective and sustainable integrated care.

Organization and Governance: Leadership. Mission is critical to support the shift to integrated care. Successful safety net provider organizations that are practicing integrated care identified this as essential to forging agreement about care integration and making necessary operational changes to support the new direction. When these organizations look at missions that target improvements in health status and quality of life for individuals who depend on the safety net, many of whom have multiple health risks and/or chronic conditions, and look at the needs manifesting in their patients, the rationale for and benefits of integrated care are hard to deny. Missions that reflect not only a commitment to the safety net, but also a patient-centered approach to serve the whole person support integration of behavioral health and primary care. Among the scanned organizations, the role of leadership in driving change varied by organization, ranging from charismatic leaders who were early adopters, actually "early crafters" of integrated care, to more entrepreneurial leaders determined to respond to unmet community need by adding primary care services to behavioral health services in parts of states that otherwise lacked access to care.

Organizational and Staff Culture. The commitment of safety net organizations to high-risk and medically complex individuals supports board, senior management and clinical leadership in tackling practice culture, program operations, and resource development challenges to adopt integration as a better fit for meeting their patients' needs. Effective program operations are built on a cohesive organizational design that defines leadership and accountability structures as well as a clinical department or division structures, grouping employees to align with organizational and service delivery goals. Integrating care will likely require changes in team structures and reporting relationships to facilitate implementation of new clinical pathways, adoption of collaborative practice protocols, and changes in organizational culture as staff and organizations alike adapt. Despite shared values and a common patient population in the safety net, behavioral health and primary care developed as distinct and siloed fields, with different policies, procedures, incentives, and practice cultures. For example, work and productivity patterns are different. PCPs typically see multiple patients per hour, accommodate walk-in and emergent care demands in office, consult with colleagues and specialists during the patient visit, record more measures, and have less narrative documentation in the record. Behavioral health specialist typically see one to two patients per hour, do not handle emergent or walk-in cases on a routine basis, consult with collaborators in separate meetings, and are burdened with more record documentation. The common wisdom among profiled organizations is that several strategies are key to forming an integrated culture: leadership that articulates the value and rewards participation; a focus on the patients and their needs which makes obvious the purpose and value of integrated care; cross-training to educate respective parties on the other professional service legacy culture and on shared methods for integrated care; and shared physical space or "collocation" so that practitioners are working side-by-side on a daily basis.

Workforce development for both primary care and behavioral health care professionals to understand the complex health problems and needs of patients, as well as the practices and processes of the other practice field, is identified as a critical obstacle to adequately staffing integrated care programs and meeting demand for care. Workforce development initiatives that build mutual understanding of complex needs and effective care protocols are similarly critical to bridging the cultural gaps between primary and specialty behavioral health care to produce a well-informed and truly integrated care delivery system. For example, there is a need to focus on care management rather than case management, which has been the tradition in behavioral health programs, while there is a need to move away from the "patient for a day" view traditionally held in primary care practices to build a long-term patient/practitioner medical home partnership. In order to adapt to these changes, behavioral health case managers will need to expand their knowledge of general health issues. Through this transition from case managers to care managers, the broader skill set acquired in training may allow the care team to address health issues from a whole body perspective; assessment in this model will put more emphasis on the relationship between physical health and behavioral health.

Clinical Systems and Protocols. As the Bauhaus architects preached, "form follows function" and in integrated care, function follows a redesigned response to complex client need. The challenge of service delivery redesign varies depending on the legacy structure of the initiating organization, CHC/FQHC or CMHC/CBHO. Conceptual frameworks and practice models, while informative, will not alone ensure sound implementation. Emerging evidence, although mostly drawn from private health sector endeavors, indicates that effective integrated care results from service delivery redesigns that incorporate the following components: use of evidence-based assessment and treatment protocols, properly designed clinical and operational pathways, and joint behavioral and primary care management. One of five high-level metrics for one model of integrated care includes a team that incorporates primary care and behavioral health professionals with a shared population and mission (Miller, Kessler, Peek, & Kallenberg, 2011). The team should use a clinical system and should be supported by an office practice and financial system that maintains continuous quality improvement processes and measures effectiveness (Miller et al.).

Once an organization determines the direction of its service line expansion, integrated clinical pathways must be designed from point of intake. Service delivery methods need to be built on team-based, patient-centered care structured with evidence-based practices that are deployed with fidelity to establish standards defining staff configuration, practice methods, and protocols. Integrated service delivery needs support of a robust team communications infrastructure composed of routine clinical and care management meetings and a shared, preferably electronic, health record. Patient navigation systems are an effective complement to integrated care and reinforce a partnership between patients and the care team. Finally, redesigned physical plant configurations that minimally colocate and better "collocate" staff produce better and more efficient communication and collaboration on shared patient care.

Practice Management and Financial Systems. As underscored by the profiled organizations, safety net programs are heavily dependent on foundation and government grants to fill gaps in health care reimbursement to support their behavioral health and primary care integration work. This is not a sustainable arrangement as foundation and government program priorities shift over time.

Peter Drucker is credited with the statement "what gets measured gets done," but more fitting to safety net health systems challenges in integrating care is John E. Jones' statement, "What gets measured gets done, what gets measured and fed back gets done well, what gets rewarded gets repeated." Within safety nets particularly, organizations must deliver services that can be reimbursed. So, the latter portion of Jones' statement is both a source of concern in the world of safety net financing with its state-by-state variation, and a source of hope should more cohesive and consistent financial models for integrated care emerge as a result of ACA reforms. As discussed earlier, the HRSA Section 330 grants confer considerable financial advantages on FQHCs and remain an important component of adequate financing for integrated care. FQCH grants are a significant element in the reimbursement mix with Medicaid and Medicare payments, including those derived from Rehab or Case Management options covering case management services, and capitation payments covering care management functions in PCMHs or health homes.

The ACA, as discussed earlier, contains provisions that provide supports and incentives for states and health care providers to adopt integration practices. For patients, this may translate into improved, more coordinated care that fosters better health outcomes and improved quality of life. For systems, effectively delivered integrated care can bend the cost curve and produce savings. In particular, the ACA changes what services will be available to individuals with mental health and substance use disorders, requiring benefit packages that include behavioral health treatment, prescription medications, rehabilitative, habilitative and prevention and wellness services by Fiscal Year 2014. However, a significant ruling in the recent Supreme Court decision upholding the ACA eliminates the mandatory aspect of the extension of Medicaid benefits to single adults up to 133 % of federal poverty level. States are free to elect or decline this provision of the ACA. Since a substantial portion of those single individuals are uninsured and have serious health conditions, they will remain dependent on the safety net without insurance coverage.

Practice-Based Quality Improvement and Evaluation

Improved quality is an implicit assumption underlying the integration of behavioral health and primary care, however few of the surveyed organizations reported being directed to systematic quality improvement practices that support integrated care objectives. Some organizations adopt quality improvement efforts to align with external review organizations' standards, including those from the Joint Commission and the National Commission on Quality Assurance (NCQA). In particular, the NCQA Physician Practice Connections Patient Centered Medical Home (PPC-PCMH) certification, based on the Wagner Chronic Care Model, recognizes practices that systematically employ information technology and operational processes to improve care quality. The NCQA standards are instructive, covering ten elements that include: use of written standards and data tracking to account for patient access and patient communication; use of charting tools to organize clinical information; use of data to identify significant diagnoses and conditions to better target practice and interventions; active efforts to support patient self-management; systems for tracking test results and efforts on actionable findings; tracking of critical referrals; measurement of clinical and service performance; physician and cross-practice service reporting. Perhaps most important to heed is the advice of Jurgen Unutzer, MD, "deliver measures driven care" (J. Unutzer, June, 2012, personal communication).

Summary and Conclusion

The behavioral health and primary care fields are experiencing a rapid rate of change, accelerating now that the Supreme Court has upheld most provisions of the ACA. Several ACA provisions contain service delivery and payment method reforms that serve to promote integration of behavioral health and primary care, including creation of health homes and accountable care organizations and use of bundled rates, pay-for-performance, and gain-sharing associated with value-based purchasing. The focus on care integration as a solution to system fragmentation, patient morbidity and mortality, and growing costs will increase as integration holds significant promise for achieving the Triple Aim of improving the quality, outcomes, and cost of health care.

Although the bidirectional relationship of behavioral and other health conditions is acknowledged and the high prevalence of comorbid conditions is well established, acting on this knowledge remains a challenge for many siloed care settings. The majority of care delivered in the USA continues in siloed fashion, missing critical opportunities for prevention in primary care settings where the majority at risk and in need first appear for care, and in specialty settings where patients with serious and persistent mental illnesses in particular die early due to preventable yet unaddressed health conditions. However, a number of safety net organizations are tackling the task of integration. Despite several frameworks and models for integration, provider organizations on the front lines are adapting and creating models to respond to perceived patient needs, contend with operational constraints in their current environments, and manage within local reimbursement rules and opportunities. There is a substantial risk in the current strategy of perpetuating an inconsistent approach to care, even if integrated care. Broad scale implementation of effective, accountable, and sustainable behavioral health and primary care integration requires public policy changes to support scientific, broadly disseminated and supported measures-driven integrated care approaches. Evaluation and research efforts emerging from recent integration efforts should shape practice redesign and encourage practitioners to set aside cultural differences in favor of the opportunity to deliver more effective care. Disparate practice cultures and workforce challenges aside, low reimbursement rates and fragmented and complicated reimbursement policies are the greatest barrier to universal adoption of integrated behavioral health and primary care in the safety net. Data documenting improved patient satisfaction, clinical and cost outcomes will support policy, coverage and reimbursement changes needed to sustain integration as standard practice.

References

AIMS Center. (2012). Retrieved September 30, 2012 from http://uwaims.org/prorams.html

Alegria, M., Chatterji, P., Wells, K., Cao, Z., Chen, C. N., Takeuchi, D., et al. (2008). Disparity in depression treatment among racial and ethnic minority populations in the United States. *Psychiatric Services, 59*, 1264–1272.

Begley, C., Hickey, J., Ostermeyer, B., Teske, L., Vu, T., & Rowan, P. (2008). Integrating behavioral health and primary care: The Harris County Community Behavioral Health Program. *Psychiatric Services, 59*, 356–358.

Butler, M., Kane, R., McAlpine, D., Kathol, R., Fu, S., Hagedorn, H., et al. (2008). Integration of mental health/substance abuse and primary care. *Evidence Report/Technology Assessment, 173*, 1–362.

Chapa, T. (2011, May). *An approach to eliminating disparities in racial and ethnic minority populations through the integration of behavioral and primary healthcare: Recommendations and strategies.* Presented at the Policy Summit to Address Behavioral Health Disparities within Health Care Reform, San Diego, CA.

Croghan, T. W., & Brown, J. D. (2010). *Integrating mental health treatment into the patient centered medical home.* Prepared by Mathematica Policy Research Under Contract No.

HHSA2902009000019I TO2. (AHRQ Publication No. 10-0084-EF). Rockville, MD: Agency for Healthcare Research and Quality.

Finegold, K., Wherry, L., & Schardin, S. (2004). Block grants: Historical overview and lessons learned. *New Federalism, A-63*, 1–7. Retrieved September 30, 2012 from http://www.urban.org/uploadedPDF/310991_A-63.pdf

Foley, H. A., & Sharfstein, S. S. (1983). *Madness and government: Who cares for the mentally ill?* Washington, DC: American Psychiatric Press.

Frequent Users of Health Services Initiative. (2008). *Summary report of evaluation findings: A dollars and sense strategy to reducing frequent use of hospital services.* Oakland, CA: The California Endowment and the California Health Care Foundation.

Garret, B., Holahan, J., Cook, A., Headen, I., & Lucas, A. (2009). *The coverage and cost impacts of expanding Medicaid.* Retrieved September 30, 2012 from http://www.kff.org/medicaid/upload/7901.pdf

González, H. M., Croghan, T., West, B., Williams, D., Nesse, R., Tarraf, W., et al. (2008). Antidepressant use in black and white populations in the United States. *Psychiatric Services, 59*, 1131–1138.

Green, S., Singh, V., & O'Byrne, W. (2010). Hope for New Jersey's city hospitals: The Camden Initiative. *Perspectives in Health Information Management, 1*, 71d.

Health Resources and Services Administration. (2010). *HRSA national health center data—2010 national report.* Retrieved September 30, 2012 from http://bphc.hrsa.gov/uds/doc/2010/National_Universal.pdf

Hunkeler, E., Katon, W., Tang, L., Williams, J., Kroenke, K., Lin, E., et al. (2006). Long term outcomes from the IMPACT randomised trial for depressed elderly patients in primary care. *British Medical Journal, 332*, 259–263.

Insel, T. (2008). Assessing the economic costs of serious mental illness. *The American Journal of Psychiatry, 165*, 663–665.

Institute of Medicine (IOM). (2001). *Crossing the quality chasm: A new health system for the 21st century.* Washington, DC: National Academy Press.

Jones, A. S., & Sajid, P. S. (2009). *A primer on health care safety nets.* Princeton, NJ: Robert Wood Johnson Foundation.

Kaiser Commission on Medicaid and the Uninsured estimates based on MSIS 2007/2008.

Katman, S., Pauk, J., & Alter, C. L. (2011). Meeting the mental health needs of low-income immigrants in primary care: A community adaptation of and evidence-based model. *The American Journal of Orthopsychiatry, 81*, 543–551.

Katon, W., Lin, E., Von Korff, M., Ciechanowski, P., Ludman, E., Young, B., et al. (2010). Collaborative care for patients with depression and chronic illnesses. *The New England Journal of Medicine, 363*, 2611–2620.

Katon, W., Robinson, P., Von Korff, M., Lin, E., Bush, T., & Walker, E. (1996). A multifaceted intervention to improve treatment of depression in primary care. *Archives of General Psychiatry, 53*, 924–932.

Katon, W., Rutter, C., Ludman, E., Von Korff, M., Lin, E., Simon, G., et al. (2001). A randomized trial of relapse prevention of depression in primary care. *Archives of General Psychiatry, 58*, 241–247.

Kessler, R. C., Berglund, P., Demler, O., Jin, R., Merikangas, K. R., & Walters, E. E. (2005). Lifetime prevalence and age-of-onset distributions of DSM-IV disorders in the National Comorbidity Survey Replication. *Archives of General Psychiatry, 62*, 593–602.

Kessler, R., Demler, O., Frank, R., Olfson, M., Pincus, H. A., Walters, E. E., et al. (2005). Prevalence and treatment of mental disorders, 1990 to 2003. *The New England Journal of Medicine, 352*, 2515–2523.

Kessler, R. C., Heeringa, S., Lakoma, M., Petukhova, M., Rupp, A., Schoenbaum, M., et al. (2008). Individual and societal effects of mental disorders on earnings in the United States: Results from the National Comorbidity Survey Replication. *The American Journal of Psychiatry, 165*, 703–711.

Levit, K., Kassed, C., Coffey, R., Mark, T., Stranges, E., Buck, J. A., et al. (2008). Future funding for mental health and substance abuse: Increasing burdens for the public sector. *Health Affairs, 27*, 513–522.

Mark, T. L., Levit, K. R., Coffey, R. M., McKusick, D. R., Harwood, H. J., King, E. C., et al. (2007). *National expenditures for mental health services and substance abuse treatment, 1993–2003.* Rockville, MD: Substance Abuse and Mental Health Services Administration.

Marr, A., Pillow, T., & Brown, S. (2008). Southside medical homes network: Linking emergency department patients to community care. *The Official Journal of The National Association of EMS Physicians and The World Association For Emergency and Disaster Medicine In Association With The Acute Care Foundation, 23*, 282–284. Prehospital and Disaster Medicine.

Mental Health Weekly. (2008). Groundbreaking depression initiative expands to 10 Minnesota clinics. *Mental Health Weekly,* 18.

Miller, T., & Hendrie, D. (2008). *Substance abuse prevention dollars and cents: A cost-benefit analysis* (DHHS Publication No. SMA 07-4298). Rockville, MD: Center for Substance Abuse Prevention, Substance Abuse and Mental Health Services Administration.

Miller, B. F., Kessler, R., Peek, C. J., & Kallenberg, G. A. (2011). *A national agenda for research in collaborative care.* Papers from the collaborative care research network research development conference (AHRQ publication no. 11-0067). Rockville, MD: Agency for Healthcare Research and Quality.

National Center for Primary Care, Morehouse School of Medicine. (2008). *Making it real: Integrating primary care and behavioral health in community-based settings,* November 18th–19th, 2008. Atlanta, GA.

National Council for Community Behavioral Healthcare. (2009). Healthcare payment reform and the behavioral health safety net: What's on the horizon for the community behavioral health system. *The National Council.* Retrieved September 30, 2012 from http://www.thenational-council.org/galleries/policy-file/Healthcare%20Payment%20Reform%20Full%20Report.pdf

O'Connell, M. E., Boat, T., & Warner, K. E. (2009). *Preventing mental, emotional, and behavioral disorders among young people: Progress and possibilities.* Washington, DC: National Academies Press (US).

Reiss-Brennan, B., Briot, P., Savitz, L., Cannon, W., & Staheli, R. (2010). Cost and quality impact of Intermountain's mental health integration program. *Journal of Healthcare Management/ American College of Healthcare Executives, 55*, 97–113.

Rosenbaum, S., Zakheim, M. H., Leifer, J., Golde, M.D., Schulte, J. M., & Margulies, R. (2011). Assessing and addressing legal barriers to the clinical integration of community health centers and other community providers. *The Commonwealth Fund.* Retrieved September 30, 2012 from http://www.commonwealthfund.org/Publications/Fund-Reports/2011/Jul/Clinical-Integration.aspx

Rost, K., Pyne, J., Dickinson, L., & LoSasso, A. (2005). Cost-effectiveness of enhancing primary care depression management on an ongoing basis. *Annals of Family Medicine, 3*, 7–14.

SAMHSA-HRSA Center for Integrated Health Solutions. (2012). *SAMHSA PBHCI program.* Accessed May 5, 2012, from http://www.integration.samhsa.gov/about-us/pbhci

Section 330 of the Public Health Service Act, 42 U.S.C.S. § 254b.

Sharfestein, S. S. (2000). Whatever happened to community mental health? *Psychiatric Services, 51*, 616–620.

Substance Abuse and Mental Health Services Administration. (2012). *Mental health, United States, 2010* (HHS publication no. (SMA) 12-4681). Rockville, MD: Author.

Substance Abuse and Mental Health Services Administration. (2011, March). *Leading change: A plan for SAMHSA's roles and actions 2011–2014* (Rep. No. SMA11-4629). Rockville, MD: Author..

Unutzer, J., Ya-Fen, C., Hafer, E., Knaster, J., Shields, A., Powers, D., et al. (2012). Quality improvement with pay-for-performance incentives in integrated behavioral health care. *American Journal of Public Health, 102*, e41–e45.

Urban Institute and Kaiser Commission on Medicaid and the Uninsured. (2010). *Health insurance coverage of the nonelderly population by race/ethnicity.* Retrieved September 30, 2012 from http://facts.kff.org/chart.aspx?ch=365

Wang, P. S., Berglund, P., Olfson, M., Pincus, H. A., Wells, K. B., & Kessler, R. C. (2005). Failure and delay in initial treatment contact after first onset of mental disorders in the National Comorbidity Survey Replication. *Archives of General Psychiatry, 62*, 603–613.

Wang, P. S., Demler, O., & Kessler, R. C. (2002). Adequacy of treatment for serious mental illness in the United States. *American Journal of Public Health, 92*, 92–98.

Wang, P., Lane, M., Olfson, M., Pincus, H., Wells, K., & Kessler, R. (2005). Twelve-month use of mental health services in the United States: Results from the National Comorbidity Survey Replication. *Archives of General Psychiatry, 62*, 629–640.

Wang, P., Simon, G., & Kessler, R. (2003). The economic burden of depression and the cost-effectiveness of treatment. *International Journal of Methods in Psychiatric Research, 12*, 22–33.

Chapter 8
The Financial History and Near Future of Integrated Behavioral Health Care

Jennifer Hodgson and Randall Reitz

Abstract Most programs that integrate physical and behavioral health struggle with financial sustainability. The growth and development of mechanisms for supporting grass-roots integration highlight the creativity and sheer will of communities, states, and health care systems to innovate their way to health. And now, for the first time, national-level funding initiatives have begun to directly or indirectly support integration. This chapter will highlight funding mechanisms at the state, foundation, payer, and federal levels. It will provide a historical and future-oriented primer of the various mechanisms for advancing and sustaining integration.

The Financial History and Near Future of Integrated Behavioral Health Care

> If care is clinically inappropriate it fails. If care is not operationalized properly, it also fails. If care does not make reasonable use of resources, the organization, its patients, or society eventually go bankrupt and thousands of patient-clinician relationships are disrupted.
>
> -The Three-World View of Healthcare (Peek, 2008)

President Kennedy's focus in the 1963 Community Mental Health Center Act was to "return mental health care to the mainstream of American medicine" (Kennedy, 1963). Then again in 1979, the US Surgeon General Julius B. Richmond argued in

J. Hodgson, Ph.D., LMFT (✉)
Departments of Child Dev't & Family Relations and Family Medicine,
East Carolina University, Greenville, NC 27858, USA
e-mail: hodgsonj@ecu.edu

R. Reitz, Ph.D., LMFT
St Mary's Family Medicine Residency, St Mary's Regional Medical Center,
2698 Patterson Road, Grand Junction, CO 81506, USA
e-mail: reitz.randall@gmail.com

M.R. Talen and A. Burke Valeras (eds.), *Integrated Behavioral Health in Primary Care: Evaluating the Evidence, Identifying the Essentials*, DOI 10.1007/978-1-4614-6889-9_8,
© Springer Science+Business Media New York 2013

his report for the integration of medical and mental health services. However, achieving and sustaining their shared goal has proven elusive.

As with most major changes in health care services, integrated behavioral health care began with a clinical theory that evolved into an operational model and only later took into serious consideration the financial infrastructure to support and grow it. In fact, in 1993, when the intellectual founders of integrated behavioral health care initially met to create strategy to develop integrated behavioral health care, they intentionally left financial considerations out of their vision statement: "No matter how financed, what should a thoroughly modern health care delivery system look like at the clinical level?" (Collaborative Family Healthcare Association [CFHA], 2012). While probably inevitable, the decision to focus on clinical services and operational models before financial sustainability was in place has deeply shaped the evolution and growth of integrated behavioral health care in the US health system.

This book's operational definition for integrated behavioral health care was provided by C.J. Peek in Chap. 2 of this book. Integrated behavioral health care is "a team with a shared population and mission using a clinical system supported by an office practice and financial system and continuous quality improvement and effectiveness measurement." This chapter will focus almost exclusively on the "financial system" of this definition. We will start with a historical context of public health funding and analyze the development of integrated behavioral health care across several states. We will then examine financial aspects of integrated behavioral health care in vertically integrated and nationwide systems. We will finish this chapter by highlighting the impact of very recent initiatives that might sustain integrated behavioral health care and how they might rollout in the near future.

Historical Perspective on Divergent Funding and Reimbursement Between FQHCs and CBHOs

By D. Mauch and J. Bartlett (See Chap. 7, *Integrated Behavioral Health in Public Health care Contexts: Community Health and Mental Health Safety Net Systems*).

Financing and reimbursement have long posed barriers to the integration of behavioral health and primary care. While FQHCs (Federally Qualified Health Centers) and CBHOs (Community Behavioral Health Organizations) share payer mix profiles that are similar in their heavy concentration of persons with public insurance, there are significant differences in the methods and rates of free care, Medicaid, and Medicare reimbursement available to these respective safety net entities. CBHOs now depend largely on state contracts (that may include federal substance abuse and mental health block grant funds) and Medicaid reimbursement rates, which vary from state to state and are

(continued)

often set at rates well below cost with discounted fee for service (FFS) and managed care reimbursements. By contrast, FQHCs have significant financial advantages pursuant to provisions of the Section 330 legislation. FQHC grants not only cover the costs of uncompensated primary health care, but also provide enhanced reimbursement under the prospective payment system (PPS) or other state-approved alternative payment methodologies that cover FQHC costs. FQHCs also qualify for PPS-type reimbursement from the Medicare program for the "first dollar" of services rendered to Medicare beneficiaries, with the deductible waived. Again this is in contrast to CBHOs that are not only reimbursed for Medicare recipients at negotiated rates (that often do not cover costs), but provide behavioral health services that until 2010, carried twice the deductible as other health services (Mauch, Pozniak, & Pustell, 2011). This deductible for low income persons who were not dually eligible for Medicaid, tended to fall into the category of free or uncompensated care. Services were provided free of charge unless providers or their patients had access to state-funded patient assistance programs covering co-pays for eligible low income persons. Moreover, FQHCs are protected under safe harbor provisions of the federal anti-kickback statute to waive co-payments associated with care to patients whose incomes are below 200% of the federal poverty level (FPL).

FQHCs enjoy other financing advantages, including access to federal loan guarantees for capital and information technology (IT) improvements, costs of developing and operating managed care and practice management networks or health plans, and access to favorable drug pricing from manufacturers under Section 340B of the PHS Act (42 USCS § 256b). Unlike CBHOs, FQHCs can avoid the cost of malpractice insurance because they have access to coverage for the CHC and its professional staff under the Federal Tort Claims Act (FTCA). Other provisions conferring advantages on FQHCs meeting certain qualifications include access to providers from the National Health Service Corps and to training and technical assistance from HRSA's BPHC. Under terms of the ACA, FQHC funding nearly triples over a 5-year period, from $2.98 billion in FY 2010 to $8.33 billion in FY 2015 (ACA, 2010). The ACA includes an estimated $11 billion for FQHCs (Rosenbaum et al., 2011).

Financing Collaboration at the State Level

Although the 1979 US Surgeon General, Julius B. Richmond, highlighted in his report a national interest in integration, much of the energy has remained at the local and state levels, until recently. State foundations and local nonprofits realized that waiting for private payer and federal support would not respond to communities' needs quickly enough. While examples of all states are not included in this chapter, some of the more prominent programs and pilots (also reviewed in Butler et al., 2008; Collins, Hewson, Munger, & Wade, 2010) are included to provide a sampling of the power of community influence and the critical backing of local and state foundations to support advancements in health care. The local perspective is important because of the following features:

- Most aspects of the American health care system still vary widely by state.
- Medicaid rules allow for considerable cross-state flexibility and state-dependent rules.
- Most commercial insurances offer state-specific plans to accommodate local laws and preferences.
- Health care networks and private practices adapt to meet the requirements of state laws and preferences of local patients.
- Most philanthropic grant support comes from foundations that target specific states or regions.

In this milieu, integrated behavioral health care has also developed in state-specific patterns. In order to allow for both a deep and broad presentation of state-level variation, an in-depth integrated behavioral health care history from one state (Colorado) will be presented, followed by an analysis of common developmental themes across multiple states.

Colorado. Grand Junction, Colorado, is named after the confluence of the mighty Colorado and Gunnison Rivers near the city's artsy downtown. However, in Colorado's integrated behavioral health care circles, Grand Junction is known more for pioneering the merger of medical care and mental health care. The history of integrated behavioral health care in Colorado begins with the leaders of a little-known safety net clinic whose vision went viral across the state.

In 1998, Marillac Clinic (Mauksch et al., 2001) was a small medical center in the heart of rural western Colorado. In an attempt to better meet the high psychosocial needs of their patient population, the Executive Director, Janet Cameron, serendipitously invited a family friend, Larry Mauksch, to come out for a sabbatical. Unbeknownst to her, Larry was a faculty member in the University of Washington's medical school who had published widely on collaborative care. Marillac Clinic proved to be an ideal laboratory for him to train clinicians and test his models. At the end of his nine months in Grand Junction, Larry was awarded a grant from Robert Wood Johnson Foundation, which, along with a local match, provided sufficient funds to hire a collaborative care supervisor, two collaborative counselors, and a case manager. This team was in place by 2000 (full disclosure: Randall Reitz, coauthor of this chapter, was the first hire of the RWJ grant).

From the outset, Marillac's staff and leadership maintained a missionary zeal for sharing the model. They created a countywide collaborative care consortium, presented frequently at the Collaborative Family Healthcare Association conference, and published research on their findings (Mauksch et al., 2007). Representatives from many other Colorado clinics traveled to Grand Junction to see the model and attempt integration in their settings. By 2004, collaborative projects were increasingly common throughout Colorado.

At the same time, a group of five Colorado foundations pooled funds to assess the current status of mental health treatment in Colorado. Their 2003 report identified "lack of integration" as one of the largest barriers to improving mental health services (TriWest Group, 2003). These same foundations funded a five-year statewide mental health integration project beginning in 2005. This initiative heralded collaborative care as a Colorado standard and jump-started many other initiatives. Increasingly, the rise of collaboration was spurned by the rise of The Colorado Health Foundation (TCHF). The foundation was formed in 1995 and has since grown to be one of the largest health foundations in the United States. Most of Colorado's collaborative clinics have benefitted from TCHF support.

In 2008, the Collaborative Family Healthcare Association held their national conference in Denver. This event included a policy summit, which convened leaders from around the state to coordinate a plan to advocate for necessary changes. The conference also highlighted the work of the Salud Clinics and other large Federally Qualified Health Centers in the Denver area.

In 2011, TCHF partnered with the Collaborative Family Healthcare Association to create the Colorado Promoting Integrated Care Sustainability (PICS) project. Through PICS, these organizations conducted an assessment of collaborative care in Colorado and promoted policy changes to financially sustain collaborative services. Fifty-six integrated sites completed an online survey, and 29 sites participated in key informant interviews. While these sites represent only a percentage of the collaborative care sites in Colorado, their data provide a clear picture of collaboration in the state. Findings include the following:

- Collaborative care sites span many health care sectors, including safety net medical settings, specialty behavioral health settings, for-profit primary care offices, government clinics, school-based clinics, addictions treatment centers, and specialty pediatric settings.
- Despite the diversity of settings, the vast majority (about 60–70 %) of integrated behavioral health care clinics are nonprofit primary care offices.
- Collaboration occurs in small towns and large cities: 40 % urban, 26 % rural, 17 % suburban, and 17 % inner city.
- There is great diversity in the size of the programs, with treatment visits per month for the clinics ranging from 100 to 31,000 (mean=3,700). Of these services, the range offered by the integrated behavioral health staff was from 15 to 3,000 (mean=340).
- Fifty percent of the offices have had integrated behavioral health staff for 5 years or longer.
- Most have developed chronic disease treatment models for illnesses such as depression (98 %), diabetes (73 %), obesity (71 %), and tobacco cessation (63 %) (The Colorado Health Foundation, 2012).

The PICS project assessed financial barriers and made recommendations for financial next steps. The researchers discovered that, while there is great diversity in

Colorado's collaborative clinics, there is considerable uniformity in the financial obstacles that still limit the growth of integrated behavioral health care and its movement into the sustainable mainstream of health care services. The PICS assessment of collaboration revealed the following:

- Seventy percent of patients in integrated behavioral health care settings are either uninsured or have a governmental insurance for people of low income.
- Revenue from insurance billing and patient payments cover only 21 % of the costs for collaboration, with the difference being made up through grant funding (47 %) and writing off the expense (32 %).
- Seventy-eight percent of the sites reported receiving grant funds to help with collaborative costs.
- When asked about the largest obstacles to better financial sustainability for collaborative care, three stated obstacles were endorsed by greater than 50 % of the respondents:

  - Sixty-eight percent were concerned about the inability for medical and behavioral health providers to bill for the same patient on the same day (e.g., same-day insurance billing).
  - Fifty-six percent described the need for more grant funds.
  - Fifty-two percent were concerned that behavioral health clinicians could not bill insurance "Health and Behavior Codes".

Key informant interviews provided additional richness to the quantitative data. The PICS project manager conducted recorded interviews with key staff from 29 clinics that participated in the initial survey. Analysis of the interviews corroborates the findings of the survey. Many respondents expressed concern over the insurance practice of "carving-out" mental health coverage as a disincentive to integration. Interviewees expressed a high level of interest in scrapping traditional fee-for-service insurance models in exchange for other models that they hoped would align incentives to support integrated behavioral health care (i.e., patient-centered medical home [PCMH] enhanced payments, pay-for-performance, capitation, and case rate models).

Based on the survey and interview findings (The Colorado Health Foundation, 2012), leaders of the PICS project proposed five recommendations for enhancing the financial sustainability of integrated behavioral health care:

1. Clarify the current billing regulations and train staff in integrated care sites to optimize existing revenue sources to provide cost-efficient, medically necessary care
2. Resolve confusion about same-day billing restrictions and pursue efforts to reduce administrative barriers
3. Examine the viability of paying for Health and Behavior Assessment codes under insurance plans
4. Test and analyze the viability of global funding strategies to financially sustain integrated care services
5. Plan and implement a standardized statewide data collection system to document financial, operational, and clinical outcomes and costs of integrated care services

The PICS group asserted that the first three recommendations were short-term fixes that would provide initial financial support for integrated behavioral health care. However, they would be wholly insufficient without the systemic changes envisioned in recommendations four and five.

Perhaps the most important success story from the Colorado legislature was the 2011 passage HB 1,242. This law reads, "(c)urrent reimbursement policies for providers providing physical and behavioral health care services on the same day are complicated and the policies create a barrier to the seamless integration of these services for the well-being of the patient." The law mandates that the Colorado Medicaid office review state policies that create obstacles to integration and propose solutions to them in 2012. The law specifically identifies the PCMH model and Accountable Care Organizations as possible solutions.

Other state-level successes. The growth of integrated behavioral health care and the development of its financial supports across the United States share many similar themes from Colorado's story. All states with highly developed collaborative models reflect several of these core elements: pioneering clinics and foundations, legislative victories, frequent convening, and a supportive commercial insurance environment. The following sections highlight these themes from multiple states.

Pioneering clinics and foundations. State successes in pioneering behavioral health integration in primary care share two categorical things in common: a variety of funding mechanisms for support and a variety of models for implementation. In just about every case, their voyage into the unknown of integrated behavioral health care was financed by a philanthropic foundation that provided the financial resources to jump-start these initiatives. For Colorado, it was Marillac Clinic, the Robert Wood Johnson (RWJ) Foundation, and later a consortium of foundations. As noted in the Colorado section, many Colorado clinics continue to require foundation support for ongoing collaborative operations. The fact that integrated behavioral health care services are not self-sustaining presents one of the largest financial obstacles to the model.

State Pioneers

Maine. The health care system in Maine has benefitted from a pairing between clinical sites and the Maine Health Access Foundation (MeHAF). Based on early pilots with Penobscot Community Health Care, Maine Medical Center, and TriCounty Mental Health, the foundation invested $10 million in integrated care initiatives starting in 2007. These funds benefited over 43 projects covering 100 different sites (B. Boober, personal communication, March 29, 2012). Another entity, MaineHealth, the largest health care system in Maine, has been a recipient of MeHAF grants for integration (N. Korsen, personal communication, April 24, 2012). MaineHealth is a nonprofit integrated health care delivery system serving 11 counties in rural Maine (www.mainehealth.org). MaineHealth is supporting a service line, which helps practices implement and sustain integrated services. The health system currently funds services such as care management through a mixture of sources, including departmental funding, PCMH-incentive dollars, and direct patient care (J. Schirmer, personal communication, May 11, 2012). To this end, MaineHealth integration staff has worked with a variety of types of practices, including hospital-owned practices, FQHCs, rural health clinics, and private practices. While some practice types have reimbursement rates that are more favorable for integrated services, MaineHealth's financial models suggest that not only can integration be financially sustained in any of these practices and pay for itself with a reasonable expectation for productivity; it can also generate funds to support its service line.

California. Several California clinics have integrated care for decades. The Haight-Ashbury Free Clinics and Walden House function as a combined FQHC. This system has over 200 paid staff and 500 volunteers providing services to over 15 facilities and 19,000 clients, with some facilities specifically designed for integrated care. The vast majority of their revenues come from state and local government general funds, with most of it being public health community behavioral health service funding (Butler et al., 2008; K. Linkins, personal communication, April 24, 2012). California has an organization, Integrated Behavioral Health Project (IBHP)—which has the financial backing from the California Endowment and is a project of the Tides Center. IBHP is a nonprofit organization dedicated to accelerating and elevating integrated behavioral health care throughout California (www.ibhp.org). IBHP's initial goal was to accelerate integrated care by providing training and grants to primary care clinics to broaden their behavioral health services and increase intra-clinic collaboration. To date they have funded three rounds of initiatives. In 2007, phase I supported "vanguard clinics" that had co-location of BH and primary care. Phase II funded a larger group of "learner clinics" to train and guide enable those that were newly embarking on integration. In Phase III, with the availability of federal and Mental Health Services Act grants in California, the public mental health sector rather than the primary care centers have been more active with integration initiatives. Most of their efforts, though, have focused on collaborating with primary care to ensure identification and treatment of chronic physical problems for their populations with serious mental illness. Many local mental health departments have also provided psychiatric consultation for local primary care clinics. Thus, to simplify the movement in this state, the thrust of primary care has been to expand the mental health services they provide internally to their patients and the thrust of mental health has been to secure physical health services to their own clients. Both systems seem to prefer to operate on their own turf (B. Lurie Demming, personal communication, May 24, 2012). The funding criteria and funded projects are listed on their website (www.ibhp.org).

Texas. The Hogg Foundation for Mental Health began their investment in integrated care in 2006 by funding 2.6 million in three-year grants to bring the "collaborative care" model of integrated health care to several clinics in Texas (L. Frost, personal communication, April 16, 2012). In 2009, a staff member from the Hogg Foundation was appointed to the Texas Integration of Health and Behavioral Health Workgroup created by House Bill 2,196 to recommend best practices in policy, training, and service delivery to promote the integration of health and behavioral health services in Texas. Members were appointed by the Texas Health and Human Services' executive commissioner and represent stakeholders, such as consumers, family members, advocacy groups, providers, health care workers, and state agencies. In 2012, the foundation launched a second round of grants to promote integration, focusing on 1-year planning grants and 2-year implementation grants for agencies across Texas. The Hogg Foundation continues to commit funding to the advancement of integration of health and behavioral health and has become a national figure in advocacy and public policy efforts.

New Jersey. Since 2009, The Nicholson Foundation has provided the state of New Jersey with grants and technical assistance to develop and maintain collaborative care sites (The Nicholson Foundation, 2011). The most well known among them is their support of the Camden Coalition of Health care Providers. This organization leads the "hotspotting" health care model of Jeffrey Brenner, M.D., which has been shown to reduce health care costs and improve health outcomes for very high utilizers of health care services. Resulting Nicholson-supported initiatives include seven Family Success Centers (FSCs) located in disadvantaged areas of Newark and surrounding urban communities in Essex and Union Counties. These neighborhood-based one-stop resources are funded to promote family stability and child well-being. Following the successful implementation of the Foundation's centers, the State funded a statewide network of 37 additional FSCs. All combined, there are 44 FSCs currently operating in New Jersey.

Productive Convening. While some states blazed trails in integration using foundation support, or were inspired by pioneering nonprofit clinics and health care systems, other states pulled resources and established links across state agencies, foundations, clinics, and educational institution partners to help promote, advance, and disseminate information about integration.

An entity called The Collaborative Family Healthcare Association (www.CFHA.net) has played a key role in state-by-state convening. Each year, the Collaborative Family Healthcare Association hosts its annual conference and a policy summit in a state that has been identified as being in a developmental "sweet spot" for advancing collaborative care. That is, the integrated behavioral health care environment is primed to advance greatly by hosting a major training and policy event. This annual convening helps to advance state-level collaborative efforts in many ways:

- The planning process brings together a statewide committee who develop strategic goals for advancing collaboration.
- The policy summits highlight existing successes and develop a roadmap for the next steps in sustaining collaboration.
- A large percentage of the conference attendees are from the host state and the training sessions are their first exposure to formal integrated behavioral health care instruction, leaving a legacy of workforce development.

Many of the states/regions that currently have advanced collaborative care models benefitted from hosting a recent CFHA conference and summit, including

Minnesota (2004), Washington (2005), New England (2006), North Carolina (2007), Colorado (2008), California (2009), Kentucky (2010), Pennsylvania (2011), and Texas (2012). A few of these states are featured below. See Chap. 4 in this book for more details on policy and its influence on the past, present, and future of health care.

Minnesota. In Minnesota, the Institute for Clinical Systems Improvement (ICSI) is a nonprofit, health care quality improvement organization that helps its 55 medical groups and hospital members practice evidence-based medicine, and work toward achieving the Triple Aim of improving population health, the quality of the patient experience, and the affordability of care (G. Oftedahl, personal communication, April 4, 2012). ICSI members represent about 85 % of Minnesota's physicians, and the organization receives funding support from five major Minnesota and Wisconsin health plans.

Through a collaboration of member groups, health plans, employers, patients and the Minnesota Department of Human Services, ICSI, developed the DIAMOND (Depression Improvement Across Minnesota—Offering a New Direction; www. ISCI.org) program. Built upon the foundation of Wagner's Chronic Care model (Wagner, Austin, & Von Korff, 1996) and incorporating the main components of the University of Washington IMPACT study (Unutzer, Katon, Callahan et al., 2002), the program is unique in that it changes both how care is delivered and paid for in primary care. Participating health plans pay for the additional bundle of services provided through the DIAMOND program, most notably for a care manager and limited consulting time of a psychiatrist. They pay certified DIAMOND clinics a monthly care management fee using a single service code and fund a specific proto-col, not a general behavioral health primary care model. To avoid antitrust concerns, contracts between each medical group and health plan were negotiated individually. Finally, a pay for performance program funded through organizations such as the Buyers Health Care Action Group (BHCAG) and their Bridges to Excellence (BTE) provides financial rewards to providers who achieve optimal outcomes for patients with depression (Buyers Health Care Action Group, 2012).

Maine. The Maine Health Access Foundation conducted a lengthy stakeholder engagement process beginning in 2006. This effort guided their investment in inte-grated behavioral health care. It culminated in the 2011 creation of the Integrated Care Training Academy. Through this effort, early adopters of integrated care men-tor new start-up programs.

North Carolina. North Carolina provides an excellent example of how convening the right parties can dramatically boost the adoption and financial support for col-laboration. In 2005, the Assistant Secretary of Health and Human Services, with support from the Director of the North Carolina Office of Rural Health, enacted an idea for a statewide initiative on integrated care. The project was originally named "ICARE" and was later renamed "The North Carolina Center of Excellence in Integrated Care (COE)." The COE serves as a "think tank" for a wide array of stake-holders for the advancement of integrated care in the state (R. Dickins, personal communication, April 4, 2012). They have had several funding partners over the years supporting development, implementation, evaluation, and dissemination of integration projects across the state of North Carolina. Funding sources have included private and state entities such as: (a) The Duke Endowment, (b) Kate B. Reynolds Charitable Trust, (c) AstraZeneca, (d) North Carolina Area Health Education Centers, (e) North Carolina Department of Health and Human Services, and (f) North Carolina Foundation for Advanced Health Programs (www.icare.org). These funding sources along with other progressive statewide offices such as the Community Care of NC (CCNC) Networks and Governor's Institute on Substance Abuse have helped to clear the landscape for integration and pilot projects to advance integration. For example, there have been a variety of projects funded from SBIRT (Screening, Brief Intervention, and Referral to Treatment; see Chap. 13 for more detail) to co-location models to help clinics offset start-up costs.

Pennsylvania. In Philadelphia, Pennsylvania, a nonprofit public health organization has proven to be the model's best ally. The Health Federation of Philadelphia (HFP) was established in 1983 to coordinate and advance the services of Philadelphia area FQHC and FQHC "look alike" centers (N. Levkovich, personal communication, April 2, 2012). An important example of HFP's many achievements has been the development and expansion of primary care behavioral health integration in Philadelphia's health centers. Their numbers have grown from the initial seven primary care sites to 18, with at least five more likely by the end of 2012.

The HFP has successfully promoted local payment and policy reform to align with the practice of integrated health care. By working collaboratively with the local Medicaid payer, advocating with the State Medicaid agency, and raising the visibility of the model with private foundations, HFP has helped to increase the feasibility and sustainability of the clinical practice. The local behavioral health Medicaid plan, called Community Behavioral Health (CBH), has simultaneously worked to define billing and credentialing standards to reflect the integrated FQHC model and has established a Request for Qualifications (RFQ) process requiring any FQHC in Philadelphia County that wants to contract for services to do so using the integrated model, based on the principles of Behavioral Health Consultation, established by HFP. While further payment reform is needed to reach beyond fee-for-service models, HFP has been able to secure local commitment to primary care behavioral health integration. Using a billing code for "FQHC visit," CBH reimburses interventions provided by the behavioral health specialist, who is part of the FQHC primary care team, and the State Medicaid Office has approved same-day billing for primary and behavioral health visits in the context of this integrated model.

Currently, BHC visits are covered when provided to Medicaid beneficiaries who have a mental health diagnosis. However, many services are not currently reimbursable, including the following:

- Universal screening, preventive services, and psychoeducation
- Interventions aimed at modifying health behaviors for chronic care self-management and adherence
- Telephone follow-up with patients who initiate psych meds or are having a particularly hard time

- Psychiatry consultation (which is supported by grant funds)
- Psychiatrist review of records and curbside team consultation

Supportive Insurance Environment. As demonstrated by the data from Colorado, fee-for-service billing has not been effective as a mechanism for covering the costs of providing collaborative care services. Currently, few, if any Colorado insurances reimburse for Health and Behavioral services codes or integrated care services offered on the same day as a medical service. Additionally, clinics report little success in navigating the insurance system to obtain reimbursement for the services that are allowed. The current insurance billing protocols for mental health services were not envisioned for systems that integrate with medical services. Fortunately, there are a number of examples from other states that could prove effective at sustaining collaborative models if adopted more widely.

Tennessee. Perhaps the collaborative organization that is most frequently cited as creating and benefiting from a favorable insurance environment is Cherokee Health Systems (CHS). Discussed more in depth in other chapters, Cherokee led the way by developing a fully functioning FQHC and merging it with its community mental health operation. As a result, they have been able to secure a wider range of payment streams to support their integrated care model. Cherokee has been successful in negotiating favorable contracts, which include payment for consultation between providers and same-day billing for behavioral health and primary care services.

Cherokee has been able to mitigate limitations of the carve-out system by merging the medical Medicaid benefits of an FQHC with the behavioral health Medicaid benefits of a CMHC. As frequently happens, changes in Medicaid policy have begun to be adopted by commercial insurances in Tennessee. Blue Cross (TNCARE) and AmeriChoice negotiated "contract rates" or global rates that better support Cherokee's integration design (Takach, Purington, & Osius, 2010). CHS also partnered with the Tennessee Primary Care Association, the trade association for the FQHCs, to affect some modifications in State policies favorable for integrated care programming. They have also been successful in securing federal Health Resources and Services Administration (HRSA) funding, including the Graduate Psychology Education grant for training psychology interns and fellows in primary care psychology.

Cherokee's approach is noteworthy, not only for its clinical efficiency, but also because they found ways to remove many of the financial barriers for Medicaid and other insurances. In contrast to the structured clinical chronic care pathway approaches, Cherokee opted for supporting local flexibility and provider-directed interventions for whatever was needed for patient-centered care. The leader-champions in Tennessee have tried several different avenues for negotiating funding streams, including major insurance companies. These negotiations have been challenging and not as productive due to frequent changes in personnel, mergers with private and public organizations, and competing focus areas and vision in primary care contexts. Tennessee's success has come from throwing the funding net wide and seeing which organizations and provider groups are willing players.

Virginia. In Virginia, innovative systems like Sentara Health care in Norfolk, a not-for-profit health care system and Anthem Blue Cross Blue Shield, a for-profit system are piloting models of health care that are sensitive to the local community health care needs and result in financial savings from better management of disease (B. McFeature & C. Hudgins, personal communication, April 2, 2010). Sentra understood they would need to spend money to study how to make money while generating better health outcomes. They are working with Community Services Board in Norfolk who was awarded one of the 64 national Primary Care Behavioral Health Integration (PCBHI) grants for integrated care service development. They are gathering data for showing sustainability to Sentra, and, hopefully, reflecting better health outcomes for co-occurring disorders. Regarding Anthem and BCBS plans in Southwest Virginia, there is a strong interest in reviewing proposed PCBHI programs showing better health outcomes. Another note of importance is that Virginia is one of the states that successfully activated the evaluation and management (E&M) codes and behavioral health and substance abuse codes for same-day services.

Minnesota. Part of the reason that the Minnesota insurance system has been supportive of ICSI and the DIAMOND project is that, by law, all health insurance companies are nonprofit. These insurance companies were key in supporting the DIAMOND project and developing statewide treatment protocols. In 2009, the Minnesota Department of Health issued a report about the benefits of nonprofit health plans, including the following:

- Focusing on collaborative health care models
- Increasing support of public health
- Encouraging philanthropic endeavors (Minnesota Department of Health, 2009)

Their supportive nonprofit insurance environment has allowed for dissemination and sustainability to happen faster than what is observed in other states and regions.

Washington and Northern Idaho. Similarly, Washington state and Northern Idaho have benefited from the nonprofit health care system, Group Health Cooperative (GHC). This combined medical insurance, health care provider with approximately 568,000 enrollees, has pioneered efforts in integrating care.

GHC is an example of a staff model HMO. That is, the same company provides the insurance coverage and the health care services. The HMO owns and staffs the health care clinics. Because this approach aligns the insurance and health bottom lines, it has proven to be fertile ground for mainstream integrated behavioral health care services. For example, GHC was a key partner in the IMPACT research. That being said, the integrated model of most staff model HMOs is different than the integrated behavioral models typically identified with collaborative care. The models tend to focus more on screening, case management, and psychiatric consultation, and less on colocated psychotherapy.

Utah and Southern Idaho. Intermountain Health care (IHC) is a nonprofit integrated health care system servicing Utah and Southern Idaho and it provides over

50 % of Utah's health care. They have been providing mental health integration in primary care for over 10 years. Their care team includes PCPs, their staff, MH professionals, care management, and the patient and his or her family. The model is a fully integrated delivery system approach that extends beyond co-location to address mental health conditions in the context of other chronic illnesses (e.g., diabetes). Unlike some integration models, they also focus heavily on the patient's family context to enhance protective factors that affect quality outcomes over time. For example, positive outcomes for patients with depression included lower ED visits, better coordination of care for mental health issues, and reduced overall costs for payers. IHC is a cost-neutral system for integration, and without subsidies they have demonstrated outcomes in improved patient satisfaction, lower costs, and better quality outcomes, saving money from reductions in ER visits, psychiatric inpatient admissions, and length of stay for inpatient admissions related to other medical conditions (Reiss-Brennan, Briot, Savitz, Cannon, & Staheli, 2010).

California. California's largest nonprofit health plan, Northern California Kaiser Permanente (Kaiser), is a staff HMO that serves approximately 3.2 million Californians across 21 medical centers and 160 medical offices (K. Linkins, personal communication, April 14, 2012). Since 1996, it has focused on integrated care as part of a region-wide redesign of primary care. As one of the sites for the IMPACT study, they found that underdiagnosing and coding issues for mental health issues resulted in missed opportunities to maximize revenue from Medicare reimbursement. Funding for integration came from streamlining the way the system identified and treated behavioral and mental health issues in the medical setting. While nonprofit health plans like Northern California Kaiser Permanente may be struggling with some aspects of sustainable integration, they have a history of investment and are an example of pioneers in integration.

Legislative and Policy Movement and Victories

Over the years, many of the foundations that have provided grant support for integrated behavioral health care projects have expanded their focus to promoting policy change to create mechanisms for sustaining collaborative care across all levels of the health care system. There is considerable variation across states and health plans with respect to how reimbursement for behavioral services in primary care takes place. In 2006, SAMSHA, HRSA, and CMS convened an expert panel to discuss barriers and identify solutions for the reimbursement of mental health services in primary care settings (Kautz, Mauch, & Smith, 2008). They identified seven priority barriers:

- State Medicaid limitations on payments for same-day billing for a physical health and a mental health service/visit
- Lack of reimbursement for integrated behavioral health care and case management related to mental health services

- Absence of reimbursement for services provided by nonphysicians, alternative practitioners, and contract practitioners and providers
- Medicaid disallowance of reimbursement when primary care practitioners submit bills listing only a mental health diagnosis and corresponding treatment
- Level of reimbursement rates in rural and urban settings
- Difficulties in getting reimbursement for mental health services in school-based health center settings
- Lack of reimbursement incentives for screening and providing preventive mental health services in primary care settings (pp. 2–3)

Billing restrictions are a key barrier to furthering integrated care. As of 2010, there were 30 states that covered same-day billing for behavioral health visits on the same day as a medical visit (National Association of Community Health Centers & Substance Abuse and Mental Health Services Administration [NACHC & SAMHSA], 2010). A critical component of The Affordable Care Act signed in 2010, is reform of reimbursement to support behavioral interventions for chronic health conditions. Restrictions on same day services and specific codes needed for integrated care are not being recognized or reimbursed in many states (e.g., H&B codes). When reimbursement is permitted, and in some states it is, extensive protocols to getting reimbursed (e.g., paperwork, communicating with payers) and low reimbursement rates are disincentives. In spite of this, some states have conquered various barriers and a few are featured below for what they have done in spite of resistance and confusion at the policy and payer levels. (Note: The SAMHSA-HRSA Center for Integrated Health Solutions has a website (http://www.integration.samhsa.gov/financing/billing-tools) that is being populated with information. It will eventually provide up-to-date billing and financial worksheets for providers in each state to help primary and behavioral health care organizations successfully implement bidirectional integrated health care.)

Texas. Efforts in Texas have resulted in movement toward legislative action and hopefully policy change. In 2009, staff members from the Hogg Foundation were appointed to Texas Integration of Health and Behavioral Health Workgroup created by House Bill 2,196 recommend best practices in policy, training, and service delivery to promote the integration of health and behavioral health services in Texas. Members were appointed by the Texas Health and Human Services' executive commissioner and represent stakeholders such as consumers, family members, advocacy groups, providers, health care workers, and state agencies. The Hogg Foundation hosted meetings and provided administrative support to the workgroup. The workgroup published its report on Integration of Health and Behavioral Health Workgroup before the 82nd Legislature convened in 2011.

California. Californians helped to remedy their financial issues with mental health services when in November 2004 their state legislature passed Proposition 63 (now known as the Mental Health Services Act (CalMHSA)). This was the first opportunity in many years for the California Department of Mental Health (DMH) to increase funding, personnel, and other resources to support county mental health programs.

They established a state personal income tax surcharge of 1 % on an estimated 25,000–30,000 taxpayers with annual taxable incomes of more than $1 million. This money has helped Californians to develop innovative programs in integration otherwise not affordable or reimbursable by the existing system. One example is the California Endowment's Integrated Behavioral Health Project (IBHP), a 4-year, $3.35 million partnership with the Tides Center (an independent 501(c)(3) non-profit grant making foundation). The project's focus was to help reduce the stigma of seeing a behavioral health provider by integrating them into primary care set-tings targeting low-income and minority health care consumers with limited access. The work of IBHP is now supported by a 3-year, $3 million grant from the CalMHSA.

North Carolina. Several legislative advancements have helped highlight North Carolina as a progressive state for behavioral integration. Since the 1980s, the NC Division of Medical Assistance (DMA) has been developing policy to support the patient-centered medical home through multiple care initiatives (R. Dickens, per-sonal communication, April 24, 2012). In 1991, the Centers for Medicare and Medicaid Services (CMS) approved a 1915(b) waiver allowing mandatory enroll-ment of select Medicaid eligibility groups into "Primary Care Case Management." This was accomplished through a program called Carolina Access (renamed Community Care of North Carolina [CCNC] during an expansion in 1998). Their goal was open access to primary care, preventive services, and disease management for the entire NC Medicaid population. However, early Medicaid policy did not address the significant mental health treatment needed and provided at the primary care provider level.

According to Dickens (personal communication, April 24, 2012), in 2009, DMA updated the CCNC's contracts to include additional capitation funding for initia-tives aimed at treatment and management of behavioral health conditions at the PCP and network levels. Then in the early 2000s, DMA contracted with Local Management Entities (LMEs) to provide care management to high-cost, high-risk recipients with behavioral health needs and behavioral health referrals to any Medicaid enrollee. North Carolina began implementation of the 1915(b) Medicaid waiver with a pilot project in 2005 and in 2009, expanded the waiver statewide with the intent to establish additional LMEs as DMA vendors by 2013, providing over-sight to the specialty behavioral health care system. In 2009, they also began reim-bursing colocated mental health therapists for assessments, smoking cessation counseling, and substance abuse screening/SBIRT. In 2011, DMA submitted a State Plan Amendment to CMS to identify CCNC as the "Health Home" for Medicaid recipients with chronic conditions such as seriously and persistent mental illness.

Maine. In Maine, the Maine Health Access Foundation convened an integrated care policy committee that includes the departments of Health and Human Services (including Medicaid, Adult Mental Health, and Substance Abuse) and Labor, the Maine Health Access Foundation, employers, payers, providers, and other health care stakeholders and policymakers (B. Boober, personal communi-cation, March 29, 2012).

In Maine, a variety of strategies are used to pay for integrated services (B. Boober, personal communication, May 15, 2012). As is the case currently for most health care costs, fee for service is the most prominent. However, bundled per-member-per-month payments in incentive programs have also assisted with nonreimburseable costs, such as care/case management provided by bachelor-level personnel. Most of what is tracked is fee for service. It is tracked through the all-claims database and through FQHC records for the uninsured. Successes of this group have included the following:

- Opening of Health and Behavior Medicaid codes by Anthem, Maine's largest private sector payer. This pilot is open to all primary care practices, and committee members have assisted with providing additional promotion and clarification of the use of those codes. Anthem is analyzing the impact on patient outcomes and cost.
- The creation of an integrated care billing guide that rolled out statewide with training on its usage.
- Promotion of the inclusion of integrated care in other major health care and payment reform initiatives such as the Patient-Centered Medical Homes pilots, Health Homes, and DHHS Values-based Contracting.

National Foundations and Payers

Several national foundations and payers have stepped up to support innovations in health care service delivery. Foundations wanted a way to invest in their communities and payers wanted to save money; hence, they shared a common goal: promotion of health.

Pilot projects born out of these investments have led the way for future funding in integration. Most of the projects were crafted around targeted populations (e.g., minority groups, children) with specific conditions (e.g., depression, substance abuse). Projects have also supported provision of care management services to some of the more costly and complex chronic illness conditions.

MacArthur Foundation. The MacArthur Foundation "is one of the nation's largest independent foundations. Through the support it provides, the MacArthur Foundation fosters the development of knowledge, nurtures individual creativity, strengthens institutions, helps improve public policy, and provides information to the public, primarily through support for public interest media" (MacArthur Foundation, 2012). They have funded trials and large dissemination pilots and projects like RESPECT-D (see www.depression-primarycare.org).

Robert Wood Johnson Foundation. Another pioneering Foundation committed to integration is Robert Wood Johnson (see www.rwjf.org). Over the years, they have provided grants to health organizations to improve care for diseases such as diabetes, congestive heart failure, and depression, as well as funded projects on integration. Their mission is "to improve the health and health care of all Americans" and they have supported numerous pilot projects across the United States that improve standards of care in medicine. They are particularly focused on improving the health of vulnerable populations and support the adoption of better laws and policies that can transform America's health with a "patients first" focus. In 2010 alone, they funded $300 million in grants.

AETNA. A for-profit insurance company with a national scope, AETNA, has sought out ways to incentivize providers to initiate more mental health care screenings in primary care settings. AETNA offers a program available only to physicians called, "Depression in Primary Care Program" (AETNA Inc., 2012). While this is not a program that funds integration of personnel, they do provide online training and teach providers how to use the PHQ-9 and get reimbursed by AETNA for it. Even though this program is limited to physicians, it is a step toward recognizing that mental health issues influence and drive up costs, which can later compromise health outcomes.

HUMANA-LifeSynch. Another for-profit insurer is doing something slightly different. LifeSynch, "a wholly owned Humana subsidiary, serves more than 10 million members and offers extensive resources, including behavioral health care, employee assistance program (EAP)/work-life services, behavioral pharmacy services, health coaches and Web-based wellness tools" (LifeSynch, 2011). Integration occurs at the case manager level. They provide telephonic coaching and support (including facilitating conversations to deal with their emotional issues and to assure they are receiving the right kind of care) to Humana subscribers identified by various screening methods. Primary care physicians are notified of what is occurring but are not involved actively. The company is studying return on investment longitudinally, but its "2010 Quality Improvement End of Year Program Evaluation" report indicated it saw benefits just after one year. For example, they reported their members exceeded the national average in reported lower hospital readmissions, fewer customer complaints related to patient safety, a positive response to their wellness program (e.g., smoking cessation, weight loss), an increase in engagement between patients and case managers, and a general positive attitude about life.

Federal Agencies and Mechanisms

While funding for integration has been largely at the local, state, and not-for-profit national foundation levels, there has been a gradual movement toward federal involvement in funding integrated care projects and programs. Examples of this growth and progress are provided below. (Note: Many of the projects and programs funded using federal mechanism have had to combine their funding with other sources to effectively implement and sustain integration.)

The Veterans Administration (VA). The VA was the first governmental entity to support integration with a $23 million dollar investment (A. Pomerantz, personal communication, April 2, 2012). In 2007, the VA funded 94 facilities (out of 134 across the United States) to develop integrated care programs. These pilot programs continued with funding of another $32 million during FY 2008. Program growth occurred at additional facilities through VISN (VISN=regional Veteran integrated service networks) and local initiatives. Since then, some minor funding has occurred but most other VA facilities developed programs without special funding. Since the end of the special funding, the programs have continued to grow and have now been incorporated into the VA Patient-Centered Medical Home model of primary care.

Department of Defense. Likewise, in 2011 the Department of Defense (DoD) approved the spending of $251 million from FY2012–FY2016 to hire and train 429 full-time patient-centered medical home (PCMH) behavioral health personnel (C. Hunter, personal communication, April 2, 2012). The funds for these individuals become part of the core personnel budget; cost adjusted for inflation each year and will continue indefinitely past FY 2016. (See Chap. 9 for more information on DoD funding for integration and its financial sustainability model).

Health Resources and Services Administration (HRSA). HRSA has issued a large number of grants for workforce development and expansion of integration efforts designed to improve and expand health care services for underserved people. They have partnered with other federal entities such as SAMSHA to help promote large-scale integration efforts. Together in 2009, HRSA and SAMSHA, formed the Primary and Behavioral Health Care Integration (PBHCI) program. It was designed to support communities in their coordination and integration of primary care services into publicly funded, community-based behavioral health settings. The goal was to improve the physical health status of people with mental illnesses and addictions. Since September 2009, SAMHSA has awarded more than $26.2 million in Primary and Behavioral Health Care Integration grants to 64 organizations nationwide (http://www.integration.samhsa.gov/about-us/pbhci). SAMSHA and HRSA have also joined together to fund the Center for Integrated Health Solutions (CIHS). CIHS is run by the National Council for Community Behavioral Health care under a cooperative agreement from the US Department of Health and Human Services. It provides training and technical assistance to organizations that have received SAMHSA grants under its Primary and Behavioral Health Care Integration (PBHCI) program (see http://www.integration.samhsa.gov/).

Agency for Healthcare Research and Quality (AHRQ). AHRQ's mission is to establish a broad base of scientific research to promote improvements in clinical and health system practices (http://www.ahrq.gov/). While most programs fund implementation and design efforts, AHRQ invests in research, integration workforce competencies, and dissemination projects around payment reform and best practice for behavioral health integration. Examples of ARHQ-sponsored projects include: (a) Collaborative National Network Examining Comparative Effectiveness Trials (CoNNECT), whose aim is to use comparative effectiveness research to answer the myriad of questions that have been raised around mental health in primary care, (b) The Academy for Integrating Behavioral Health and Primary Care, designed to function as both a coordinating center and a national resource for people committed to delivering comprehensive, integrated health care (http://integrationacademy.ahrq.gov/), and (c) Technical Assistance for Effective Quality Improvement and

Evaluation in Behavioral Health-Primary Care Integration, with the purpose of developing materials and providing technical assistance that focuses on measures and measurement in QI and evaluation in mental health-primary care integration. These examples demonstrate AHRQ's strong investment in integration at the national level, as well as the independent practice levels.

National Institutes of Mental Health (NIMH). The NIMH has funded a few high profile and multimillion dollar research effectiveness studies on behavioral interventions in primary care (e.g., IMPACT, DIAMOND, and STAR-D). In 2011, NIMH released a RO1 for proposals seeking Research Project Grant applications for "Behavioral Interventions to Address Multiple Chronic Health Conditions in Primary Care" with the goal being to modify health behaviors and improve health outcomes in patients with comorbid chronic diseases and health conditions.

Center for Medicare and Medicaid Services (CMS). Momentum was growing rapidly at the Federal level in 2011 for funding integration: bigger projects, quicker turnaround times to demonstrate financial and clinical outcomes, and more funding. In fact, in 2011 CMS announced their "The Health Care Innovation Challenge" (see http://www.innovations.cms.gov/initiatives/Innovation-Challenge/index.html). Their intent was to award $1 billion to innovative projects across the country that test creative ways to deliver high-quality medical care and save money. Launched by the Department of Health and Human Services and funded by the Affordable Care Act, the Health Care Innovation Challenge's intent was to give preference to projects that rapidly hire, train, and deploy health care workers. Grants, were expected to range from $1 million to $30 million over 3 years and were awarded to applicants with the most compelling new ideas to deliver better health, improved care, and lower costs to people enrolled in Medicare, Medicaid, and the Children's Health Insurance Program, particularly those with the greatest health care needs and costs.

Patient-Centered Outcomes Research Institute (PCORI). By law, PCORI, is an independent, nonprofit organization that was established by Congress through the 2010 Patient Protection and Affordable Care Act (PPACA). It was created to conduct research to provide information about the best available evidence to help patients and their health care providers make more informed decisions. PCORI spearheaded a Pilot Projects Grant Program in 2011 to assist with ongoing development and enhancement of national research priorities for patient-centered outcomes research. Through its call for proposals, it intended to commit up to $13 million under this program during the first year in support of approximately 40 awards (http://www.pcori.org).

Summary

Does integrated behavioral health care meet the financial challenge of Peek's (2008) "Three-World View of Healthcare"? Can it be objectively asserted that integrated behavioral health care makes "reasonable use of resources"? If we define this as having revenues from the services themselves covering the expenses of providing the services, then the most accurate response to that question is "No." Compared to other health care sectors, integrated behavioral health care services require an inordinate amount of faith from foundations to provide grant support and faith from health care systems to write-off expenses. Fortunately, we are still incubating a variety of approaches to support best practices in integrated behavioral health care. It is not yet clear, however, which of these approaches may survive these embryonic stages.

Integrated behavioral health care has been more commonly implemented in safety net settings, but even in this cohort, the level of collaboration varies widely. In these settings, services are widely written off or sustained by grant funds. Integrated behavioral health care has made little penetration in the for-profit settings that are the mainstream of American health care. The primary obstacle to increased adoption is the lack of a viable, sustainable funding source to pay for the services.

In order for collaborative care to make reasonable use of resources (and move into the mainstream of health care), a system-wide and sustainable source of revenue will need to be adopted. Currently, there are a myriad of pioneering pilot approaches being implemented, which may shape a more favorable environment for financially sustaining integrated behavioral health care. As described in this chapter, these opportunities include growth in the PCMH and ACO models and innovations in Medicaid and Medicare that might spread throughout the system. If you are living in a state where you want to promote integration of behavioral health into primary care, your resources and opportunities for funding it are much better now than even 5 years ago.

In Chap. 2 of this book, Peek describes a developmental process by which health care services evolve from pilots to projects to mainstream services. From a financial perspective many integrated behavioral health care initiatives are still pilots, some are sustained programs, but few are mainstream service lines. Starting local primary care and mental health organizations and seeking foundational support has been the quintessential mechanism for getting started. Projects with momentum and strong collaborative partners can go after the bigger pots (e.g., PCORI, CMS, NIMH). Regardless, better data collection to make the argument for integration with payers is necessary. While the federal government does manage the Medicaid and Medicare purse strings, the payers of individual health plans are the ones who need the hard sell. Noting the few for-profit insurers referenced in this chapter, they too are starting to take notice that this nation has taken an unhealthy turn and integration is producing clinical, operational, and financial outcomes that indicate a way out.

References

AETNA Inc. (2012) *Depression in primary care program*. Retrieved April 3, 2012, from http://www.aetna.com/healthcare-professionals/documents-forms/depression- program.pdf

Affordable Care Act (ACA). (2010). *About the law*. Retreived from http://www.whitehouse.gov/healthreform/healthcare-overview.

Butler, M., Kane, R. L., McAlpine, D., Kathol, R. G., Fu, S. S., Hagedorn, H., & Wilt, T. J. (2008). *Integration of mental health/substance abuse and primary care* (AHRQ Publication No. 09-E003). Rockville, MD: Agency for Healthcare Research and Quality.

Buyers Health Care Action Group. (2012). *Clinic quality: Minnesota bridges to excellence.* Retrieved April 16, 2012, from http://bhcag.com/initiatives/clinic-quality/.

Collaborative Family Healthcare Association. (2012). *History of the Collaborative Family Healthcare Association.* Retrieved April 2, 2012, from http://www.cfha.net/?page=History.

Collins, C., Hewson, D. L., Munger, R., & Wade, T. (2010). *Evolving models of behavioral health integration in primary care.* New York: Milbank Memorial Fund.

Kautz, C., Mauch, D., & Smith, S. A. (2008). *Reimbursement of mental health services in primary care settings* ((HHS Pub. No. SMA-08-4324)). Rockville, MD: Center for Mental Health Services, Substance Abuse and Mental Health Services Administration.

Kennedy, J. F. (1963). *Special message to the Congress on Mental Illness and Mental Retardation,* Washington, DC. Retrieved April 4, 2012, from http://www.presidency.ucsb.edu/ws/?pid=9546#axzz1qolIcUcC.

LifeSynch. (2011). *LifeSynch mission: Changing health behaviors, improving lives.* Retrieved April 2, 2012, from http://www.lifesynch.com/about/company_information/.

MacArthur Foundation. (2012). *About us.* Retrieved April 2, 2012, from http://www.macfound.org/about/.

Mauch, D., Pozniak, A., & Pustell, M. (2011). State and Federal Standards for Mental Health Coverage. HHS Publication No. (SMA) Pending. Rockville, MD: Center for Mental Health Services, Substance Abuse and Mental Health Services Administration.

Mauksch, L. B., Reitz, R. S., Tucker, S., Hurd, S., Russo, J., & Katon, W. (2007). Improving quality of care for mental illness in an uninsured, low-income primary care population. *General Hospital Psychiatry, 29,* 302–309.

Mauksch, L. B., Tucker, S. M., Katon, W. J., Russo, J., Cameron, J., Walker, E., et al. (2001). Mental illness, functional impairment, and patient preferences for collaborative care in an uninsured, primary care population. *Journal of Family Practice, 50*(1), 41–47.

Minnesota Department of Health. (2009). *Community benefit provided by non profit health plans.* Retrieved April 27, 2012, from http://www.health.state.mn.us/divs/hpsc/hep/publications/legislative/hlthplancommbenefit.pdf.

National Association of Community Health Centers & Substance Abuse and Mental Health Services Administration. (2010). *Medicaid/medicare.* Retrieved April 24, 2012, from http://www.integration.samhsa.gov/financing/medicaid-medicare.

Peek, C.J. (2008). Planning care in the clinical, operational, and financial worlds. In R. Kessler and D. Stafford (Eds.), *Collaborative Medicine Case Studies: Evidence in Practice* (pp. 25–38). NY, NY: Springer.

Reiss-Brennan, B., Briot, P. C., Savitz, L. A., Cannon, W., & Staheli, R. (2010). Cost and quality impact of intermountain's mental health integration program. *Journal of Healthcare Management, 55*(2), 97–114.

Rosenbaum, S., Zakheim, M. H., Leifer, J., Golde, M.D., Schulte, J.M., & Margulies, R. (2011). Assessing and addressing legal barriers to the clinical integration of community health centers and other community providers. The Commonwealth Fund. Retrieved http://www.commonwealthfund.org/Publications/Fund- Reports/2011/Jul/Clinical-Integration.aspx.

Takach, M., Purington, K., & Osius, E. (2010). *A tale of two systems: A look at state efforts to integrate primary care and behavioral health in safety net settings.* Washington, DC: National Academy for State Health Policy.

The Colorado Health Foundation. (2012). *The Colorado blueprint for promoting integrated care sustainability.* Retrieved April 27, 2012, from http://www.coloradohealth.org/studies.aspx.

The Nicholson Foundation. (2011). *Improving healthcare for vulnerable populations: Executive summary.* Retrieved April 2, 2012, from http://www.thenicholsonfoundation-newjersey.org/programs/sub/.

TriWest Group. (2003). *The status of mental health care in Colorado.* Denver, CO: Mental Health Funders Collaborative.

Unützer, J., Katon, W., Callahan, C. M., Williams, J. W., Jr., Hunkeler, E., Harpole, L., et al. (2002). Collaborative-care management of late-life depression in the primary care setting: A randomized controlled trial. *The Journal of the American Medical Association, 288,* 2836–2845.

Wagner, E. H., Austin, B. T., & Von Korff, M. (1996). Organizing care for patients with chronic illness. *The Milbank Quarterly, 74,* 511–543.

Chapter 9
Department of Defense Integrated Behavioral Health in the Patient-Centered Medical Home

Christopher L. Hunter

Abstract The Department of Defense (DoD) is integrating 470 full-time behavioral health personnel in every military treatment facility patient-centered medical home with 1,500 or more enrollees. This chapter provides an overview of the DoD military health system's integrated behavioral health efforts. Areas including staffing and service delivery model, population served, finance, policy, and program evaluation are discussed. DoD efforts have broad applicability to other systems and can serve as a guide to developing and implementing integrated behavioral health care services in primary care.

Introduction

Integrating behavioral health services into primary care is not a new concept. Since the 1990s, both nonfederal (e.g., Katon et al., 1996) and federal health systems have been integrating behavioral health personnel into primary care. Over the last 15 years, the United States Air Force, Army, and Navy have developed, implemented, and evaluated different integrated behavioral health care service models (Hunter, Goodie, & Dobmeyer, 2012). These experiences have informed the recent development and implementation of a coherent set of Department of Defense (DoD) service

Disclaimer: The views expressed herein are those of the author and do not necessarily represent the official policy or position of the Department of Defense (DoD), the Military Health System, TRICARE Management Activity, the United States Department of Health and Human Services, or the United States Government.

C.L. Hunter, Ph.D., ABPP (✉)
DoD Program Manager for Behavioral Health in Primary Care,
Office of the Chief Medical Officer, TRICARE Management Activity,
Defense Health Headquarters, Falls Church, VA, USA
e-mail: Christopher.hunter@tma.osd.mil

M.R. Talen and A. Burke Valeras (eds.), *Integrated Behavioral Health in Primary Care: Evaluating the Evidence, Identifying the Essentials*, DOI 10.1007/978-1-4614-6889-9_9,
© Springer Science+Business Media New York 2013

delivery practices and standards that apply uniformly to all three military medical Services. This chapter details these efforts that, although specific to the military health care system, also have broad applicability and can serve as a guide to other health care systems as they develop and implement integrated behavioral health care services in primary care.

Sometimes there is confusion about the differences and similarities between the DoD and Veterans Health Administration (VHA) health care services and benefits and there may be benefit in delineating the differences before describing integrated behavioral health care in the DoD. The DoD and the VHA are two separate health care systems, with separate funding streams, policy, leadership, and populations served. The DoD provides health care for active duty Service members, retired active duty Service members (e.g., served 20 years and are getting retirement pay), and their families. The VHA provides services for individuals who are retired active duty service members, those who have served but not long enough to earn a retirement (e.g., completed initial 4-year commitment and decide not to reenlist), and the family members of disabled or deceased veterans. A more detailed description of the differences can be found at: http://www.kaiseredu.org/Issue-Modules/Military-and-Veterans-Health-Care/Background-Brief.aspx.

Department of Defense Military Health System

Over 9.7 million active duty and retired Service members and their families are eligible for DoD Military Health System (MHS) services. These services are delivered through military treatment facilities (MTFs) and through local regionally managed civilian networks. Of these eligible beneficiaries, 3.3 million are enrolled to receive primary health care services in MTF primary care clinics. This chapter focuses on the model of care delivered through MTFs. Contrary to the commonly held idea that MTFs primarily take care of young active duty Service members, a relatively even number of male and female enrollees ranging in age from birth to over 65 years of age receive services in these clinics.

The MHS is focused on creating integrated medical teams that provide optimal health care services. Improving population health, experience of care, cost management, and mission readiness (the Quadruple Aim Table 9.1) are prime areas of focus in pursuit of cutting-edge health care. The implementation of the patient-centered medical home (PCMH) in all MTFs is the primary model being used to achieve Quadruple Aim goals (TRICARE Management Activity, 2011).

Integrating behavioral health personnel as full-time PCMH team members has been an important focus of the PCMH implementation. From 2012 to 2016, the MHS plans to integrate 470 behavioral health personnel to work as full-time team members in PCMHs. Integrating behavioral health personnel is expected to result in: (1) better identification and management of those at risk for suicide, (2) decreased use of emergency services for behavioral health concerns, (3) improved PCMH staff and patient satisfaction with health care, (4) increase in the percentage of

Table 9.1 Quadruple aim

1.	Readiness	Ensuring that the total military force is medically ready to deploy and that the medical force is ready to deliver health care anytime anywhere in support of the full range of military operations, including humanitarian missions
2.	Population health	Reducing the generators of ill health by encouraging healthy behaviors and decreasing the likelihood of illness through focused prevention and the development of increased resilience
3.	Experience of care	Providing a care experience that is patient and family centered, compassionate, convenient, equitable, safe, and always of the highest quality
4.	Responsibly managing the total health care cost	Creating value by focusing on quality, eliminating waste, and reducing unwarranted variation; considering the total cost of care over time, not just the cost of an individual health care activity

family members receiving behavioral health services in the MTF that were previously provided in the civilian network of care, (5) lower per-year health care cost per member, (6) improved evidence-based care for anxiety and depression, (7) increased percent of enrollees engaged in healthy behaviors (e.g., quit smoking, weight management), and (8) increased behavioral health-screening (e.g., major depressive disorder, post-traumatic stress disorder, suicide risk), referral, and engagement.

HOW: PCMH Team Composition

DoD PCMH team composition varies among Army, Navy, and Air Force, but generally a PCMH team consists of 3–5 primary care providers (PCPs) supported by approximately four full-time equivalent (FTE) support staff per PCP. Support staff per PCP includes .65 registered nurse, 2.3 medical/nurse assistants, .65 administrative/clerk support, .25 health educator/disease manager, and .15 clinic manager. Integrated behavioral health care staffing is based on the number of enrollees to a PCMH team.

PCMH teams with between 1,500 and 7,499 enrollees are required to have a minimum of one full-time behavioral health provider. The range came from a working group that included members from the Army, Navy, Air Force, and Public Health Service; from a range of professional backgrounds (e.g., family physicians, psychologists, psychiatrists, and social workers), and solicited expert input from nine different organizations/projects (Department of Veterans Affairs, Cherokee Health, HealthPoint Community Health Centers, Integrated Behavioral Health Project, Mountain Area Health Education Center, Maine Health, DIAMOND Project, Hogg Foundation, and Intermountain Health Care). We decided a good upper limit was 7,499 based on military and others experiences. Most of the primary care clinics that are small have about 3,000–3,600 enrollees (Hunter & Goodie, 2010).

Systematic Clinical Approaches: Integrated Care Service Delivery

Primary Care Behavioral Health Model

In the DOD, the behavioral health provider working in the PCMH provides services using a Primary Care Behavioral Health model of service delivery. This is a population-health-based model of care where the medical team and behavioral health provider share information regarding patients using a shared electronic health record (EHR), treatment plan, and standard of care (Hunter & Goodie, 2010). The behavioral health provider is embedded (works in the primary care clinic as a full-time team member) with the PCMH team and serves as a consultant to the PCP in the assessment, intervention, and health care management of the full spectrum of concerns patients bring to the clinic. In addition to common mental health concerns, the behavioral health provider engages with the patient and PCP on problems usually addressed by clinical health psychologists and behavioral medicine specialists (e.g., chronic pain, headache, health risk behavior, medical non-adherence, sleep disturbance, smoking cessation, weight management). Consistent with a consultation model, the behavioral health provider operates within a scope of practice and a standard of care that is consistent with PCMH primary care and differs from the scope of practice and standard of care for a specialty outpatient mental health clinic (e.g., no separate mental health record, no signed informed consent about the limits of confidentiality). The behavioral health provider typically sees patients in appointments that are 30 min or less, documents patient appointments in the shared medical record, and typically provides feedback the same day to the PCP regarding the assessment, intervention started, and recommendations regarding how the PCP might manage, support, or monitor a "behavioral health provider"-initiated plan. This feedback typically takes place through verbal discussion, secure email, alerting the PCP to review EHR note, or some combination based on PCP preference. Behavioral health providers deliver care in the primary care clinic where patients are seen by PCPs. The goal is to have a team-based approach to care where PCPs and patients are given direct access to behavioral health provider services/consultation when a need is identified.

HOW: Blended Model

Clinics that have multiple PCMH teams with 7,500 or more enrollees will have a minimum of one full-time behavioral health provider and one full-time care facilitator who assists with depression and anxiety treatment monitoring and functions as a clinical care manager. The behavioral health provider and care facilitator work in a Blended Model of care (Zeiss & Karlin, 2008) which combines the Primary Care Behavioral Health Model with a Care Management model of service delivery. A Care Management model is a population-based model of care focused on a specific clinical problem (e.g., major depressive disorder, post-traumatic stress disorder, diabetes). The Care Management model incorporates the use of specific clinical practices (e.g., set screening and assessment measures used as specific intervals of treatment) that systematically and comprehensively address how behavioral health problems are managed in the primary care setting. Typically the care facilitator and behavioral health provider have some form of systematic interface (e.g., weekly case review and treatment change recommendations) with a behavioral health specialist with prescriptive privileges (e.g., psychiatrist, psychiatric nurse practitioner, prescribing psychologist, or another provider credentialed for independent practice who can prescribe medication and has specialty training in the use of psychotropics). In a Blended Model, the PCP, behavioral health provider, and care facilitator share information regarding patients using a shared medical record, treatment plan, and standard of care. In over 90 Army clinics, a care management model for depression and PTSD has been implemented, and there are weekly meetings with a care facilitator and psychotropic prescriber to discuss new patients and patients not responding to treatment. The goal is for the behavioral health provider to join these weekly team meetings in the Blended Model of service delivery.

The minimum staffing requirements for the Blended Model of service delivery are based on DoD and civilian staffing experiences (Hunter & Goodie, 2010) that suggest this is the minimum number of behavioral health providers and care facilitators needed to meet the generic needs of a given number of enrollees. The age and health status of enrollees vary across MTFs. As such, some larger clinics may have greater chronic health condition and/or behavioral health problem prevalence and might benefit from additional behavioral health provider and care facilitator staffing. However, since this system rollout is new, the determination on the benefit of mandating additional behavioral health provider or care facilitator personnel for larger clinics could not be determined yet. Staffing requirements were set to minimize excessive personnel cost as a result of overstaffing. It should be noted that the minimum staffing requirements are not iterative. For example, in a clinic with 15,000 enrollees, the minimum staffing is still one behavioral health provider and one care facilitator, not two behavioral health providers and two care facilitators. A clinic can integrate staffing into larger clinics if the need exists.

Identified Patient Population: Who Gets Care?

Anyone who is at least 18 years old who is enrolled with a provider in a PCMH can receive integrated behavioral health care. Anytime a PCP desires, he or she can bring in a behavioral health provider (or care facilitator in larger clinics for a circumscribed set of actions) to assist with behavioral health screening, assessment, intervention, or recommendations regarding the need for specialty behavioral health services. A patient can request to see the behavioral health provider without going through the PCP first, but this is rare. There is effort on the part of the PCP and the behavioral health provider to engage the patient in shared patient-centered decision making, but there is no set system or protocol on how this process takes place. This is primarily an individual-PCP-driven process based on clinical judgment rather than a structured systems-based protocol for everything except depression and post-traumatic stress disorder, where screening, training, and protocol for intervention and referral exist. This clinical protocol is in place for the Army and is expected to be in place for the Air Force and Navy over the next 2–3 years. Preferences and care options related to bringing in the behavioral health provider to assist with care are discussed with the patient. The goal is to assist the patient in making informed decisions about their health care.

Patient care in the PCMH for "nontargeted," clinician-identified patients may focus on a range of concerns—behavioral and mental health conditions (e.g., major depressive disorder), psychophysiological symptoms (e.g., headache, insomnia), medical conditions (e.g., diabetes), and complex cases regardless of disease. There is no behavioral health condition that is being systemically targeted in all PCMHs at this time. However, there are individual clinics within each Service that are specifically screening, assessing, and initiating integrated behavioral health care services interventions for individuals who have specific problems like diabetes, obesity, or tobacco dependence. Future plans for all three Services to include universal screening for Major Depressive Disorder with a Patient Health Questionnaire-2 (every patient at every appointment) and anxiety disorder screening, likely with the two-item Generalized Anxiety Disorder Scale are being reviewed, but a final decision on the screening instruments has not been reached. Currently, there is no systematic data collection using these measures.

Program Maturity

Integrated behavioral health care in the DoD is a standard mainstream service. However, this did not happen quickly or easily. Since 2000, the United States Air Force, Navy, and Army have independently implemented Primary Care Behavioral Health or Care Management Models of service delivery (Hunter et al., 2012). In 2008, the DoD launched a concerted effort to develop clinical, administrative, and operational standards for integrated care across the MHS. After a 22-month process that involved primary care providers, psychologists, psychiatrists, and social workers, the group finalized a set of evidence-informed (e.g., Bower, Gilbody, Richards, Fletcher, & Sutton, 2006; Butler et al., 2008; Cigrang, Dobmeyer, Becknell, Roa-Navarrete, & Yerian, 2006; Craven & Bland, 2006; Engel et al., 2008; Unutzer et al., 2002) approaches to integrated care. These approaches served as the foundation for five recommendations that are guiding the integration of behavioral health providers and care facilitators into primary care (see Table 9.2).

Table 9.2 Recommendations for integrating behavioral health personnel into primary care

1. Minimum behavioral health staffing ratios based on number of primary care enrollees

    7,500+ enrollees   1 full-time PCBH provider **and** 1 care facilitator

    1,500–7,499   1 full-time PCBH provider, **or** 1 full time care facilitator, **or** 1 full time
    enrollees   BHP providing PCBH and care facilitator services

2. The primary care clinic owns the PCBH personnel positions. These individuals will not engage in outpatient specialty behavioral health care

3. PCBH personnel will incorporate the following for the detection, assessment, and treatment of Major Depressive Disorder and Anxiety Disorders
   a. Evidence-based screening
   b. Evidence-based treatment guidelines
   c. Systematic follow-up assessment and focus on continuity of care
   d. Patient education and use of patient self-management strategies
   e. Supervision for care facilitators by a behavioral health specialist
   f. Consultation with psychiatry on psychotropic medication

4. Standards for integrated behavioral health programs shall include, but are not limited to:
   a. Administrative, procedural and operational standards for behavioral health providers, care facilitators, and psychiatric medication consultation and recommendations
   b. Core competencies, skills, and standards for those who serve as expert trainers of behavioral health providers and care facilitators
   c. Core competencies, skills, and standards that behavioral health providers and care facilitators must meet to be credentialed for integrated behavioral health care practice
   d. Minimum Service-wide standards that adapt current evidence-based DoD/VA clinical practice guidelines
   e. Service and clinic assessment of fidelity of Service integrated behavioral health care standards and symptom and functional outcomes of patient care
   f. Service and clinic assessment of fidelity of Service integrated behavioral health care standards and symptom and functional outcomes of patient care

5. Service-level oversight of integrated behavioral health care PCBH model and CMM programs. Oversight responsibilities shall include, but are not limited to:
   a. Advising senior Service staff on a range of programs and services required to fully implement and sustain integrated behavioral health care
   b. Assisting with planning strategies to support implementation and administration of Service-wide programs; establishing and altering Service-level goals and measures as appropriate
   c. Assisting with ongoing Service-level program evaluation plans for components and models of integrated-collaborative behavioral health services in primary care
   d. Guide Service-level evaluations through resources such as reports, site visits, process reviews, studies, and surveys
   e. Participating in Tri-Service efforts to create and maintain Service-level data bases, reporting procedures, and data displays that permit the integration of Service databases, and create common implementing practices that permit cross-service comparisons of programs
   f. Establish feedback mechanisms to ensure ongoing information is received from all relevant stakeholders

(continued)

Table 9.2 (continued)

g. Making recommendations on implementation, alteration, or discontinuation of components and models of integrated-collaborative behavioral health services in primary care
h. Developing Services-level quality assessment to assess fidelity to administrative, operational, and clinical component standards of integrated behavioral health care
i. Providing Service representation to an ongoing DoD IBHC committee, headed by Health Affairs, which will coordinate, facilitate, and assess IBHC efforts at the DoD level and among each Service

BHP behavioral health provider, *CMM* Care Management Model, *DoD* Department of Defense, *IBHC* integrated-behavioral health care, *MHIWG* Mental Health Integration Working Group, *PCBH* primary care behavioral health, *VA* veterans affairs

SUPPORTED BY: Practice Design

It was clear from past efforts at the individual Service level that if the MHS was going to have fidelity to a service delivery model, each Service needed a program manager and a clinical, administrative, and operational practice standards manual that set the standards for behavioral health provider and care facilitator work. Setting these benchmarks improves the chances of fidelity to the service delivery model, and provides a mechanism to objectively evaluate that clinic services are being delivered consistently. Each of the Services is working on creating a blended model practice standards manual based on the Air Force Behavioral Health Optimization Manual (BHOP) for behavioral health providers (United States Air Force, 2011) and the Army's RESPECT-Mil Manual for care facilitators (Uniformed Services University, 2008). These comprehensive documents serve as the reference guide on how services are delivered.

In addition to the practice manuals, behavioral health providers and care facilitators are trained by experts prior to seeing patients. Expert trainers must meet a set of standards before their Service can designate them as such (see Department of Defense, 2012 for standards). Development of a common training procedure across all three Services is in the final stages of development and will include didactic training on clinical and administrative standards and core competencies. This is augmented by another level of training that includes observation of video and/or role-play demonstration of standards and competencies by the expert trainer and expert trainer role-play observation and feedback with the behavioral health provider and care facilitator. Once the behavioral health provider or care facilitator begins work in a clinic, the expert trainer observes their services in the clinic and provides feedback and training to ensure minimum core competencies can be demonstrated in a real-world setting (see Appendix A from the Air Force BHOP manual for an example of behavioral health provider core competencies). The Air Force has been using benchmarked competencies in training for behavioral health providers since 2000. To date, over 250 individuals have been trained to meet these competencies. Although this type of training requires an expert trainer to spend time in the clinic modeling appropriate competencies and observing and giving feedback on observed behaviors to meet competencies, it ensures that a minimum competency standard for the important components of the Primary Care Behavioral Health Model of service delivery model are being met.

Office Management and Financial Sustainability

Unlike civilian health care systems, funding for behavioral health provider and care facilitator services are part of the overall budget for all PCMH staffing and is not a fee for service model. This funding was secured based on the evidence suggesting that integrating behavioral health providers and care facilitators into primary care would produce a return on investment on the variables outlined in Table 9.3. Behavioral health provider and care facilitator service delivery gets coded with a current procedural technology (CPT) or an evaluation and management (E&M) health and behavior codes as a way to track the value of services delivered, but "billing" for those services does not occur. This frees the behavioral health providers and care facilitators from the financial, administrative, and bureaucratic entanglements that limit service delivery in other health systems.

Practice-Based Quality Improvement and Program Evaluation

Currently, there are no quality improvement reports that have been generated to document or evaluate the impact of a behavioral health provider and a care facilitator on quality care indicators. However, there is a strong commitment to building a system to collect and use practice data to evaluate the impact of behavioral health provider and care facilitator services. A plan to examine outcome and process metrics is well underway (see Table 9.4 for metrics being considered). The current infrastructure of the MHS EHR does not allow for centralized collection of most of the process and outcome metrics under consideration. Work has begun on developing behavioral health provider and care facilitator note templates for the EHR that will include standardized data fields and screening and assessment measures for all initial and follow-up appointments. Common data fields and documentation will

Table 9.3 Expected impact of behavioral health integration in the PCMH

1.	Better identification and management of those at risk for suicide
2.	Decreased use of emergency services for behavioral health concerns
3.	Improved PCMH staff and patient satisfaction with health care
4.	Recapture family member behavioral health services from purchased network care
5.	Lower per-member per-year health care cost
6.	Improved evidence-based care for anxiety and depression
7.	Increased percent of enrollees engaged in healthy behaviors (e.g., quit smoking)
8.	Increased behavioral health screening, referral, and engagement

PCMH Patient-Centered Medical Home

Table 9.4 Evaluating the impact of integrating behavioral health personnel into the PCMH

Quadruple aim	Potential performance measures
Improved Readiness To Deploy	**Anxiety**
	1. % Enrollees screened for an anxiety disorder (e.g., GAD-7)
	2. % Screening positive for an anxiety disorder
	3. % Diagnosed with an anxiety disorder
	4. % Positive managed in PCMH only
	5. % With symptoms and functioning improvement pre/post (use of a general measure [e.g., Duke Health Profile, Behavioral Health Measure-20] and/or specific anxiety measure)
	6. % Attending initial behavioral health in PCMH appointment by beneficiary category
	7. % Referred to specialty outpatient behavioral health
	8. % Attending initial specialty outpatient behavioral health appointment
	Depression
	1. % Enrollees screened for major depressive disorder and suicidality (Patient Health Questionnaire-2 and suicide question # 9 from Patient Health Questionnaire-9)
	2. % Screening positive for a Major Depressive Disorder
	3. % Diagnosed with Major Depressive Disorder
	4. % Positive managed in PCMH only
	5. % With symptoms and functioning improvement pre/post (general measure [e.g., Duke Health Profile, Behavioral Health Measure-20] and/or specific depression measure (e.g., Patient Health Questionnaire-9)
	6. % Attending initial behavioral health in PCMH appointment by beneficiary category
	7. % Referred to specialty outpatient behavioral health
	8. % Attending initial specialty outpatient behavioral health appointment
Population Health Impact	**Obesity (overlaps with readiness)**
	1. % Enrollees with BMI $\geq$ 30
	2. % Enrollees screened for obesity (BMI $\geq$ 30)
	3. % Screening positive for obesity
	4. % Working with PCMH behavioral health for intensive behavioral weight counseling and BMI change from 12 months post treatment initiation
	5. Average BMI change for all enrollees with a BMI over 30
	Tobacco Use (overlaps with readiness)
	1. % Enrollees who smoke
	2. % Enrollees screened for tobacco use
	3. % Screening positive for tobacco use
	4. % Diagnosed with tobacco dependence (TD)
	5. % Diagnosed with TD Working with PCP and behavioral health in PCMH based cessation program
	6. % Treated remaining tobacco free 12 months post quit date
	7. % Diagnosed with TD getting cessation services out of PCMH

(continued)

Table 9.4 (continued)

Quadruple aim	Potential performance measures
	Alcohol Use (overlaps with readiness)
	1. % Enrollees screened for alcohol use
	2. % Screening positive for alcohol problems (AUDIT-C)
	3. % Diagnosed with alcohol abuse or engaged in risky drinking
	4. % Working with PCP and behavioral health in PCMH-based treatment
	5. % Referred to specialty outpatient alcohol treatment
	Chronic Pain (overlaps with readiness)
	1. % Enrollees with chronic pain condition
	2. % Enrollees referred to PCMH behavioral health for screening/assessment as part of standard of care for all chronic pain patients
	3. % With significant anxiety/depression or functional impairments that might benefit from cognitive/behavioral pain management skills training
	4. % Working with PCP and behavioral health in PCMH-based pain management program
	5. % After treatment with clinically and statistically significant changes in depression/anxiety symptoms, functioning and quality of life
	6. % With appropriate medication use
	7. % That receive an invasive procedure
	Diabetes
	1. % Enrollees with HbA1C < 7
	2. % Enrollees with HbA1C > 7 referred to PCMH behavioral health for screening/assessment to improve diabetes management
	3. % That work with PCMH behavioral health for weight loss, increased physical activity, improved monitoring, and management of mood
	4. % After treatment with significant decrease in HbA1C, blood pressure, lipids, weight loss
Experience of Care	1. Same day access to PCMH behavioral health appointment
	2. Time to same day available new and 3rd return open appointment for PCMH behavioral health
	3. % Who desire same day PCMH behavioral health who receive it
	4. Patient satisfaction with getting timely behavioral health care
	5. % of family members seen by PCMH behavioral health (potentially recaptured network care)
	6. Primary care staff satisfaction with behavioral health services
Health care Costs	1. Annual percent increase in per capita costs
	2. Emergency room visits per 100 enrollees per year for anything
	3. Emergency room visits per 100 enrollees per year for behavioral health presentation

BMI body mass index, *HbA1C* hemoglobin A1C, *PCP* primary care provider, *PCMH* Patient Centered Medical Home

facilitate centralized data collection as the EHR data pull capabilities evolve. Standardized data fields will also make data collection easier as evaluation in the near future will likely be done through discreet program evaluation studies with select clinics through record review data pulls.

Recommendations and Conclusions

Developing and initiating an integrated behavioral health care service is an evolutionary process. A great deal of work has been and is still left to be done in the DoD with hiring and training personnel and developing standardized data collection and evaluation. There are several recommendations based on our experience that systems may consider when developing and launching integrated behavioral health care.

1. Solidify an evidence-based rationale for integrated behavioral health care that takes into account the financial and operational barriers that need to be addressed.
2. Identify a primary care and/or behavioral health lead who can champion program development and speak the language of management, personnel, and finance. A strong advocate can facilitate coordinated movement of the clinical, financial, and operational worlds in a way that can improve the chances of successful program launch and sustainment.
3. When developing a service delivery model, include relevant health care professionals (e.g., PCPs, psychiatrists, psychologists, and social workers) and key management, personnel, and finance individuals. Having all the "players in the game" from the start ensures the agreed-upon plan can be funded, can be supported by leadership, and can improve acceptance of a new service delivery paradigm throughout the system.
4. Define the unique concepts and terminology used (e.g., integrated behavioral health care, PCBH Model, Care Management Model). Unique concepts and language mean different things between and within professions and, if not clarified, can slow down or derail program development and implementation. For instance, referring to specific service delivery models (e.g., Primary Care Behavioral Health model) instead of a generic term like "integrated care" can facilitate agreement on supporting scientific evidence for a given model and the components needed for success. The proposed lexicon in this book can be used as a foundation to facilitate the use of a common set of defined terms when developing, initiating, and evaluating models of service delivery.
5. Develop a manual with descriptions of clinical, administrative, and operational standards that are observable and can be enforced. Create a strategy to train this new workforce to benchmarked standards in the manuals to enhance fidelity of service delivery.
6. Determine the metrics that will demonstrate the desired impact of integrated behavioral health care services. Incorporate the metrics when possible into standard clinical practice in the medical record and determine a method for extracting and evaluating the data in a manner that is scientifically robust.

Appendix A: Training Core Competency Tool

Dimension	Element	Attribute	Skill rating (1 = low; 5 = high)					Comments
			1	2	3	4	5	
I. Clinical Practice Knowledge and Skills	1. Role definition	Says introductory script smoothly, conveys the BHC role to all new patients, and answers patient's questions						
	2. Problem identification	Identifies and defines the presenting problem with the patient within the first half of the initial 30-min appointment						
	3. Assessment	Focuses on current problem, functional impact, and environmental factors contributing to/maintaining the problem; uses tools appropriate for primary care						
	4. Problem focus	Explores whether additional problems exist, without excessive probing						
	5. Population-based care	Provides care along a continuum from primary prevention to tertiary care; develops pathways to routinely involve BHC in care of chronic conditions; understands the difference between population-based and case-focused approach						
	6. Biopsychosocial approach	Understands relationship of medical and psychological aspects of health						
	7. Use of empirically supported interventions	Utilizes evidence-based recommendations/interventions suitable for primary care for patients and PCPs						
	8. Intervention design	8.a. Bases interventions on measurable, functional outcomes and symptom reduction						
		8.b. Uses self-management, home-based practice						
		8.c. Uses simple, concrete, practical strategies based on empirically supported treatments for primary care						

(continued)

Appendix A: (continued)

Dimension	Element	Attribute	Skill rating (1 = low; 5 = high)					Comments
			1	2	3	4	5	
	9. Multi-patient intervention skills	Works with PCMs to provide classes and/or groups in format appropriate for primary care (e.g., drop-in stress management class, group medical visit for a chronic condition)						
	10. Pharmacotherapy	Can name basic psychotropic medications; can discuss common side effects and common myths; abides by recommendation limits for nonprescribers						
II. Practice Management Skills	1. Visit efficiency	30-min visits demonstrate adequate introduction, rapid problem identification and assessment, and development of intervention recommendations and a plan						
	2. Time management	Stays on time when conducting consecutive appointments						
	3. Follow-up planning	Plans follow-up for 2 weeks or 1 month, instead of every week (as appropriate); alternates follow-ups with PCMs for high-utilizer patients						
	4. Intervention efficiency	Completes treatment episode in four or fewer sessions for 85 % or more of patients; structures behavioral change plans consistent with time-limited treatment						
	5. Visit flexibility	Appropriately uses flexible strategies for visits: 15 min, 30 min, phone contacts, secure messaging						
	6. Triage	Attempts to manage most problems in primary care, but does triage to mental health, chemical dependency, or other clinics or services when necessary						
	7. Case management	Utilizes patient registries (if they exist); takes load off PCM (e.g., returns patient calls about behavioral issues); advocates for patients						
	8. Community resource referrals	Is knowledgeable about and makes use of community resources (e.g., refers to community self-help groups, Airmen and Family Readiness Center resources)						

III. Consultation Skills	1. Referral clarity	Is clear on the referral questions; focuses on and responds directly to referral questions in PCM feedback
	2. Curbside Consultations	Successfully consults with PCMs on-demand about a general issue or specific patient; uses clear, direct language in a concise manner
	3. Assertive follow-up	Ensures PCMs receive verbal and/or written feedback on patients referred; interrupts PCM, if indicated, for urgent patient needs
	4. PCM education	Delivers brief presentations in primary-care staff meetings (PCM audience; focus on what you can do for them, what they can refer, what to expect, how to use BHC optimally, etc.)
	5. Recommendation usefulness	Recommendations are tailored to the pace of primary care (e.g., interventions suggested for PCMs can be done in 1–3 min)
	6. Value-added orientation	Recommendations are intended to reduce physician visits and workload (e.g., follow-up with BHC instead of PCM)
	7. Clinical pathways	Participates in team efforts to develop, implement, evaluate, and revise pathway programs needed in the clinic
IV. Documentation Skills	1. Concise, clear charting	Clear, concise notes detail: • Referral problem specifics • Functional analysis • Pertinent history • Impression • Specific recommendations and follow-up plan
	2. Prompt PCM feedback	Written and/or verbal feedback provided to PCM on the day the patient was seen
	3. Appropriate format	Chart notes use SOAP format

(continued)

Appendix A: (continued)

Dimension	Element	Attribute	Skill rating (1 = low; 5 = high)					Comments
			1	2	3	4	5	
V. Administrative Knowledge and Skills	1. BHOP policies and procedures	Understands scheduling, templates, MEPRS codes for PC work, criticality of accurate ADS coding						
	2. Risk-management protocols	Understands limits of existing BHOP practices; can describe and discuss how and why informed consent procedures differ, etc.						
	3. KG ADS (coding) documentation	Routinely and accurately completes coding documentation						
VI. Team Performance Skills	1. Fit with primary care culture	Understands and operates comfortably in fast-paced, action-oriented, team-based culture						
	2. Knows team members	Knows the roles of the various primary care team members; both assists and utilizes them						
	3. Responsiveness	Readily provides unscheduled services when needed (e.g., sees patient during lunch time or at the end of the day, if needed)						
	4. Availability	Provides on-demand consultations by beeper or cell phone when not in the clinic; keeps staff aware of whereabouts						

Use a rating scale of 1 = low skills to 5 = high skills to assess current level of skill development for all attributes within each dimension. Check in the column corresponding to the rating that best describes the trainee's current skill level. *Competency Tool*: Behavioral Health Consultant (BHC) mentor rates the BHC trainee based on their observations for each dimension (verbal feedback is also strongly recommended). A rating of 3 or higher is considered satisfactory for training

References

Bower, P., Gilbody, S., Richards, D., Fletcher, J., & Sutton, A. (2006). Collaborative care for depression in primary care: Making sense of a complex intervention: Systematic review and meta-regression. *The British Journal of Psychiatry, 189*, 484–493.

Butler, M., Kane, R. L., McAlpine, D., Kathol, R. G., Fu, S. S., Hagedorn, H., et al. (2008). *Integration of mental health/substance abuse and primary care* (AHRQ publication no. 09-E003). Rockville, MD: Agency for Healthcare Research and Quality.

Craven, M. A., & Bland, M. (2006). Better practices in collaborative mental health care: An analysis of the evidence. *Canadian Journal of Psychiatry, 51*, 1S–72S.

Cigrang, J. A., Dobmeyer, A. C., Becknell, M. E., Roa-Navarrete, R. A., & Yerian, S. R. (2006). Evaluation of a collaborative mental health program in primary care: Effects on patient distress and health care utilization. *Primary Care and Community Psychiatry, 11*, 121–127.

Department of Defense. (2012). *Integration of behavioral health personnel (BHP) services into patient-centered medical home (PCMH) primary care and other primary care service settings.* Document under publication review and coordination.

Engel, C. C., Oxman, T., Yamamoto, C., Gould, D., Barry, S., Stewart, P., et al. (2008). RESPECT-Mil: Feasibility of a systems-level collaborative care approach to depression and post-traumatic stress disorder in military primary care. *Military Medicine, 173*, 935–940.

Hunter, C. L., & Goodie, J. L. (2010). Operational and clinical components for integrated-collaborative behavioral health care in the patient centered medical home. *Journal of Families Systems and Health, 28*, 308–321.

Hunter, C. L., Goodie, J. L., & Dobmeyer, A. C. (2012). *Tipping points in the department of defense's experience with psychologists in primary care.* Manuscript submitted for publication.

Katon, W., Robinson, P., Von Korff, M., Bush, L. E., Ludman, E., & Walker, E. (1996). A multi-faceted intervention to improve treatment of depression in primary care. *Archives of General Psychiatry, 53*, 924–932.

TRICARE Management Activity. (2011). *Military health system medical home guide.* Retrieved from http://www.tricare.mil/tma/ocmo/download/MHSPCMHGuide.pdf.

Uniformed Services University. (2008). *RESPECT-MIL care facilitator reference manual: Three component model for primary care management of depression and PTSD* (Military Version). Bethesda, MD.

United States Air Force. (2011). *Primary behavioral health care services practice manual: Version 2.0.* San Antonio, TX.

Unutzer, J., Katon, W., Callahan, C. M., Williams, J. W., Hunkeler, E., Harpole, L., et al. (2002). Collaborative care management of late-life depression in the primary care setting: A randomized controlled trial. *Journal of the American Medical Association, 288*, 2836–2845.

Zeiss, A. M., & Karlin, B. E. (2008). Integrating mental health and primary care services in the department of veterans affairs healthcare system. *Journal of Clinical Psychology in Medical Settings, 15*, 73–75.

Part III
Review of Collaborative Behavioral Health Clinical Services

Chapter 10
Collaborative Partnerships Within Integrated Behavioral Health and Primary Care

Tricia Hern, Aimee Burke Valeras, Jamie Banker, and Genevieve Riebe

Abstract Health care teams are increasingly utilized to provide care to patients as medicine has become more complex. Over the past decades providers have subspecialized to a greater degree and communication gaps have grown between providers of the same patient. Major health organizations now endorse the use of health care teams, and health profession education is recognizing the importance of educating its learners about how to function effectively in a health care team. The characteristics of successful health care teams are difficult to define but there are key elements associated with successful health care teams. This chapter highlights four health care teams to connect the need for quality team-based care and the practice of how to maintain functional partnerships within the team and between provider and patient.

T. Hern, M.D. (✉)
Community Group Family Medicine, 10122 East 10th Street, Suite 100,
Indianapolis, IN 46229, USA
e-mail: thern@ecommunity.com

A.B. Valeras, Ph.D., MSW
NH Dartmouth Family Medicine Residency, Concord Hospital Family Health Center,
250 Pleasant St., 03301, Concord, NH, USA
e-mail: aimeevaleras@gmail.com

J. Banker, Ph.D., MFT
California Lutheran University, The Bell House, 3263 Pioneer St. #4250,
Thousand Oaks, CA 91360-2700, USA
e-mail: jbanker@callutheran.edu

G. Riebe, M.D.
University of Arizona, Tucson, AZ, USA
e-mail: genevieveriebe@gmail.com

M.R. Talen and A. Burke Valeras (eds.), *Integrated Behavioral Health in Primary Care:*
Evaluating the Evidence, Identifying the Essentials, DOI 10.1007/978-1-4614-6889-9_10,
© Springer Science+Business Media New York 2013

Health Care Teams

The typical Medicare patient in one year sees seven different doctors, including five different specialists, working in four different practices. For vulnerable patients with multiple chronic conditions, care is even more fragmented and involves more doctors. Forty percent of the patients in our study had seven or more chronic conditions and they saw on average 11 doctors in seven practices; the upper quartile of this group saw 16 or more different doctors in nine or more different practices. (Bach, 2007, p. A17)

Background

Health care teams are increasingly utilized to provide care to patients as medicine has become more complex, providers have subspecialized to a greater degree, and communication gaps have grown between providers of the same patient. It is now more and more difficult for an individual provider to successfully care for his or her patients alone. Team-based care is one vehicle for providing safer, more effective, efficient, personalized, timely, and equitable care, as endorsed by the Institute of Medicine (IOM, 2001). A health care team is defined as two or more individuals involved in a patient's care; the team members each have specific responsibilities, and the members work together to contribute to the care of the patient (Bosch et al., 2009).

Health care teams can be categorized based on setting, such as primary care or acute care; disease state such as diabetes or stroke care; or a specific patient population such as geriatric or pediatric care (Bosch et al., 2009). Health care teams can be comprised of a combination of physicians, mid-level providers (nurse practitioners and/or physician assistants), pharmacists, nurses, medical assistants, phone or clerical staff, case managers, and social workers. Other providers, such as care managers; psychologists; nutritionists; health educators; physical, occupational, or speech therapists; and nutritionists, may also be members of the team depending on patient needs and setting. The objectives of the team can range from health promotion and improving the health of a population to direct patient care for acute or chronic disease management.

Major health organizations now endorse the use of health care teams, while health profession education is recognizing the importance of educating its learners about how to function effectively in a health care team. Health care teams can enable increased coordination of care, improved communication among providers, and pooling of expertise to make rational patient-centered decisions. Teams can ensure the completion of key components of care that a physician may not have the training or time to do (Wagner, 2000).

It is challenging to measure the effectiveness of health care teams because the many permutations of teams vary in their characteristics and dynamics. Team health can be measured by member satisfaction and member turnover. Markers of functional teams include a clear guiding vision and clear role definition for its individual members. Communication patterns and respect among team members are important features to examine when evaluating teams. Improvements in patient outcomes and patient satisfaction are also indicators that health care teams are being utilized effectively.

Leadership and Organizational Issues

Leading health care and health profession education organizations have endorsed the use of patient care teams. The Institute of Medicine points to the use of high-performing patient-centered teams as a means to achieve safer and more effective patient outcomes (IOM, 2001). The Association of American Medical Colleges (AAMC) predicts a physician workforce shortage of 63,000 physicians by 2015, an estimate that has been increasing as health reform expands coverage to many uninsured and as more of our aging population becomes eligible for Medicare (AAMC Center for Workforce Studies, 2010). This expected physician shortage necessitates novel solutions to providing patient care, and AAMC has responded by endorsing the role of health care teams. Physicians will need to increasingly rely on team members to effectively care for their patient populations.

The Patient-Centered Medical Home (PCMH) movement in the primary care arena, which originated with the American Academy of Pediatrics (AAP) in 1967, and which has since been endorsed by the World Health Organization, the Academy of Family Physicians, the American Osteopathic Association, the American College of Physicians, highlights the importance of health care teams (American Academy of Family Physicians, American Academy of Pediatrics, & American College of Physicians, American Osteopathic Association, 2007). One of the seven key elements of the PCMH model is a physician-led team of individuals who collectively care for the patients (Robert Graham Center: Center for Policy Studies in Family Medicine and Primary Care, 2007). In 2004, an expert task force in family medicine supported a "new model" of practice that utilizes a multidisciplinary team approach to care for the population served by the practice (Green et al., 2004). During the same year, a similar task force from the Society of General Internal Medicine supported general internists as leaders of health teams, with the physician leader having responsibility for the care provided by the team (Larson et al., 2004).

Patient care teams have been endorsed by leading health service organizations; however, implementing the educational framework to teach health professionals how to function in teams has lagged behind the reality of practice. Teamwork skills have historically been learned "on the job" (Leggat, 2007). Recently, leading health education organizations joined together to form the Interprofessional Education Collaborative (IPEC) and in May of 2011 published an expert panel report describing the core competencies for interprofessional collaborative practice. IPEC sponsors included leading organizations in nursing, medicine, dentistry, pharmacy, and public health, but notably, behavioral and mental health specialties were not represented. The IPEC report highlighted the importance of having a health care workforce that is ready to practice effective teamwork and team-based care, and charges the individual disciplines to "move beyond these profession-specific educational efforts to engage students of different professions in interactive learning with each other" (Interprofessional Education Collaborative Expert Panel report, 2011).

These recommendations have lead to the development and revision of many health care teams around the country. One way to examine the factors involved in the health care teams is to observe teams currently in practice. Four health care teams will be highlighted in this chapter as a way to connect the need for health care teams with the practice of how to create functional partnerships. These featured health care teams are: The IMPACT (Improving Mood-Promoting Access to Collaborative Treatment) depression care program at a University of Washington (UW)-affiliated safety net primary care clinic, Crozer-Keystone Center for Family Health, Concord Hospital Family Health Center team, and University of California San Diego Family Medicine Residency team. These health care teams work toward two missions—meeting the needs of their patients and educating medical residents and behavioral health trainees. Patient care teams can serve as educational channels in training programs, and can role model team functioning for use in future practice. Health care teams also serve as a practical vehicle for patient care in training settings, where transitions of providers occur more frequently.

Factors and Qualities of Partnership

There are many identifiable elements of health care team formation and functioning that can be studied, including team structure, team processes, and team effectiveness. Team structure is the composition and skill mix. Team processes involves the communication and information flow among the team members. Team effectiveness is the output of the team (Bosch et al., 2009). Teamwork is also influenced by members' various skills, knowledge, traits, and motives (Leggat, 2007).

Team structure varies depending on the patient care setting, and can be as small as two individuals, such as a physician and a medical assistant, or could be a larger team of physicians, nurse practitioners, therapists, nurses, case managers, and social workers operating in a particular setting. A core team of ten or fewer members allows everyone to have a say and tends to work more efficiently than a larger team, but it is key to have a balance between heterogeneity and homogeneity of members' skills and backgrounds (Michan & Rodger, 2000). In a study of primary health care team effectiveness, there was no association between team effectiveness and team structure characteristics (such as team size, team tenure/experience, or financial status) (Poulton & West, 1999).

Case Examples

The AIMS Center at the University of Washington (UW) is an example of an organization that provides training and consultation to health care teams across the country to implement integrated mental health programs, including the IMPACT model of depression care. One example is a primary care clinic run by a UW-affiliated county hospital that serves a safety net population. Clinic staff received consultation, training, and implementation support from the AIMS Center, implemented the program in 2008, and has since served over 400 clients with depression and other common mental disorders. Within the clinic the integrated behavioral health team includes the patient, primary care provider (PCPs), and behavioral health care coordinator (CC; a licensed clinical social worker). A consulting psychiatrist (CP) meets weekly with the care coordinator to review patients who are not improving and to make treatment recommendations. The CP is also available to the PCP and the CC or to see occasional patients who are not improving as expected in direct consultation. This team serves about 150 patients a year, 75 of which are active at any given time.

Crozer-Keystone Center for Family Health is the clinical office of their Family Medicine Residency Program, in Delaware County, Pennsylvania, and sees 20,000 patient visits per year. Their providers include family medicine residents and faculty physicians, a psychologist, a pharmacist, and a nurse care manager, who assist with population health management and chronic disease management.

The Concord Hospital Family Health Center (CHFHC) is a community health center in Central New Hampshire that both serves to meet the primary care needs of a under- or uninsured population and to train approximately 24 family medicine resident physicians through the New Hampshire Dartmouth Family Medicine Residency (NHDFMR). The clinic serves 16,000 patients and their teams consists of six Medical Assistants, three Registered Nurses, one Integrated Behavioral Health Clinician (social worker), two faculty physicians, and six resident physicians. University of California San Diego Division of Family Medicine (UCSDDFM), which is within the Department of Family and Preventive Medicine, is an academic health care system that works through three primary care clinics and one inpatient care facility in the San Diego area. The Division of Family Medicine houses the UCSD Family Medicine Residency Program, which is composed of over 40 clinical faculty physicians and 27 family medicine residents. Each clinic provides between 120 and 160 patient encounters each day. The UCSDDFM system is an academic training program, which is composed of family medicine, pharmacy, and behavioral health providers who attend and supervise family medicine residents, marriage and family therapy trainees and interns, psychology interns, and pharmacy interns. Team members include the patient, primary care provider, behavioral health specialists (Licensed Clinical Health Psychologist and Licensed Marriage and Family Therapist), pharmacist, care manager (RNs), medical assistant, and consulting psychiatrist.

Team processes are the ways in which the team handles communication, coordination of care, conflict and change, leadership, and decision-making (Lemieux-Charles & McGuire, 2006). To achieve high-functioning team processes, interpersonal trust must be cultivated and nurtured. Such trust first comes from team members acting knowledgeably and skillfully in their own discipline and secondly from members caring about and working to promote the best interests of others. When both of these happen, team members can reliably bring their best work to the team and to promote the best work of others. Teams with high interpersonal trust work together like a jazz band or a basketball team, that is, each member skillfully carries out their own function while collectively working for the good of the team. Interpersonal trust creates safety to voice all views. High-functioning teams possess positive communication patterns, low levels of conflict, high levels of participation, shared decision-making, and cooperation. These positive team processes are associated with a perception of greater team effectiveness (Lemieux-Charles & McGuire, 2006). Health care teams have to establish unique and distinctive team processes to make their team successful within the context in which they function. The UW-affiliated safety net primary care clinic, CHFHC team, and UCSDDFM team have developed specific roles to structure their teamwork, which are all distinctly different from one another but effective for their individual practices. The following are examples of how these teams have organized themselves.

The UW AIMS Center guided the UW primary care clinic in a step-wise approach to fully integrate the integrated behavioral health model into their practice. First, a patient population was identified that would benefit from the model—Medicaid patients with a diagnosis of depression, anxiety, substance abuse, or post traumatic-stress disorder (PTSD). The PCPs are responsible for identifying patients through systematic screening and clinician-based identification during routine care. The patient is at the center of care and is given treatment choices including medications prescribed by the PCP and/or counseling from the CC. All patients are tracked in a web-based registry tool, which summarizes quality indicators by clinics, teams, and patients and identifies opportunities for improvement. The CP uses the registry to identify patients who need to be discussed in consultation because their symptoms are not improving as expected. A program manager at the county hospital regularly reviews the panel- and clinic-specific quality indicators and can consult with experts at the AIMS Center about opportunities to improve the overall program. The primary care team collaborates and communicates through informal hallway consultation and through more formal channels by sending tasks and messages using the electronic health record (EHR). Decision-making is meant to be by consensus between the patient, CCs, and their PCP in consultation with the CP as needed.

The CHFHC team reports that communication between the three team members is essential to their success, and thus they make a significant time commitment for this purpose—including a one-hour leadership meeting (exclusively the PCP, BH clinician, and nurse supervisor) and a one-hour pod meeting weekly (the larger team of providers and staff). Patient information exchange occurs through mostly informal processes, in meetings or on the fly, depending on the urgency of needs. All members of the pod document in shared electronic health records, so team members often communicate requests and information through chart "flags" or documents. This shared utilization also allows for an efficient way of triggering reminders to include other necessary members of the team.

The UCSDDFM team describes their operation as a medical home model where the personal physician coordinates a fully integrated whole-person family-centered integrated behavioral health practice incorporated across the entire UCSD Health care system. In addition to the team-based approach to general patient care, specific clinical markers (A1c, LDL, and Positive Depression Screen) are used to identify, monitor, intervene, and improve quality health outcomes throughout the entire patient population. Care managers are used to identify and engage patients within physician panels that would benefit from additional monitoring and management. T-CARE therapists, primarily MFT trainees and interns and pharmacy interns, identify potentially high-risk patients during clinic sessions on a provider's schedule and collaborate with the PCP and other team members to address identified concerns. The care team actively utilizes information technology to support and coordinate patient care.

One example of their integrated behavioral health model is their method of assessing all patients for depression. All patients arriving for a primary care visit are asked to complete a PHQ-2. The Targeted Collaborative-integrative Assessment Response and Empowerment model (T-CARE) is used to clinically manage patients who report moderate to severe depressive symptoms based on the PHQ-2 and the more extensive PHQ-9. When a patient comes into the clinic and screens positive on the PHQ-2, the care team's medical assistant then administers the PHQ-9 and enters the score into the EHR for the physician to review before the visit. If the patient scores 20 or higher on the PHQ-9 or endorses the desire to hurt themselves, the T-CARE therapist is informed and provides an initial assessment. The T-CARE therapist then consults with the PCP and develops a clinical management plan for the patient, which may include a referral to the consulting psychiatrist, integrated behavioral health program (co-located psychotherapy services), physician medication management, and/or brief behavioral intervention by the T-CARE therapist.

Health service managers have identified certain skills, knowledge, traits, and motives as being present in the most effective team members and the teams that show improved team performance. Leadership skills, knowledge of organizational goals and strategies, and respect for others are key characteristics of effective team members. Strong team members show commitment to working collaboratively, commitment to the organization, and commitment to a high-quality outcome (Leggat, 2007.)

There are important steps that should occur when a health care team is initiated. Vision setting, role definition, and a culture of respect should be established early in team development. The team at Crozer-Keystone Center for Family Health spent the necessary time to clarify and solidify the roles of the team prior to operation. The initial set up of their team began when their leadership team embraced the concepts of the chronic care management model and secured funding to implement this new model of care. Through an immense investment of time and resources by the supervisory multidisciplinary leadership, a team was created and molded through participating in a learning community session, which originally outlined the goals and objectives for the NCQA and Improving Performance In Practice (IPIP) initiatives.

The team met for over a year to design their system of care. As specific tasks and roles were delineated, different team members were included in goal-setting and meetings. Usually the leadership group identified a targeted quality improvement goal, such as increasing monofilament exams with diabetic patients. They then drafted a protocol for managing the intervention and rolled out the new protocol to a pilot group. This test group worked out the initial "bugs" and tweaked the process before it went "live" with the larger group of clinic providers and staff. The teams met weekly to review these Plan-Do-Study-Act (PDSA) cycles, gauge their level of improvement, identify obstacles or communication roadblocks, and brainstorm solutions. This continual process of reviewing and improving is familiar to the team.

Effective health care teams have a shared purpose that team members can identify and articulate. Each team member needs to understand his or her roles and responsibilities, and understand team processes and how to operate within the framework of the team. Members need to feel valued and respected by other team members, particularly by the team leader or leaders. Shared accountability, shared problem solving, and shared decision-making are important elements of a functioning health care team (Interprofessional Education Collaborative Expert Panel, 2011).

Time should be set aside for the team to reflect on the changes they have implemented as a whole. The team can adapt to the changing nature of practice and to unforeseen events or untended consequences in response to previous actions when team members ask in open dialogue: What is going well? What is not going well? What do we know now that we did not know before? What needs to change in our implementation processes? In addition to taking the time necessary to develop a clear vision, the Crozer-Keystone Center for Family Health team also implemented several strategies to help reflect as a group on successes or unforeseen events. First, they hosted a variety of educational sessions for team work, such as day-long quarterly retreats over several years and monthly "lunch and learn" sessions, which helped educate providers and staff about the importance of new patient-care initiatives and opportunities for quality improvement approaches. This process helped "connect the dots" so that each team member understood how their task contributed to better patient care. When staff and providers understood the importance of their role within the whole, it helped with accountability and ownership of patient care. Second, every month, graphs and charts were used to provide feedback on improvement or declines on targeted quality improvement indicators. This helps with buy-in, staying "on message," and cheerleading successes. Using the data as a feedback tool offers opportunities for gaining top-down and bottom-up perspectives on adjusting the system of care toward a common goal. Lastly, the team felt supported by a collaborative leadership team that empowers team members to have a voice and a role in the process of change. For example, clinical teams have been given the opportunity to train the leadership team on their successes in PDSA cycles. Highlighting team members' accomplishments has added to sustainability of staff employment and satisfaction.

There are many potential barriers on the journey to effective health care team functioning. Physicians and other care providers who have traditionally functioned autonomously may not be comfortable moving into a role where the care of their patients is shared among a group. When the AIMS Center began working with the UW-affiliated primary care clinic, some PCPs viewed the program as a referral resource for mental health. PCPs made referrals to the CC and did not feel they needed to continue participation in the patient's mental health care. The AIMS Center and the CC worked with the PCPs to help them understand that the PCP plays an integral role in the IMPACT integrated behavioral health model; everyone must be an active member of the team for integrated behavioral health to work well. The AIMS Center has found that conflicts like these are best worked out by encouraging team members to communicate directly with each other, but occasionally, the clinic leadership and/or the CC and PCP's supervisors help mediate discussions.

Team members need to be able to trust each other's professional competence to effectively rely on each other. Trust, and thus team functioning, can be enhanced when the time and resources are provided for all team members to be clear in their roles and responsibilities (Wagner, 2000). The UCSDDFM team reports that the success of their team is based on role clarification, communication through the EHR, and relevant responses. When team members are acknowledged and receive responses to their requests, they can begin to trust each other and feel supported. Response time and quality of the response are necessary components of their teamwork.

If a practice's organizational structure and limits do not allow staff to be available to serve in a designated team role, then the team is unlikely to be successful. Without clear role definition, important work may be overlooked when no particular team member feels ownership of a given task. Team members can falsely presume someone else is taking care of a certain piece, when no one is. The opposite consequence of unclear role definition is duplication of efforts and responsibilities. Members may not know that someone else will complete a given task, and more than one member ends up completing the same task.

Interdisciplinary teamwork can be especially challenging in light of the entrenched medical model in which they work. Often integrated behavioral health primary care teams are functioning under the premise of a paradigm shift away from the medical model, striving to invite and appreciate all members' contributions (Nembhard & Edmondson, 2006). Yet, the hierarchy that exists in medicine remains palpable, and if a team leader is named, it is often the physician. Financial incentives are not always aligned among the team members, leading to competing interests. Perceived inequalities in status, competing objectives, separate lines of control can limit the effect of teamwork. These themes can create a rigid environment, which can lower morale or inhibit the fluid and flexible responses a health care team often needs to make (Poulton & West, 1993).

The CHFHC team acknowledged this paradigm shift when they began organizing their teams (pods). Their initiative began approximately five years ago to create a Pod Leadership Team consisting of a physician, nurse and social worker triad, who would comprise a three-pronged "leadership" team of the entire pod for patient care, issues with clinical staff, education of residents, and general workflow concerns. The interdisciplinary team interviewed for this chapter has been working together since the inception of Pod Leadership. All three members of this team agreed that working together in the face of the medical-model hierarchy required a personal and professional cultural shift. They describe being "thrown together without a lot of direction and without the necessary tools," which resulted in both conflict between the three leaders and presented a struggle for the pod members. The physician, for example, had difficulty sharing the workload, citing the medical school indoctrination that a "good doctor" is being everything to every patient and asking for help is a sign of weakness. Letting go of this notion took time and experience. This team reports that working as an effective team has not come easy, all three members agree, and they still struggle for truly having equal voices. Ultimately, this team agrees, it has taken them a full five years to create a shared vision of what patient-centered care looks like and means, how to work with each other's personalities and role definitions, how to prioritize patient's needs, and how to respond to patient complexity. The CHFHC's Organizational Development consultants has helped give their team the tools for development and evaluation, including trainings on how to work best with various personality types, on conflict resolution, and on giving and receiving feedback.

While pay differences and financial incentives may lead to competing interests, the health care team members at the UW-affiliated primary care clinic are paid separately for their services and the team has remained stable and cohesive since its inception in 2008. The clinic receives payment for a portion of the CCs salary based on the size of her active caseload. The psychiatrist receives payment for 3 hours/week for his availability to the CC and the PCPs and is able to bill for his consulting services when he sees the patients in clinic, and the PCP is paid for on a fee-for-service basis. Everyone is incentivized to collaborate to improve patient outcomes because the contracted health insurance company increases payments to the clinic when monthly quality indicators are met (Unützer et al., 2012). The AIMS Center also receives payment for its training and general consultation services through a consulting services agreement with the health plan supporting the program.

There are other potential drawbacks to team-based care. Teams may take longer to reach decisions, in comparison to decisions made by an individual provider. There can be abuses of power, competition among team members, and pressure for individual team members to conform to the wishes of the team (Michan & Rodger, 2005). Communication patterns can be dysfunctional, leading to an "in group" and an "out group", where the "in group" makes the key decisions, and the "out group" is not meaningfully included in those discussions.

Transitions in care are a safety risk for any health care team. With each transition of care, information can be misinterpreted or omitted, leading to inaccurate perceptions about the patient's care. Handoffs of care between team members should be standardized for the sake of patient safety. The UCSDDFM team operates in an educational format, training graduate behavioral health interns and medical residents, and they face both advantages and challenges. On the one hand, the trainees are learning together and from each other, and in this sense, collaboration is a part of the professional orientation from this next generation's very first practice-based experiences. On the other hand, faculty members are pulled in many directions serving both as educators and clinicians, so and competing time pressures can create miscommunications related to the urgency of a situation.

Sustainability and Continuity of Care

The sustainability of health care teams is also an area with little research. Sustaining the relationships within a health care team is likely to be fostered by regular open communication among team members, whether in the form of daily huddles, weekly administrative session, or monthly case conferences or open, frequent, and familiar communication channels.

Although there is quite a bit written about health care teams and their processes and effectiveness, published studies do not provide a clear direction on how to create or maintain high-functioning health care teams (Lemieux-Charles & McGuire, 2006). Health care teams with multiple members are subject to disruptions in continuity. Little literature has been generated on continuity in primary care teams. In fact, there is no clear recommendation about what the optimal size is for a well-functioning health care team. Larger teams bring more disciplines and greater expertise, although teams that are too large can be perceived as being less effective and individual team members may participate less. The patient will probably not have a continuity relationship with all members of the team, so it is vitally important that each team member understand his or her role in communicating the recommendations and decisions of the team to the patient.

Patients may begin to feel connected to their team rather than just one provider. According to the CHFHC team, the most ideal and effective form of collaborative communication is when they conduct a team-patient visit—the patient and two or more team members meet together in the same room at the same time. This serves multiple purposes; patients tell their story only once and feel "heard" by multiple members of the health care team, thus interpreting the team as not only the physician, but also the nurse and the social worker, and/or the medical assistant. When this is reinforced over time, the patients feel known by this enhanced team and trust various members to meet their needs, rather than only their doctor. Their care, in effect, becomes more patient-centered and comprehensive. Additionally, each team member is enabled to see their colleagues doing what they do best. This enhances their respect for each other's expertise and encourages them to rely on each other in the future. Over time, this "flow" results in each team member using his or her time most wisely, stepping in and out of the visit as necessary, with minimal interruption. In this setting, when a care plan is created with patients, the physician leader is always a contributor and other team members play various roles, depending on which needs are most pressing—medical, psychological, or social. That being said, often the nurse or social worker spends the most amount of time with the patient creating and carrying out the negotiated goals outlined in the care plan.

A Team-Oriented Tool

By Lora Council, MD, Dominic Geffken, MD & Aimee Valeras, Ph.D.

Patient-centered care plans (PCCP) are a constantly evolving communication tool for all team members, and include space for the patient's voice in the medical record (Council et al., 2012). PCCPs were developed in a quality improvement initiative at a CHFHC in an effort to improve communication, teamwork, pro-active health care, patient- and family-centered care, and patient involvement (Council et al.). The PCCP differs from traditional care plans that involve problem-based protocols, in that they rely on input from all disciplines and include negotiated plans based on the patient and family's goals.

The PCCP emerged from the frustration experienced by this multidisciplinary health care team including physicians, nurses, behavioral health staff, medical assistants, and business staff through interacting with patients on a daily basis without understanding the context of the patient's life and circumstances (Council et al., 2012). As they developed the PCCP, they realized this tool also helps address each of the joint principles of the Medical Home:

- Personal medical home: The PCCP documents individuals, their situations, priorities, and needs in a way that allows a customization of care for the individual.
- Continuity: The PCCP allows for improved continuity by providing a tool for communication between providers. Given the part-time status of every provider in this system, continuity with a personal physician is not possible. A plan that remains the same despite seeing multiple providers may improve patient's perception of continuity and continuity of care.
- Comprehensiveness: The PCCP addresses multiple quadrants of care—medical, social, behavioral, functional—and allows each team member to contribute to the overall care of the patient.
- Physician-led team: The PCCP clearly identifies team members, clarifies their roles, and assigns responsibilities in writing, helping the physician understand who is on the team and thus improves intra-team communication.
- Whole person orientation: Given that a PCCP addresses multiple quadrants of care, the patient is addressed as a whole person. Issues of acute, chronic, preventive, and palliative care can be customized for an individual in a PCCP.
- Coordinated care across a complex system: The PCCP provides the tool to record patient assessment, planning, and goals. By documenting roles and responsibilities, care plans create the foundation for coordinating care.
- Patient-centered care: PCCPs are patient centered when they incorporate patient values in addition to patient needs and wants. Patient's cultural and family values help direct the plan.

(continued)

(continued)

Thus, through creating care plans, all aspects of medical home care were enhanced. The PCCP is three "pages" within the EHR (see Fig. 10.1). It was designed to be a living document: one that is gradually completed at each interaction over time, rather than all at once. The information in the PCCP includes demographic information, information releases, and a list of collateral providers. It also includes a Patient Snapshot, which provides an opportunity for the patient to let the care team know what is important to them and for the provider to communicate important information to the care team, allowing for personalization and customization of care. The PCCP also provides space for a description of personal strengths, supports, and assets, which allows the patient identify strengths so that goal-setting and problem-solving can work from this perspective. A Medical Summary with a Problem list is included with suggested actions, continuum of care information, and an urgent plan of action, which communicates both medical and psychosocial information necessary for appropriate cross coverage or nurse phone triage. Lastly, the PCCP includes patient priorities and goals, and has a built-in section that prompts the use of motivational interviewing. It also helps sort out what needs to be done next by the patient and/or health care team. The traditional "problem/plan" form is also used, but the difference is that problems are now addressed in the context of the patient's goals and priorities. That is, the plan for the medical need, hopefully, now matches with the patient's goals.

Ultimately, the PCCP is a useable, electronic document that enables the health care team to care *for* the patient by providing the right interventions for the right person at the right time, to care *about* the patient by providing a system of care where each patient or family feels known, heard, and valued; to assign roles and responsibilities to the patient and team members; and to address goals and priorities. By using the PCCP, team functioning and patient care are enhanced (Council et al., 2012).

Quality of Evaluation and Strength of Research Evidence

Health care teams are ultimately formed to improve patient outcomes. There is a body of evidence showing that multidisciplinary team care leads to better patient health outcomes compared to usual care, although identifying which particular element of team care leads to improved outcomes is challenging. Bosch et al. (2009) examined literature on the effectiveness of health care teams on patient outcomes revealing that teams with improved coordination demonstrated positive effects on patient outcomes; however, the effects of the teams were limited in terms of costs and use of resources.

PART 1: MEDICAL SUMMARY

Name: _____ Nickname _____ DOB _____

Address: _____

Phone # (preferred)_____ (Blocked?❒ Y ❒ N) Best time to reach_____

How do you prefer to be contacted:_____

E-mail_____ Alternate Phone _____

Emergency Contact_____Phone _____ Relationship _____

Health Insurance/Plan _____ Identification #_____

Emergency Plan? ❒ Yes ❒ No   **Advance Directives?** ❒ Yes ❒ No

Allergies/reaction:

Medications/dose/purpose:

PCP _____ **Phone**_____ **Fax**_____ **E-Mail**_____

Care Manager_____**Phone**_____ **Fax**_____ **E-Mail**_____

Team RN _____ **Phone**_____ **Fax**_____ **E-Mail**_____

Medical Synopsis/Sign-out:

Who else is involved in your care? (specialists, nurses, outside agencies)

#1 Name Clinic/Hospital Phone	Other (fax, e-mail, etc.):
	Release? ❒ Y ❒ N
#2 Name Clinic/Hospital Phone	Other (fax, e-mail, etc.):
	Release? ❒ Y ❒ N
Who are the most important people in your life? *(family members, a partner, friends, coworkers, people you live with)*	

Who can we talk to about your care?	
#1 Name Relation Phone	Other (fax, e-mail, etc.):
	Release? ❒ Y ❒ N
#2 Name Relation Phone	Other (fax, e-mail, etc.):
	Release? ❒ Y ❒ N

Fig. 10.1 Outline of a typical patient-centered care plan (PCCP)

PART 2: SNAPSHOT

Snapshot: What do you want your health care team to know about you? (This can include your most important medical and/or emotional concerns. You can also include information about what you like to do in your free time, what you do for work, what your spiritual or religious affiliations are, what your financial situation is, what your unique talents or hobbies are, and what makes you happy.)	
My provider wants my care team to know:	
Urgent Plan of Care: *Do you have any recommendations for how your health care team should respond if you are in a crisis?*	

PART 3: ACTION PLAN

Patient goals		Provider goals	
Short-term			
Long-term			
Negotiated goal	Action Plan	Person responsible	Time Frame
1.			
2.			

Fig. 10.1 (continued)

There are specific examples from the literature where team-based care has been shown to improve patient outcomes. Collaborative, interdisciplinary teams can reduce inpatient mortality (Aiken, Smith, & Lake, 1994; Knaus, Draper, Wagner, & Zimmerman, 1986; West et al., 2002), functional outcomes after surgeries (Borrill, West, Shapiro, & Rees, 2000; Gittell et al., 2000; Shortell et al., 2000; Uhlig, Brown, Nason, Camelio, & Kendall, 2002), care efficiencies (Borrill et al., 2000;

Gittell et al., 2000). Heart failure care teams have been shown to reduce morbidity, enhance compliance, reduce rehospitalization, and prolong survival (Grady et al., 2000). Homebound chronically or terminally ill elderly managed by a home care team of physicians, nurse practitioners, and social workers had fewer hospitalizations, nursing home admissions, outpatient visits, and were more often able to die at home if this was their wish (Zimmer, Groth-Juncker, & McCusker, 1985). Patients with stage-three chronic kidney disease and comorbid diabetes and/or hypertension managed by a multidisciplinary team showed slower rates of decline in their renal function (Bayliss, Bhardwaja, Ross, Beck, & Lanes, 2011).

In addition to patient care outcomes, improved teamwork has lead to improved staff satisfaction and multiple studies now correlate improving staff satisfaction to improved patient satisfaction (Argentero, Dell'Olivo, & Ferretti, 2008; Borrill et al., 2000; Garman, Corrigan, & Morris, 2002; Hiss, 2006; Yang & Huang, 2005). Additionally, the work of nonphysician team members improves cancer-screening rates, office efficiency and care coordination, as well as patient and staff satisfaction (Anderson & Halley, 2008; Hudson et al., 2007; McAllister, Presler, & Cooley, 2007). Teams with higher levels of staff burnout have been shown to have significantly lower levels of patient satisfaction (Garman, Corrigan, & Morris, 2002).

Interprofessional education might also contribute to improved patient health outcomes, but the number of studies conducted in this area is limited and educating health professionals to work as a team has not clearly been associated with improved patient care outcomes. The limited number of studies found on this topic indicates that this is an area of opportunity for future research (Reeves et al., 2008).

Summary and Conclusion

The role of health care teams in patient care has expanded as complexity increases and as the number of diverse providers involved increases. Health care team members are wise to rely on the skills, expertise, and abilities of their fellow members, as an individual care provider is no longer able to effectively manage all the care needs of a single patient, particularly for those with more medically or socially complex concerns. Leading health and health education organizations support the important role of health care teams.

The characteristics of successful teams are difficult to define, but certainly there are key elements that are associated with team health. Many of these key elements are seen in the example health care teams in the section (The AIMS Center, Crozer-Keystone team, Concord Hospital Family Health Center team, University of California San Diego Family Medicine Residency team). Clear role definition, inclusive leadership, open communication, and a culture of respect for fellow team members are important characteristics of effective teams.

Collaborative partnerships: and initiatives	Vision, purpose, rationale	Health care context	Partnerships factors and qualities	Sustainability and continuity of partnerships	Evaluation/research evidence	Benefits and obstacles
Health care teams	Coordinate care, improve patient care decision making	Various settings: acute care, primary care, disease oriented, population oriented	Leadership inclusive-ness vision communication respect	Variable continuity and sustainability	Evidence supports health care teams improving patient care outcomes	Benefits: less duplication of efforts

References

AAMC Center for Workforce Studies. (2010). *Physician shortages to worsen without increases in residency training.* Retrieved April 15, 2012 from April, 2012 https://www.aamc.org/download/150584/data/physician_shortages_factsheet.pdf

Aiken, L. H., Smith, H. L., & Lake, E. T. (1994). Lower Medicare mortality among a set of hospitals known for good nursing care. *Medical Care, 32*(8), 771–787.

American Academy of Family Physicians, American Academy of Pediatrics, American College of Physicians, American Osteopathic Association. (2007). *Joint principles of the patient-centered medical home.*

Anderson, P., & Halley, M. D. (2008). A new approach to making your doctor-nurse team more productive. *Family Practice Management, 15*(7), 35–40.

Argentero, P., Dell'Olivo, B., & Ferretti, M. S. (2008). Staff burnout and patient satisfaction with the quality of dialysis care. *American Journal of Kidney Disease, 51*(1), 80–92.

Bach, P. B. (2007, June 21). Why we'll never cure cancer. *The Wall Street Journal*, p. A17.

Bayliss, E., Bhardwaja, B., Ross, C., Beck, A., & Lanes, D. (2011). Multidisciplinary team care may slow the rate of decline in renal function. *Clinical Journal of the American Society of Nephrology, 6*, 704–710.

Borrill, C., West, M. A., Shapiro, D., & Rees, A. (2000). Team working and effectiveness in health care. *British Journal of Health Care, 6*(8), 364–371.

Bosch, M., Faber, M., Cruiisberg, J., Voerman, G., Leatherman, S., Grol, R., et al. (2009). Effectiveness of patient care teams and the role of clinical expertise and coordination: A literature review. *Medical Care Research and Review, 66*(6), 5S–35S.

Council, L. S., Geffken, D., Valeras, A. B., Orzano, A. J., Rechisky, A., & Anderson, A. (2012). A medical home: Changing the way patients and teams relate through patient-centered care plans. *Family, Systems, and Health, 30*, 190–198.

Garman, A. N., Corrigan, P. W., & Morris, S. (2002). Staff burnout and patient satisfaction: Evidence of relationships at the care unit level. *Journal of Occupational Health Psychology, 7*(3), 235–241.

Gittell, H., Fairfield, K. M., Bierbaum, B., Head, W., Jackson, R., Kelly, M., et al. (2000). Impact of relational coordination on quality of care, postoperative pain and functioning, and length of stay: A nine-hospital study of surgical patients. *Medical Care, 38*(8), 807–819.

Grady, K., Dracup, K., Kennedy, G., Moser, D., Piano, M., Warner, S. L., et al. (2000). Team management of patients with heart failure: A statement for healthcare professionals from the Cardiovascular Nursing Council of the American Heart Association. *Circulation, 10*, 2443–2456.

Green, L., Graham, R., Bagley, B., Kilo, C., Spann, S., Bogdewic, S., et al. (2004). Task Force 1. Report of the task force on patient expectations, core values, reintegration, and the new model of family medicine. *Annals of Family Medicine, 2*(1), S33–S50.

Hiss, S. S. (2006). An underestimated synergy: The workplace environment, staff morale, and patient satisfaction. *Journal of American College of Radiology, 3*(3), 164–166.

Hudson, S. V., Ohman-Strickland, P., Cunningham, R., Ferrante, J. M., Hahn, K., & Crabtree, B. F. (2007). The effects of teamwork and system support on colorectal cancer screening in primary care practices. *Cancer Detection and Prevention, 31*(5), 417–423.

Institute of Medicine. (2001). *Crossing the quality chasm: A new system for the 21st century.* Washington, DC: National Academy Press.

Interprofessional Education Collaborative Expert Panel. (2011). *Core competencies for interprofessional collaborative practice: Report of an expert panel.* Washington, DC: Interprofessional Education Collaborative.

Knaus, W. A., Draper, E. A., Wagner, D. P., & Zimmerman, J. E. (1986). An evaluation of outcome from intensive care in major medical centers. *Annals of Internal Medicine, 104*(3), 410–418.

Larson, E., Fihn, S., Kirk, L., Levinson, W., Loge, R., Reyonlds, E., et al. (2004). The future of general internal medicine: Report and recommendation from the society of general internal medicine (SGIM) task force on the domain of general internal medicine. *Journal of General Internal Medicine, 19*, 69–77.

Leggat, S. (2007). Effective healthcare teams require effective team members: Defining teamwork competencies. *BMC Health Services Research, 7*(17), 1–10.

Lemieux-Charles, L., & McGuire, W. (2006). What do we know about health care team effectiveness? A review of the literature. *Medical Care Research and Review, 63*(3), 263–300.

McAllister, J. W., Presler, E., & Cooley, W. C. (2007). Practice-based care coordination: A medical home essential. *Pediatrics, 120*(3), e723–e733.

Michan, S., & Rodger, S. (2000). Characteristics of effective teams: A literature review. *Australian Health Review, 23*, 201–208.

Michan, S., & Rodger, S. (2005). Effective health care teams: A model of six characteristics developed from shared perceptions. *Journal of Interprofessional Care, 19*(4), 358–370.

Nembhard, I., & Edmondson, A. (2006). Making it safe: The effects of leader inclusiveness and professional status on psychological safety and improvement efforts in health care teams. *Journal of Organizational Behavior, 27*, 941–966.

Poulton, B., & West, M. (1993). Effective multidisciplinary teamwork in primary health care. *Journal of Advanced Nursing, 18*, 918–925.

Poulton, B., & West, M. (1999). The determinants of effectiveness in primary health teams. *Journal of Interprofessional Care, 13*(1), 7–18.

Reeves, S., Zwarenstein, M., Goldman, J., Barr, H., Freeth, D., Hammick, M., et al. (2008). Interprofessional education: Effects on professional practice and health care outcomes. *Cochrane Database of Systematic Reviews, 1*. doi:10.1002/14651858.CD002213.pub2.

Robert Graham Center: Center for Policy Studies in Family Medicine and Primary Care. (2007). *The patient centered medical home: History, seven core features, evidence and transformational change.*

Shortell, S. M., Jones, R. H., Rademaker, A. W., Gillies, R. R., Dranove, D. S., Hughes, E. F., et al. (2000). Assessing the impact of total quality management and organizational culture on multiple outcomes of care for coronary artery bypass graft surgery patients. *Medical Care, 38*(2), 207–217.

Uhlig, P. N., Brown, J., Nason, A. K., Camelio, A., & Kendall, E. (2002). John M. Eisenberg Patient Safety Awards. System innovation: Concord hospital. *The Joint Commission Journal on Quality Improvement, 28*(12), 666–672.

Unützer, J., Chan, Y. F., Hafer, E., Knaster, J., Sheilds, A., Powers, D., et al. (2012). Quality improvement with pay-for-performance incentives in integrated behavioral health care. *American Journal of Public Health, 102*(6), e41–e45.

Wagner, E. (2000). The role of patient care teams in chronic disease management. *British Medical Journal, 320*, 569–572.

West, M. A., Borrill, C., Dawson, J., Scully, J., Carter, M., Anelay, S., et al. (2002). The link between the management of employees and patient mortality in acute hospitals. *International Journal of Human Resource Management, 13*(8), 1299–1310.

Yang, K. P., & Huang, C. K. (2005). The effects of staff nurses' morale on patient satisfaction. *Journal of Nursing Research, 13*(2), 141–152.

Zimmer, J., Groth-Juncker, A., & McCusker, J. (1985). A randomized controlled study of a home health care team. *American Journal of Public Health, 75*(2), 134–141.

Chapter 11
Identification of Behavioral Health Needs in Integrated Behavioral and Primary Care Settings

Mary R. Talen and Aimee Burke Valeras

Abstract Assessing behavioral health aspects of health in the context of primary care ranges from supporting and encouraging patient's healthy protective behaviors (e.g., self-efficacy, goal-setting, action-focused coping) to screening for and diagnosing mental health and substance abuse signs, to identifying those patients with intertwined, complex medical and psychosocial needs. Identification of patients' behavioral health functioning is an essential first step in primary care integration, and, yet, it covers a wide range of psychosocial functioning. The behavioral health needs of patients can be organized on several dimensions: (1) promoting healthy behaviors and wellness, (2) identifying mental health and substance abuse risk factors and symptoms, (3) identifying medical conditions that are intertwined with behavioral health functioning, and (4) complex, intertwined biomedical and psychosocial functioning. The identification of patients within these areas takes on variety of forms—ranging from ad hoc to systematic population-based screening tools. This chapter offers a schematic template for the various methods of behavioral health identification along with specific examples of population-based tools for patients' behavioral health strengths and needs in primary care settings.

M.R. Talen, Ph.D. (✉)
Northwestern Family Medicine Residency, Erie Family Health Center,
2570 W. North Ave., Chicago, IL 60647, USA
e-mail: mary.talen@gmail.com

A.B. Valeras, Ph.D., MSW
NH Dartmouth Family Medicine Residency, Concord Hospital Family Health Center,
250 Pleasant St., 03301, Concord, NH, USA
e-mail: aimeevaleras@gmail.com

M.R. Talen and A. Burke Valeras (eds.), *Integrated Behavioral Health in Primary Care:*
Evaluating the Evidence, Identifying the Essentials, DOI 10.1007/978-1-4614-6889-9_11,
© Springer Science+Business Media New York 2013

Introduction

Assessing behavioral health aspects of health in the context of primary care falls along a broad continuum. It ranges from supporting and encouraging patient's healthy protective behaviors (e.g., self-efficacy, goal-setting, action-focused coping) to screening for and diagnosing mental health and substance abuse signs, to identifying those patients with intertwined, complex medical and psychosocial needs. Like preventive primary care where patients are assessed for a range of system functioning (e.g., cardiac, pulmonary, digestive), patient's behavioral health functioning should also be assessed. Identifying patients' functioning on different levels—cognitive, emotional, family relationships, community-cultural context—are important processes for addressing holistic health care.

Purpose of Identification of Behavioral Health Issues in Primary Care

The overarching principles for identifying patients and patient populations that might benefit from the prevention, acute care, and chronic/complex health care needs in primary care are an essential initial phase in any integrated system of care. Identifying individuals who can benefit from a variety of behavioral health support, integrated care plans, and treatment is a complex process. Identification of patients' behavioral health functioning is an essential first step in primary care integration and, yet, it is a broad and robust concept. The behavioral health needs of patients can be organized on several dimensions: (1) promoting healthy behaviors and wellness, (2) identifying mental health and substance abuse risk factors and symptoms, (3) identifying medical conditions that are intertwined with behavioral health functioning, and (4) complex, intertwined biomedical and psychosocial functioning. The identification of patients within these areas takes on a variety of forms—ranging from ad hoc to systematic population-based screening tools. The detection of behavioral health functioning of individuals also varies depending on different categories such as stages of the life cycle, gender, sexual orientation issues, or other physical health diagnoses (e.g., diabetes, asthma, HTN). For example, some parents may be identified as needing coaching on parenting skills with their toddler while other individuals may be identified as ready to quit smoking and in need of motivational interviewing to support their behavior change. In primary care, the detection of behavioral health factors in primary care is done in a variety of ways.

First, detection of behavioral health needs is often done on a case-by-case basis. Individuals can be identified by health care providers or staff as needing some sort of behavioral health support through a variety of clinical situations, such as patients who make many repeat visits for the same condition, frequent and lengthy calls, switches from doctor to doctor, or patients who have higher than usual billing claims. Just asking providers, medical assistants, nurses, and front desk about which patients are continually "needing something more" can generate a list of patients who could benefit from behavioral health integrated into their medical care. This method of detecting patients for behavioral health intervention is usually individually focused, not population-based, and tailored to the unique context of a clinical setting.

Detection includes those who may benefit from behavioral health interventions, even if they do not have a mental health or substance abuse condition. Common examples include patients who complain of fatigue or pain with few "physical findings," who suffer delayed recovery from injuries, who do not respond as expected to typical medical treatments, who have strained relationships with providers, who are "frequent attenders" to primary care practices without a pattern of medical conditions that would normally explain the frequent visits, or who are regularly seeking new tests, procedures, specialists, or new doctors, or whose care is extremely fragmented or characterized by "non-compliance." Some of these patients may have distinct diagnosable mental health or substance abuse conditions underlying these complaints, but many others may be distressed, demoralized, discouraged, fearful, distrustful, and unhappy without discrete mental health conditions or are at "subclinical" levels. The purpose of detection in primary care is not to "find and treat a new disease" but to apply the kinds of expertise commonly found in behavioral health professionals to the overall understanding of these patients. Their care can then be coordinated by integrating the care across participating professionals and facilities and addressing the emotional, behavioral, and social aspects that drive the distress, whether these are mental health diagnoses, effective emotional coping strategies, or otherwise. Other information such as visit data, claims data, and clinical indicators might also be used to identify patients who may benefit from behavioral health services (C. J. Peek, personal communication, August 25, 2012).

A second method for detecting behavioral health issues is through screening. Screening individuals for behavioral health is a subset of the more case-based identification process and the distinctions between identification and screening need to be defined. Screening is typically something you do with patients using one or more validated screening tools. Identification of those who can benefit from integrated behavioral health through formal screening tools has been applied to population-based approaches for detecting patients at risk for substance abuse or mental health conditions.

It is also useful for health care professionals to identify specific patient populations that are at risk for mental health concerns and should be the focus of provider's attention. A population-based approach can identify broad risk categories or subpopulations for more standardized screening (e.g., PHQ-9), follow-up assessment, and then specific treatment protocols. For example, diabetics, post partum patients, or seniors may be identified as specific population groups where focused behavioral health screening, assessment, and perhaps treatment guidelines are implemented (See Chaps. 12, 13, and 14).

When behavioral health concerns are detected, using either individual or patient-population-based screening for further behavioral health assessment is the next essential step. The follow-up assessment process and interventions can be divided into four major categories: (1) health promotion, protective factors, and wellness, (2) mental health and substance abuse, such as depression and alcohol misuse,

(3) clinical situations where physical symptoms such as pain, fatigue, and headaches or perplexing patient presentations that may be addressed with both biomedical and psychosocial approaches, or (4) patients with chronic conditions who would benefit from behavioral health coaching and life-style changes, such as diabetes, obesity, and smoking, where healthy life-style counseling and behavior changes can improve functioning. (See Table 11.1, which illustrates the scope of integrated behavioral health that depicts these categories for identifying individuals for a range biopsychosocial care plans).

Strategies for Initial Detection of Behavioral Health Needs in Primary Care

Patient Engagement, Quality of Life, and Social Support

Promoting prevention and wellness are cornerstones for primary care health systems, and many who present with chronic diseases or health conditions such as fatigue, insomnia, or chronic pain could benefit from integrated behavioral health. Patients with tobacco abuse, diabetes, obesity, asthma, chronic pain, insomnia, or dementia are commonly seen in primary care settings and may benefit from behavioral health interventions such as motivational interviewing, resiliency training, or problem-solving skills. Yet, there are no well-established standardized identification tools that alert providers to behavioral health interventions that may enhance a patient's ability to manage or cope with a life stressor, health condition, or disease, much less enhance wellness and resiliency.

Currently, screening is primarily focused on mental health or substance abuse and chronic disease. The few existing standardized screening tools that assess the patient's quality of life, readiness for change, level of engagement in their health care, social support, optimism, and self-efficacy have not been systematically used or evaluated in primary care settings. Consequently, we have few guidelines and many opportunities to expand our understanding of the relationship between different types of behavioral health screening and health conditions or health promotion. The following list provides examples on the types of identification tools that may help shape the direction of these integrated care clinical interventions that range from promoting healthy habits to intervening in complex biopsychosocial care strategies.

Patient Activation Measurement (PAM). The PAM assessment tool and its shorter 17-item version (PAM-17) identifies a patient's level of engagement with the health care system and the level of self-efficacy in his/her own health care by gaging knowledge, skills, and confidence to manage one's own health and health care (Hibbard, Stockard, Mahoney, & Tusler, 2004; Hibbard, Mahoney, Stockard, & Tusler, 2005). PAM scores predict health care outcomes including medication adherence, ER utilization, and hospitalization and can help providers match their

Table 11.1 Areas of application for integrated behavioral health in primary care: examples of screening, assessment, and treatment (Adapted from MRT by CJP 8-25-12)

Area of application for integrated behavioral health	Promoting healthy behavior and protective factors	Mental health and substance abuse conditions	Medical conditions with intertwined behavioral health factors	Complex situations: clinical, health system and patient factors needing team-based care
A. Identification or screening	*Promotion* of health behavior change in chronic disease or prevention; *Behavioral risk assessment* for health and functional status. Methods: health risk assessments; behavioral/wellness checklists; developmental screening	*Screening* for MH/SA conditions that can be understood and treated more or less independently of other health concerns. Methods: basic MH/SA screening tools	*Screening* for complicated/uncontrolled medical conditions intertwined with MH/SA conditions. Methods: basic MH/SA screening tools in context of medical condition treatment	*Identification* of pts with physical symptoms or common PC complaints not fully explained via disease processes. Methods: • General sx checklists • Problem lists • Recurring visits • Basic MH screening. *Detection* of care delivery patterns in records and claims associated with: • Over utilization • Unfocused utilization • Unplanned visits, ER, hosp, urgent care • Many failed services • Distrustful pt-clin rel • Pt unhappiness with care—feeling stuck • Provider feeling stuck
B. Assessment	Interview and planning by nurse, BH consultant, physician, care coordinator, health coach	Referral to BH consultant for evaluation	Synchronized medical and BH care planning and goal-setting	Incorporation of BH consultant with physician in evaluation and care planning. Reading records with patterns above to find out what is going on; involve patient as appropriate
C. Treatment	Self-management plan guided by motivational interviewing or other adjusted goal-setting	BH treatment in or outside PC clinic—with or without close involvement from physician	Carrying out single coordinated care plan in shared EHR with treatment adjusted to targets	BH treatment in close coordination with physician or jointly. Carrying out single coordinated care plan in shared EHR with treatment adjusted to targets

interventions with patients' varying levels of engagement in their health care. This tool holds strong psychometric properties but is not easily accessible for primary care health centers due to its cost and restrictions.

Health Related Quality of Life Scales (HRQOL). HRQOL focuses on general well-being with questions about perceived physical and mental health and function, which are important components of health assessment and are generally considered valid indicators for identifying patient needs, targeting interventions, and evaluating outcomes. Self-reported quality of life health status has also been a more powerful predictor of mortality and morbidity than many objective measures of health (Fiellin, Reid, & O'Connor, 2000). Medical Outcomes Study Short Forms (SF-12 and SF-36), the Sickness Impact Profile, and the Quality of Well-Being Scale are some of the measures that assess HRQOL and functional status. The SF-36, for example, is used to evaluate the quality of care in managed care plans and other health care applications. While these measures have been widely used and extensively validated in clinical settings and special population studies, their length often makes them impractical to use in population surveillance.

Social Support Measures. Social support measures like the Duke Health Profile or Holmes Rahe Social Support could help providers to incorporate social determinants of health into the assessment and health care plan. Health and Psychosocial Instruments (HaPI) is a database that provides access to information on approximately 15,000 measurement instruments (i.e., questionnaires, interview schedules, checklists, coding schemes, rating scales, etc.) in the fields of health and psychosocial sciences. This resource gives a wealth of information on a wide range of measurement and survey tools including the history of the instrument, reliability and validity evidence, the history of an instrument over time, and information on how to obtain the instrument.

Clinical Example of Identification of Behavioral Health Needs

At one community health center, which also houses a family medicine residency, a group of integrated behavioral health clinicians (M. Chase Levesque, Psy.D., Aimee Valeras, Ph.D., Joni Haley, M.S. and William Gunn, Ph.D.) developed an "Integrated Care Assessment Tool" (ICAT) as a way of identifying people who are struggling with a variety of psychosocial stressors and/or mental health disorders. The ICAT is meant to serve two purposes: (1) to identify which patients should have comprehensive screening tools administered to better detect mental health disorders or substance use disorders and (2) to triage patient's needs to deliver the most appropriate level of behavioral health interventions.

The ICAT is a 24-question, one double-sided page that briefly assesses psychosocial stressors across a range of areas (See Fig. 11.1). It includes gaps in basic need resources, like financial stress, housing, food, and transportation, relationship stressors including grief, violence, abuse, and trauma, history of mental health diagnoses and treatments tried, current symptoms of depression, anxiety, mania, substance use, and lastly, personal strengths and coping mechanisms.

How did you get referred to an Integrated Behavioral Health Clinic (IBHC)?

⊓ Medical assistant   ☐ Other:

⊓ self   ⊓ Psychiatrist   ⊓ Community mental health center

⊓ IBHC   ⊓ ER

⊓ Provider   ⊓ Inpatient psychiatric team   ⊓ State hospital past therapist

⊓ Nurse

Primary Care Physician:

What is the problem most distressing to you right now?

How has your health been in general during the past 4 weeks?

⊓ Excellent   ☐ Good   ⊓ Fair   ☐ Poor

Are you currently employed?

⊔ Yes   ⊔ No, recv unempl.   ⊔ Satisfactory   ☐ Other:

⊔ No, no benefits   ⊔ No, recv disability   ⊔ Stressful situation

Do you currently have housing?

⊓ Yes   ⊓ No, shelter   ⊓ Stable   ⊓ Satisfactory

⊓ Living w/ friends   ⊓ No, on streets   ⊓ Unstable   ⊓ Stressful situation

Who do you currently live with?

Do you have access to enough food to feed yourself and your family?

⊓ Yes   ⊓ Receives food stamps   ☐ Utilizes food pantries / soup kitchens   ⊓ Needs additional food resources

Do you have any current legal involvement?

⊓ No   ⊓ Yes, minor   ☐ Yes, significant

Do you have problems with transportation in getting to medical appointments?

⊓ No   ⊓ Yes, but I can find a way   ⊓ Yes, I have no options

Are you experiencing any problems with the people closest to you right now?

⊓ No   ⊓ Yes

Do you have any reason to be frightened in any of your relationships?

⊓ No   ⊓ Yes

Fig. 11.1 Integrated Care Assessment Tool (ICAT) (Developed by Aimee Valeras, Ph.D., M. Chase Leveseque, Psy.D., Joni Haley, M.S., William Gunn, Ph.D. as a tool to triage behavioral health needs in a primary care setting)

Have you recently experienced any loss or grief?
     ◻ None   ◻ Mild   ◻ Significant

Over the past 2 weeks, have you felt down, depressed or hopeless?
    ◻ Not at all   ◻ Some days ◻ Most days ◻ Nearly every day

◻   ◻

Over the past 2 weeks, have you had little interest or pleasure in doing things?
    ◻ Not at all   ◻ Some days ◻ Most days ◻ Nearly every day

Do you have thoughts of hurting yourself or that you would be better off dead?
(If answer is affirmative, complete full suicide assessment)
    ◻ Not at all   ◻ Some days ◻ Most days ◻ Nearly every day

During the past 6 months, how often have you been bothered by excessive worry and anxiety and had difficulty controlling the worry?
    ◻ Not at all   ◻ Some days ◻ Most days ◻ Nearly every day

In your life have you had an upsetting, frightening, or horrible experience, which was out of the ordinary realm of life?
    ◻ No   ◻ Yes

Has their ever been a period of time when you were not your usual self and you felt so good or so hyper that other people thought you were not your normal self or you were so hyper that you got into trouble?
    ◻ No   ◻ Yes

How often do you have a drink containing alcohol?
  ◻ Never ◻ Monthly or less ◻ 2-4 times/month ◻ 2-3 times/week ◻ 4 or more times/wk

How many drinks containing alcohol do you have on a typical day?

  ◻ 1 or 2 ◻ 3 or 4 ◻ 5 or 6 ◻ 7 to 9 ◻ 10 or more

Do you use other drugs?
    ◻ No   ◻ Yes

Have you been diagnosed with a mental health disorder in the past?
    ◻ No   ◻ Yes:

  If yes, what treatments were tried?
    ◻ None   ◻ Couples therapy ◻ Medication ◻ Alternative modes
    ◻ Indiv therapy   ◻ Hospitalization ◻ Other
         ◻ Family therapy
         ◻ Group therapy

What helps you cope? What are your strengths? What resources do you have access to?

Fig. 11.1 (continued)

Delivering quality integrated care includes providing the right treatment to the right person at the right time (Clancy, 2008). The ICAT helps clinicians understand the contextual environment in which a person functions to help determine what the "right" and most appropriate behavioral health intervention to offer to one particular patient (see Chap. 13 on implementing clinical interventions). The spectrum of behavioral health interventions can range from assisting a patient to access resources that meet their basic needs, collaborating with community providers and external medical providers to reduce duplication of services and fragmentation of care, addressing challenging behaviors, providing crisis intervention, health behavior change support, facilitating family and/or team meetings, assisting with conflict resolution, to traditional therapy. The ICAT includes brief questions about mental health disorders e.g., PHQ-2 that indicate a need for further screening in these areas.

References

Clancy, C. (2008) *Measuring healthcare quality* [online tutorial]. Menlo Park, CA: KaiserEDU, Henry J. Kaiser Family Foundation. Accessed September, 2012, from http://www.kaiseredu.org/tutorials/quality/player.html

Fiellin, D. A., Reid, M. C., & O'Connor, P. G. (2000). Screening for alcohol problems in primary care: A systematic review. *Archives of Internal Medicine, 160*(13), 1977–1989.

Hibbard, J. H., Mahoney, E. R., Stockard, J., & Tusler, M. (2005). Development and testing of a short form of the patient activation measure. *Health Services Research, 40*(6 Pt 1), 1918–1930. doi:10.1111/j.1475-6773.2005.00438.x.

Hibbard, J. H., Stockard, J., Mahoney, E. R., & Tusler, M. (2004). Development of the Patient Activation Measure (PAM): Conceptualizing and measuring activation in patients and consumers. *Health Services Research, 39*(4 Pt 1), 1005–1026. doi:10.1111/j.1475-6773.2004.00269.x.

Chapter 12
Screening Measures in Integrated Behavioral Health and Primary Care Settings

Mary R. Talen, Joane G. Baumer, and Misty M. Mann

Abstract Screening is the process of measuring and detecting the signs and symptoms of a disorder before the disorder has progressed. While the evidence on the effectiveness and quality of mental health screening tools is advancing, the application of these tools into standard clinical practice has lagged behind due to implementation barriers in primary care settings. The goal of this chapter is to address the range of screening tools for specific patient populations and to address the barriers for incorporating these standardized tools into primary care. This chapter provides descriptions of reliable and valid screening tools for preschoolers, school-age children, adolescents, adults and older adults—men and women—and older adults. There are also descriptions of how screening tools are used in a clinical setting by defining roles and responsibilities for team members, identifying practice management and financial considerations, and describing relevant opportunities for quality improvement.

M.R. Talen, Ph.D. (✉)
Northwestern Family Medicine Residency, Erie Family Health Center,
2570 W. North Ave., Chicago, IL 60647, USA
e-mail: mary.talen@gmail.com

J.G. Baumer, M.D.
Department of Family Medicine, JPS Health Network, Tarrant County Hospital District,
1500 South Main Street, Fort Worth, TX 76102, USA
e-mail: jbaumer@jpshealth.org

M.M. Mann, Psy.D.
The Chicago School of Professional Psychology, Chicago, IL, USA
e-mail: mistymann@gmail.com

M.R. Talen and A. Burke Valeras (eds.), *Integrated Behavioral Health in Primary Care:*   239
Evaluating the Evidence, Identifying the Essentials, DOI 10.1007/978-1-4614-6889-9_12,
© Springer Science+Business Media New York 2013

Introduction

Screening is the process of measuring and detecting the signs and symptoms of a disorder before the disorder has progressed. This is one area of integrated care practice that rests on epidemiological, population-based research and straddles research-based initiatives and clinical approaches (Ansseau et al., 2004). While the evidence on the effectiveness and quality of mental health screening tools is advancing, the application of these tools into standard clinical practice has lagged behind due to implementation barriers in primary care settings. The goal of this chapter will be to address the range of screening tools for specific populations and to address the barriers for incorporating these standardized tools into primary care. We will describe how they are used in a clinical setting by defining roles and responsibilities for team members, identifying practice management and financial considerations, and describing relevant opportunities for quality improvement (see Peek, Chap. 2).

Background of Behavioral Health Screening in Primary Care

Screening for medical or behavioral health conditions within a population is a relatively new prevention initiative in health care. The U.S. Preventative Services Task Force (2010), which is now under the auspices of Agency of Healthcare Research and Quality (AHRQ)'s Prevention and Care Management Portfolio, makes health care recommendations based on the support of an Evidence-based Practice Center, which conducts systematic reviews of the evidence on specific topics in clinical prevention. These recommendations are meant to prevent complications from advanced disease processes and to help contain health care costs. Over the past 20 years, USPSTF's screening recommendations have increased. Initially starting with recommendations against smoking and for mammogram screenings, but recognizing the need for further preventive screenings, it has expanded to 45 recommendations in 2010.

Behavioral health screening in primary care is an even newer phenomenon than physical preventive health screenings. Behavioral health counseling interventions are seen as important within primary care, but the empirical evidence for supporting and implementing these interventions is still in the early stages of development. Presently, the USPSTF reviews evidence for all age groups and makes recommendations based on developmental stages: infants, preschool, school-age, adolescents, young adults, adults, and aging/older adults. Current standardized screening recommendations, organized by patients' age, gender, and current health status, are listed at the USPSTF website.

Criteria for screening. There are several requirements for instituting behavioral health screening measures in primary care (AHRQ, 2010):

- The clinical situation must be sufficiently common within a target group to merit screening.
- There must be well-supported methods for applying behavioral health expertise to mitigate the situation in an effort to improve the health outcome and use of health care and patient resources.
- Screening must result in the situation being recognized at an earlier stage when intervention is more effective.
- Screening must have high specificity, meaning that the mechanism is likely to detect the accurate clinical situation (low rate of false positives).
- Screening must have high sensitivity, meaning that the tool is unlikely to detect patients who are not in that situation (low rate of false negatives).
- The screening test must be feasible in that it: (a) can be done relatively easily (b) with little additional expense relative to the costs incurred in letting these clinical situations persist and worsen and (c) is easy and acceptable for the patient.

There are currently no Grade A screening recommendations for behavioral health and only four USPSTF screening recommendations that meet the Grade B criteria (health care providers should offer or provide this service) for behavioral health screening. They are: (1) alcohol misuse, (2) depression, (3) obesity, and (4) smoking. There are a number of behavioral health areas, such as illicit drug use, family violence, healthy lifestyles, or speech and language where there is insufficient evidence to support screening recommendations. Table 12.1 outlines the USPSTF recommendations for behavioral-health-oriented screening and counseling (AHRQ, 2010).

The gold standards for preventive health care screenings based on population-based studies have been set by USPSTF; however, they are not the only organization that offers behavioral health screening recommendations. The Center for Disease Control (CDC), American Association of Pediatrics (AAP) (2001), American College of Obstetricians and Gynecologists (ACOG), American Association of Family Physicians (AAFP), American College of Physicians (ACP), The National Commission on Prevention Priorities (NCPP), The Canadian Task Force on Preventative Care, and the Institute of Medicine (IOM) have outlined other recommendations that are unique for primary care populations. Internationally, the National Institute for Health and Clinical Excellence (NICE) (2012) is the UK's organization that manages a national health care data base, offers a wealth of evidence-based recommendations, and provides clinical algorithms.

Embedding Screening in the Context of Health Care Delivery Practices

Screening and detection of any disorder that requires further assessment is a complex process. Screening protocols assume that (a) detection will lead to early intervention, which can prevent a mental health or substance abuse disease process from advancing, and that (b) improved health outcomes and/or cost-effectiveness result from clearly defined screening guidelines, according to epidemiological studies and

Table 12.1 USPSTF behavioral health screening and counseling recommendations

Behavioral health screening	Date of recommendation	Description
Alcohol misuse screening; (Drinking, risky/hazardous) adults and pregnant women	Screening and counseling 2004	Grade B[a] Offer or provide this service
Depression screening for adults (>18) and adolescents (12–18)	2009	Grade B[a] Offer or provide this service when staff-assisted depression care supports *are in place*
Depression screening for adults (>18)	2009	Grade B[a] Offer or provide this service when staff-assisted depression care supports *are not in place*
Obesity screening and counseling: children and adults	2003 (Adults) 2010 (Children)	Grade B[a] Offer or provide this service
Smoking screening and tobacco cessation counseling	Counseling and interventions 2009	Grade A[b] Offer or provide this service
Dementia (Alzheimer's disease)	Screening	I[c]
Drug use, illicit	Screening 2008	I[c]
Family violence	Screening 2004	I[c]

[a]B: The USPSTF recommends the service. There is high certainty that the net benefit is moderate or there is moderate certainty that the net benefit is moderate to substantial
[b]A: USPSTF highly recommends the service
[c]I: The USPSTF concludes that the current evidence is insufficient to assess the balance of benefits and harms of the service. Evidence is lacking, of poor quality, or conflicting, and the balance of benefits and harms cannot be determined. If the service is offered, patients should understand the uncertainty about the balance of benefits and harms

evidence-based research. Therefore, sufficient evidence is needed to support the use of behavioral health screening measures for a specific population in a primary care setting.

Screening is not a diagnostic litmus test, but an indicator that further assessment is needed. Screening for mental health conditions, consequently, is not a diagnosis of a mental health condition. And, clinical situations where a patient may require behavioral health expertise does not confirm or sufficiently describe which behavioral health intervention is needed. Clinical interviewing, judgment, and decision-making processes of the provider are not replaced but augmented by standardized screening. Screening tools supplement the provider-patient relationship, with the understanding that unique patient needs, style, cultural and family backgrounds, and other factors may influence the validity of a screening tool. Choosing the appropriate tool among the many screening tools and assessment instruments is just one of the initial steps in implementation. The larger health care context plays a significant role in the effective use of screening.

Using screening tools goes beyond choosing a measurement and "sending patients off" and expecting something to change. Incorporating screening tools into clinical practice is a process that may begin with identifying the target population or condition, choosing reliable tool(s), and then implementing and nurturing a system of care to achieve expected benefits and outcomes. It requires the entire practice to adapt and embrace the incorporation of this process. These questions and tasks are described in Fig. 12.1, using the integrated care practice "lexicon" (See Chap. 2; Peek, 2011) as the framework.

In this chapter, valid and reliable screening tools for primary care will be described using the what, how, and supported by parameters of integrated care: (1) defining the team members' level of training, roles and tasks, and communication between providers about the screening results; (2) identifying the patient population and rationale for screening—life stages and/or specific patient group with particular

Defining clauses (In common for all integrated care)	Parameters (What might vary from practice to practice)	Questions, issues, tasks for implementing screening	Examples
HOW: A team	1. Team composition	Which team members are involved in screening? (e.g. PCP, nursing, medical assistant, care coordinator, behavioral health professional) • What are their roles/responsibilities in the screening process? • What is the necessary training for each in screening process?	PCP, medical assistant and behavioral health provider
	2. Level of collaboration or integration	How and how closely are team members to communicate about screening results and follow-up? • Coordinated: basic collaboration at a distance • Co-located: basic collaboration on-site • Integrated: shared space, systems, care plans, culture	PCP, MA and Behavioral Health provider huddle 3 times/week routinely to identify appropriate screening tools for adult diabetic patients scheduled for clinic.
With	3.		

Fig. 12.1 Questions, tasks, and examples for embedding screening effectively in practice (See Chaps. 2 and 11)

a shared population and mission	B. Life stage	What age group population is to be screened? Pre-school, School-age, Adolescents, Adults, Seniors, Life-limiting illness.	Adult diabetic patients who have established care in PCMH and are scheduled for follow-up visit
	C. People with identified conditions or situations	What are you screening for? • Mental health or substance abuse conditions. • Behavioral / emotional factors interfering with chronic illness care, e.g., diabetes, cardiovascular, asthma. • Behavioral health risk to success of planned or routine situations, e.g., pregnancy, surgical procedures, preventive care, transitions of care • Behavioral / emotional /social factors in chronic pain, recovery from illness or injury, over-utilization of services, unhappiness or non-engagement with care or providers, social factors interfering with care. Some combination of these?	Screening for depression and anxiety with adult diabetic patients
	4. Method for screening patient population	What are the best screening tools to identify your target population? • Specific tool for a patient population? Universal screening tool? • System indicators, e.g. visit data, claims data,	PHQ-2 and GAD-2 with new and established patients with DM II diagnosis

Fig. 12.1 (continued)

attention to the cultural, socioeconomic, and gender issues; (3) describing the clinical screening tools, including the primary purpose and function of the standardized screening tools along with its specificity and sensitivity, (4) outlining the office management process and financial systems for effectively using screening tools

		registries? Provider or patient? • Some combination of these?	
Using a systematic clinical system	5. Program scale or maturity	What is the expected scope or scale for screening process at this point? • Pilot—a circumscribed test or demonstration in one or two places • Project—a larger scale, but still limited program within certain bounds • Mainstream—full-scale implementation across entire practice or organization	Project: Consistent project with a designated team—PCP, MA, BH, and a targeted panel of diabetic patients seen on consistent days (e.g. Mon, Wed, Fri) but with limited number of days/week
	6. Level of patient engagement	How are patients involved in the screening process and follow-up care? • A background function they may or may not be aware of or data entry • A prominent feature of the patient-clinician interaction? Patient self-scoring tools • Explicit shared decision-making. or mostly provider decision-making	Diabetic patients with positive screening meet with Behavioral Health provider (15-20 minutes) for assessment and follow-up shared care plan Options for follow-up counseling, group visits, and/or medication discussed.
	7. Level of practice reliability / standardization	How consistent, reliable, and standardized are screening processes? • Informal—individual clinician identification—variability across clinicians • Some processes consistent or standardized	Schedule same continuity team (e.g. PCP, MA, BH) on the consistent clinic days (e.g. Mon, Wed, Fri, AM) PCP tags diabetic adults for MA to handout PHQ-2 and GAD-2 prior to medical visit. BH scores, documents/reports results to PCP and Patient. BH follows up with positive

Fig. 12.1 (continued)

such as cost, time, and billing; and (5) using a data collection system to track individual and/or clinical population trends and identifying quality improvement methods. Since there are a host of resources, such as Health and Psychosocial Instruments (HaPI database) for mental health and behavioral health assessment

		• Most or all screening processes consistent, reliable, standard	results.
SUPPORTED BY: Office practice and financial system	8. Business model / billing system	How is screening made a sustainable part of business model? • Billing codes for screening. Specified part of bundled services payments. • Expected as normal part of clinic processes paid in usual manner. • Some combination of these.	Billing for screening: 96110 with .59 modifier A level 3 office visit in which three developmental screening instruments were administered, scored and interpreted: 99213: Evaluation and Management 96110: Screening Tool: ASQ 96110-59: MCHAT Bill Health and Behavior codes (CPT 95801) when behavioral health provider meets with patients with a positive screening and assesses patient more fully.
	9. Practice-based data collection, analysis, and actual use	What processes are in place for routinely collecting, analyzing, and using screening data to improve care, quality, and effectiveness? • How is practice data used to guide changes in team-based care and clinical processes? • For individual patients, entire practice panel, community trends	Team of PCP, MA, BH meets monthly to review patients with positive screening results. Review follow-up with panel of depressed, diabetic patients. Review and track follow-up screening results for panel of patients.
With ongoing QI and effectiveness measurement		• QI feedback to teams on quality measures.	PDSA cycles implemented (Plan, Do, Study, Act) using PHQ9

Fig. 12.1 (continued)

instruments, the focus of this chapter is not to provide an exhaustive list of behavioral health screening tools, rather to focus on the most common standardized tools used in primary care settings and, more importantly, address the components within the health care setting that are needed to effectively embed these tools for patient-centered care.

Health Care Team: Defining Roles, Responsibilities, and Communication in Screening

One of the first steps in effectively implementing screening tools is defining the roles and responsibilities of each team member—physicians, nurses, medical assistants, behavioral health providers, and support staff. The team has the responsibility of making a number of screening decisions, such as who gets screened and with what screening tools. The responsibility of administering, scoring, reporting results to the patient or family, and managing follow-up care needs to be discussed and delegated among team members. Without clearly defined tasks and communication pathways, information from screening tools are often not completed, reviewed or discussed with patients much less become part of the clinical monitoring system for follow-up care (Hayutin, Reed-Knight, Blount, Lewis, & McCormick, 2009; Herman-Staab, 1994; Pinto-Martin et al., 2005).

Patient Populations and Clinical Screening Tools

Pediatric Screening Tools

Developmental screening for children seen in primary care has been an important and growing area of interest in our primary care system (Tolan & Dodge, 2005). The purpose of screening children is to identify those who should receive more intensive assessment or diagnosis for potential developmental delays. Screening can promote earlier detection of developmental delays, which is correlated with improved prognosis and healthier outcomes for children who receive early intervention thereby improving child health and well-being (Borowsky, Mozayeny, & Ireland, 2003; Center for Disease Control and Prevention [CDC], 2011; Glascoe, 2005; Richardson, Keller, Selby-Harrington, & Parrish, 1996; Sheldrick, Merchant, & Perrin, 2011).

Well-child checkups in primary care are a natural venue for direct contact with parents and their children and an opportunity for systematic continuity of developmental screening. Primary care providers are in a unique position to provide developmental assessments within the context of the physician–family relationship to support normal development and identify and intervene when children exhibit early warning signs of risks. It is estimated that 17 % of children have a developmental disability or behavioral disorder (Glascoe, 2005). However, studies have indicated consistently that infants and young children who have clinically significant developmental delays are not adequately detected in pediatric primary care (Drotar, Stancin, Dworkin, Sices, & Wood, 2008; Richardson et al., 1996). Only a fraction (30 %) of the children who have a developmental disability (17 %) are identified in the health care settings (Polaha, Dalton, & Allen, 2011; Sand et al., 2005). Consequently, critical opportunities for early intervention are lost.

Routine screening for developmental delays, mental health, and psychosocial problems in pediatrics has also become a matter of policy (Blanchard, Gurka, & Blackman, 2006). Medicaid, the federal health insurance program that provides health care for 20 million of the nation's economically impoverished children, implemented the Early Periodic Screening Diagnosis and Treatment Program (EPSDT) which mandates well-child visits to include screening for mental health and developmental problems (Brickman, Garrity, & Shaw, 2002; Sheldrick et al., 2011). The need to focus more attention on children's psychosocial problems has been underscored and raised to the level of policy recommendations by national benchmarking efforts like Healthy People 2010 (U.S. Department of Health and Human Services, 2000).

The American Association of Pediatricians (AAP) recommends performing developmental surveillance at every well-child visit and using a formal screening tool at the 9-, 18-, 24-, and 30-month checkups (Drotar et al., 2008) and then, annually beginning at 3 years of age (LaRosa, 2010) (See Table 12.2). In contrast, the United States Preventive Services Task Force (USPSTF) does not recommend screening for speech, language, or developmental delay in preschool children due to insufficient evidence. Despite this, AAP continues to recommend the use of screening tools to identify and describe the level of the child's risk for developmental delay as a means to systematically monitor and assess a child's developmental progression (Blanchard et al., 2006; Glascoe, 2005; Nelson, Nygren, Walker, & Panoscha, 2006; Pinto-Martin, Souders, 2005; Schonwald, Huntington, Chan, Risko, & Bridgemohan, 2009; Sheldrick et al., 2011; Williams, Klinepeter, Palmes, Pulley, & Foy, 2004).

Preschool Population

There are two recommended screening instruments for general screening during well-child visits with infants and toddlers; the Pediatric Evaluation of Developmental Status (PEDS) and the Ages and Stages Questionnaire (ASQ), including the Social and Emotional Surveys (ASQ-SE) (Drotar et al., 2008). Parents complete these surveys before office visits and the results are shared with the parents during the visit. Clinical staff—medical assistance, nurses, or physicians—may enter the information into the medical charts to track the developmental progression of the child, similar to growth chart tracking systems (Lazarus, 1999; Sices, Stancin, Kirchner, & Bauchner, 2009; Wallis & Pinto-Martin, 2008).

Pediatric Evaluation of Developmental Status (PEDS). The primary purpose of PEDS is for identification of general developmental delays based on the parent/caregiver's concerns. PEDS moderately identifies children with developmental risks (Glascoe, 2005). The ten-question tool is written at a fifth grade level, is available in multiple languages, and takes 2–5 min to complete and less than 1 min for a provider or staff member to score. The limitations of this instrument are also its strengths. As it relies on parental self-report on global areas of functioning, parents

Table 12.2 Pediatric screening tools in primary care

Patient populations	Clinical system: screening tools (sensitivity; specificity)	Administration and resources	Comments
Preschool (0–5)	Ages and Stages Questionnaire (ASQ) (.86; .85)	Parent completes 21–35 questions; results shared during office visit. Takes 15 min to complete. http://agesandstages.com/	Developmental surveillance of individual patients Facilitates systematic early detection and referral
Nontargeted screening: early childhood developmental milestones (AAP recommended at 9, 18, 24, 36, 48 months)	Pediatric Evaluation of Developmental Status (PEDS) (.74; .64)	Parent completes 7–10 questions. Takes 2–5 min to complete, less than 1 min to score. http://www.pedstest.com/	Requires coordinated, consistent use in PCMH Referral to BH and/or community resources for follow-up for pts in clinical ranges (EPPS Programs)
Specific preschool populations: Autism spectrum disorder	Checklist for Autism in Toddlers (CHAT): (.98;.18–.38)	https://www.m-chat.org/	2–5-year-olds with a positive PEDS or ASQ flagged Referral protocol for EPPS programs or CMH for assessment and treatment
Developmental delays (speech and language)	Modified CHAT (M-CHAT) (.85;.93)		
School-age children aged 6–17	Pediatric Symptom Checklist (PSC; PSC-17) (.80–.90; .70-1)	Parent completed questionnaire (age 6–17) Youth completed questionnaire (age 11–17) http://www.brightfutures.org/mentalhealth/pdf/professionals/ped_sympton_chklst.pdf	Valid and reliable tool for school age children. Useful for tracking population based data.
School-age population: ADD	Vanderbilt ADHD: (specificity: .09; sensitivity not available)	Parent, teacher, and youth complete 60–90 question form. Takes 5–35 min. (www.nichq.org/toolkits.adhd/)	
	Connors Rating Scale (CRS): (78–92 %; Specificity: 84–94 %)	Parent, teacher, and youth complete 60–90 question form. Takes 5–35 min. http://www.pearsonassessments.com	Not available to general public; purchased by only qualified buyers.

(continued)

Table 12.2 (continued)

Patient populations	Clinical system: screening tools (sensitivity; specificity)	Administration and resources	Comments
Adolescence	Guidelines for Adolescent for Preventive Services Questionnaire (GAPS) (specificity and sensitivity not evaluated)	72 item checklist on risk behaviors and mood and three semi-structure questions on strengths and self-concept. http://www.ama-assn.org/ama/pub/physician-resources /public-health/promoting-healthy-lifestyles /adolescent-health/guidelines-adolescent-preventive-services/screening-health-guidance-suicide -depression.page	Valuable resource for individual identification
	Rapid Assessment for Adolescent Preventive Services (RAAPS): (97; 74)	https://www.raaps.org/	Available to youth on the internet
	HEADSS: (specificity and sensitivity not evaluated)	http://primarycareforall.org/wp-content/uploads/ 2011/08/Adolescent-HEADSS-Assess.pdf	Less reliable and valid clinical interviewing tool for screening adolescents
Adolescent depression and anxiety	Patient Health Questionnaire—Adolescent (PHQ-A) (.75; .92) Beck Depression Inventory—Primary Care (BDI-PC): .91;91	www.phqscreeners.com/overview.aspx	Recommended by USPSTF Grade B when support systems are available
	Beck Anxiety Inventory for Youth (BYI) .74–.90 for ages 7–10, .84–.93 for ages 11–14, and .83–.93 for ages 15–18	http://www.pearsonclinical.co.uk/Psychology/ ChildMentalHealth/ChildMentalHealth/Beck YouthInventories-SecondEditionForChildren andAdolescents(BYI-II)/BeckYouthInventories-SecondEditionForChildrenandAdolescents (BYI-II).aspx	
Adolescent substance misuse	CRAAFT (.76–.92; .76; 94)	http://www.ceasar-boston.org/CRAFFT/index.php	
Adolescents with mood disorders (bi-polar)	Mood and Feelings Questionnaire (MFQ) MFQ- C (.68; .88) MFQ-P (.61;.85)		Limited evidence of specificity and sensitivity for in primary care settings

may over- or underestimate their child's development. The validity of this tool is enhanced when corroborated with clinical observation and more specific information from a clinical interview.

Ages and Stages Questionnaire (ASQ). The ASQ is a more extensive developmental screening tool for children 4 months to 5 years. This questionnaire has a reading level that ranges from third to twelfth grade and is available in four languages—English, Spanish, French, and Korean. There are 35 items in four developmental domains: cognitive, motor, self-help, and language. The Social and Emotional (SE) portion is recommended for children who have an at-risk score on any of these four primary domains. It takes approximately 15 min for parents to complete, and medical assistants or support staff may score the survey. It has high rates of sensitivity and specificity (La Rosa, 2010). This is a more comprehensive screening tool than the PEDS and has been validated in large, diverse samples including underserved families and premature babies. The form varies for different ages, carries a nominal cost, and has an EHR version.

Implementation of PEDS or the ASQ is a billable service, and codes (CPT 96110-1) can be used for more extensive screening tools and interpretive reports. The Center for Medicare and Medicaid Service (CMS) has published a relative value unit (RVU) for these services; they do not reimburse directly for the clinician's time but for office administration.

Specific Preschool Populations

Preschool children who are at biologic or environmental risk (e.g., prematurity, poverty) may require additional screening for language, speech, and autism spectrum disorders. If infants and preschoolers fail a developmental milestone based on the general screening tools, then health care providers can focus their assessment to language and/or behavioral/social development.

Checklist for Autism in Toddlers (CHAT/M-CHAT). As the rate the of children with autism spectrum disorders and pervasive developmental disorders continues to grow (Baird et al., 2000; Baron-Cohen et al., 2000; Filipek et al., 2000; Wallis & Pinto-Martin, 2008), the American Academy of Neurology and Child Neurology Society (Filipek et al., 2000) and AAP have suggested using the Checklist for Autism in Toddlers (CHAT) and the Modified Checklist for Autism in Toddlers (M-CHAT) (Baird et al., 2000; Baron-Cohen et al., 2000; Mawle & Griffiths, 2006). However, the CHAT has poor sensitivity and poor positive predictive value in primary care settings (Mawle & Griffiths; Robins, 2008). M-CHAT has limited evidence as a screening tool, but it has higher sensitivity and may be more useful in primary care settings as a secondary screening tool after the ASQ or PEDS (Robins). A positive result on these tools would indicate a referral to early assessment and intervention programs through EPSDT, the child health component of Medicaid. Follow-up assessments such as the Child Behavioral Checklist (CBCL) and the

Eyberg Children Behavioral Inventory are more expensive and require advanced levels of training and education for providers to administer these clinical assessment tools appropriately.

School-Age Children

Difficulties with psychosocial functioning is one of the leading sources of problems among school-age children (Blanchard et al., 2006; Gardner, Kelleher, Pajer, & Campo, 2003; Pagano, Cassidy, Little, Murphy, & Jellinek, 2000), and, in fact, almost half of all parent concerns at well-child visits are related to psychosocial problems (Wren, Scholle, Heo, & Comer, 2003). Using standardized tools to assess psychosocial functioning in school-age children (5–17 years), however, is the exception rather than the rule in primary care settings (Gardner, Kelleher, & Pajer, 2002; Gardner et al., 2003; Lazarus, 1999). Fewer school-age children are screened, identified, and referred for follow-up care than infants to 5-year-olds due to time constraints, limited information on validated user-friendly screening tools, lack of available mental health services, and lack of reimbursement for these assessments (Badger, Robinson, & Farley, 1999; Gardner et al., 2003; Reijneveld, Vogels, Hoekstra, & Crone, 2006; Schonwald et al., 2009).

The latency years are, however, an ideal time frame for identifying warning signs for behavioral health risks that lead to adult mental health disorders. Approximately one in ten children have a mental health disorder that affects their daily functioning (Jellinek, Little, Murphy, & Pagano, 1995; Jellinek et al., 1999; Weitzman & Leventhal, 2006), and the prevalence rates of children with a behavioral health disorder ranges from 12 % to 27 % depending on economic and cultural factors. This is higher than the prevalence of asthma or other childhood health disorders, but behavioral health concerns are routinely under-identified in primary care settings (Weitzman & Leventhal; Wren et al., 2003). Detection is often missed when physicians do not use a standardized screening tool (Simonian & Tarnowski, 2001). Consequently, a number of newer screening tools for school-age children and adolescents have been developed to address under-detection in primary care settings. The following is a list of tools that are emerging as valid and reliable screening tools in primary care settings.

Pediatric Symptom Checklist (PSC/PSC-17). The Pediatric Symptom Checklist (PSC) is a brief, reliable measurement of psychosocial-emotional functioning (Borowsky et al., 2003; Gardner et al., 2003; Gardner, Lucas, Kolko, & Campo, 2007; Jellinek et al., 1999; Jutte, Burgos, Mendoza, Ford, & Huffman, 2003; Murphy et al., 1996; Stoppelbein, Greening, Moll, Jordan, & Suozzi, 2012; Wren, Bridge, & Birmaher, 2004; Wren et al., 2003). The PSC is a one-page 35-question parent rating of a broad range of children's emotional and behavioral problems. It has a shorter version, PSC-17, and a youth self-report version for ages 11 through 17. The PSC and PCS-17 are validated for general use and for specific ethnic subgroups in the USA, including the Latino population (Stoppelbein et al., 2012;

Jutte et al., 2003; Leiner, Puertas, Caratachea, Perez, & Jimenez, 2010; Kostanecka et al., 2008; Pagano et al., 2000).

This tool has three subscale scores: Internalizing, Attention, and Externalizing behaviors, which assess a school-age child's daily functioning (Hayutin et al., 2009). A patient with scores within a clinical range should be referred for more in-depth assessment and treatment by trained behavioral health clinicians—physicians, psychologists, and social workers.

Specific School-Age Populations

Attention Deficit Disorder. Children who show signs of Attention Deficit Disorder (ADD) are commonly referred to their primary care provider for assessment. ADD and ADHD (Attention Deficit Hyperactivity Disorder) are the most common neuro-biological disorders in this age group with a prevalence of 5.5–9.3 % in the general pediatric population and 11.8 % in boys (2008). The two most commonly used screening tools in primary care for these conditions are the Vanderbilt and the Connors rating scales (Langberg, Froehlich, Loren, Martin, & Epstein, 2008; Wasserman et al., 1999).

Connors Rating Scale (CRS). The Connors rating scale, with strong psychometric properties, measures hyperactivity in children and adolescents. The Connors test is an initial step in the more complex evaluation and examination of someone with ADHD. This scale solicits input from three entities: parents, teachers, and youth self-report. Completing an ADHD Connors test takes from 5 to 30 min, depending on the short or long version of the test. Long versions of the Connors ratings scales have about 60–90 questions, while the short versions have less than 30 questions. In addition to helping diagnose ADD/ADHD, the Connors test can be used in follow-up examinations and evaluation of treatment effectiveness. Connors rating scales are not available to the general public, as they can only be purchased by qualified buyers.

Vanderbilt ADHD. The Vanderbilt is a family of screening tools for ADD and ADHD including a Parent, Teacher, and Primary Care provider forms. The AAP, Bright Futures, and NIQH recommend these tools for ADD/ADHD evaluations. It is easy to complete, designed for a third grade reading level, and has simple scoring instructions, which are consistent with the DSM-IV diagnosis. This questionnaire also functions as a screen for common comorbid conditions such as learning disabilities, depression, anxiety, and oppositional defiant disorder (Langberg et al., 2008) and works well with various populations, including parents with low reading levels. The sensitivity and specificity of these measures, however, have not yet been determined in primary care settings.

Family Psycho-social Screening. Since children's development is so closely linked to the family risk factors, screening for the level of family functioning is another area that needs to be considered in primary care. However, family functioning is rarely assessed in a systematic way in primary care settings (Gardner et al., 2001; Reitman, Currier, & Stickle, 2002). For example, the Parenting Stress Index (PSI) or its shorter PSI-S version, has strong psychometric properties for diverse cultural groups and has demonstrated utility in mental health programs, but reliability and validity in primary care settings has not been established. This screening could be beneficial for identifying the social determinants of a child's health, but a strong referral and follow-up system of care needs to be established for an effective family screening protocol (Gardner et al. 2001; Voigt et al., 2009).

Adolescent Screening Tools

Adolescents

Depression Screening for Children and Adolescents. The USPSTF recommends screening of adolescents (12–18 year olds) for major depressive disorder (MDD); however, the current evidence is insufficient to assess the benefits and harm of screening children who are younger (7–11-year-olds) (Williams, O'Connor, Eder, & Whitlock, 2009). The prevalence of MDD among adolescents is estimated at 5.6 % with a higher prevalence among girls than boys (5.9 vs. 4.6 %) and a lifetime prevalence of 20 %. Depressed youth have more difficulties in academic performance, social relationships, higher rates of pregnancy, substance abuse, physical illness and suicide, which is the third leading cause of death for 15–24-year-olds (Rausch, Hametz, Zuckerbrot, Rausch, & Soren, 2012; U.S. Preventive Services Task Force, 2010) (Williams et al., 2009).

USPTF's screening recommendation is based on sufficient evidence that early treatment of depression in adolescents is effective in improving health outcomes, but only when systems are in place to ensure accurate diagnosis, psychotherapy, and follow-up (Rausch et al., 2012; Williams et al., 2009). The benefits of early intervention on improving health outcomes or cost-effectiveness are still lacking (Sanci, Lewis, & Patton, 2010). Even when screening detects mental disorders, other factors such as readiness for care and availability of effective treatments may affect health outcomes and adolescents' engagement with treatment. The best results are obtained when screening is linked to integrated models of direct patient care and management systems. The USPTF recommends two instruments that demonstrate good sensitivity and specificity for identifying adolescents at risk for MDD in primary care settings: Patient Health Questionnaire-A (PHQ-A) and the Beck Depression Inventory-PC (BDI-PC).

Patient Health Questionnaire—Adolescent. PHQ-A is a derivative of the PHQ-9, a depression screening for adults, and also has nine questions with a moderate sensitivity and a high specificity for the adolescent population. A handful of studies have narrowed the PHQ-9 screening to two questions for adolescents, which has low to moderate rates of sensitivity and specificity (Borner, Braunstein, Victor, & Pollack, 2010; Richardson et al., 2010). As such, this brief screening measure may be more effective for identifying youth who are not at risk of depression than specifying who is at risk (Borner et al., 2010)

Beck's Depression Inventory—Primary Care. BDI-PC is a ten-item brief assessment of depression and has high rates of sensitivity and specificity with an adolescent population (Winter, Steer, Jones-Hicks, & Beck, 1999).

The Guidelines for Adolescent Depression in Primary Care. GLAD-PC is a resource for depression screening tools in primary care settings (Winter et al., 1999; Zuckerbrot & Jensen, 2006; Zuckerbrot, Cheung, Jensen, Stein, & Laraque 2007; Zuckerbrot, Maxon et al., 2007). These provide guidelines for providers and offer recommendations for screening, diagnosis, and treatment of depression and dysthymia in adolescents aged 10–21. The website provides a range of tools such as the Columbia Depression Scale (Teen Version), the Parent-Young Mania Rating Scale, Mood and Feelings Questionnaire, and Anxiety Sensitivity Index.

The Guidelines for Adolescent Preventative Services Questionnaire. The GAPS is a 72-item checklist that screens for risk behaviors (e.g., substance abuse, violence) and mood disorders (e.g., hopelessness, suicidal thoughts) (Elster & Kuznets, 1994), as well as three semi-structured questions on the adolescents' form on strengths and self-concept. This form has not been formally evaluated for sensitivity or specificity in primary care settings.

There are several other assessment tools for youth such as the Rapid Assessment for Adolescent Preventive Services (RAAPS). The RAAPS screening tool was uniquely developed with a wide base of youth input (Salerno, Marshall, & Picken, 2012), which has Internet compatibilities. CRAFFT, a mnemonic acronym for car, relax, alone, forget, friends, trouble, is a behavioral health substance abuse screening tool for use with adolescents under age 21 (Hamrin, 2010; Hamrin, Antenucci, & Magorno, 2012), and Home, Education, Activities, Drugs, Sexuality and Suicide/ Depression (HEADSS), which is a familiar clinical interviewing protocol for primary care providers to screen adolescent's psychosocial development, have no published studies on the reliability and validity of this approach in identifying MDD or other mental health disorder in adolescents (Zuckerbrot, Maxon et.al, 2007).

Adult Screening Tools

Like pediatric screening tools, screening tools for adults should be focused on identifying modifiable or treatable disorders or conditions and identifying adults who could benefit from behavioral health strategies. In addition to the recommendations of the USPSTF, other organizations, like the Veterans Administration of the

Department of Defense, the American Psychology Association, and the American Psychiatric Association, are developing guidelines for screening (Cook, Freedman, Freedman, Arick, & Miller, 1996; Engel et al., 2008). In 2009, the National Network of Depression Centers was organized to address the need for consistency in assessing and evaluating behavioral health and specifically depression in health care settings. This multi-professional group has identified a common assessment package of nine tools to measure mental health "vital signs." The purpose of this group has been to develop a standard core of assessment scales, to understand what they mean in the primary care setting, to use them regularly in clinical practice, and to use the information to facilitate communication about patient care within multidisciplinary teams (see Table 12.3 for examples).

In 2011, the National Institutes of Health in collaboration with the Society for Behavioral Medicine have joined efforts to recommend common data elements (CDEs) for patient-reported measures of health behaviors and psychosocial factors that can be used in EHRs and to identify standardized behavioral health screening tools for use in primary care settings. Their goal is to help integrate behavioral health information with other health factors, utilization reviews, and clinical outcomes and can contribute to quality improvement efforts through targeted health care initiatives in the PCMH and ACO sites.

Many integrated efforts are working toward developing consistent language, consensus of focus, and coordinated processes to synchronize behavioral health and psychosocial screenings into primary care (McGrady, Lynch, Nagel, & Tamburrino, 2010). The following review, therefore, is focused on evaluating adult behavioral health and mental health screening tools that have sufficient evidence to support their use in primary care. In this chapter, we will review screening in the three population categories:

(a) General Adult Populations: Substance Abuse and Mental Health Screening
(b) Targeted Patient Populations in Primary Care
(c) Screening for Patient Engagement, Quality of Life, and Social Support

Substance Abuse Screening

Substance abuse accounts for significant rates of morbidity and mortality among adults and warrants high priority in adult behavioral health screening and treatment. (USPSTF, AAFP, CPSTF, NCPP, 2008). There is a 10 % prevalence rate of alcohol misuse disorders in the adult population the USA, but identifying and referring at-risk patients occurs less than 10 % of the time in primary care, indicating that substance use is inadequately and inconsistently screened for. There are a substantial number of studies that support a variety of reliable and valid screening measures for alcohol misuse; however, there is insufficient evidence for brief, valid, and reliable screening tools for illicit drug use in primary care (Ansseau et al., 2004; Babor et al., 2007; Fiellin, Reid, & O'Connor, 2000; Edlund, Unutzer, & Wells, 2004; McCance-Katz & Satterfield, 2012).

Table 12.3 Brief screening tools

HEADSS:	H: Home and family
	E: Education
	A: Activities
	D: Drugs
	S: Sexual activity S: suicide/support
CRAFFT	C—Have you ever ridden in a CAR driven by someone (including yourself) who was "high" or had been using alcohol or drugs?
	R—Do you ever use alcohol or drugs to RELAX, feel better about you, or fit in?
	A—Do you ever use alcohol/drugs while you are by yourself, ALONE?
	F—Do you ever FORGET things you did while using alcohol or drugs?
	F—Do your family or FRIENDS ever tell you that you should cut down on your drinking or drug use?
	T—Have you gotten into TROUBLE while you were using alcohol or drugs?
AUDIT-C	1. How often did you have a drink containing alcohol in the past year?
	2. How many drinks did you have on typical day when you were drinking in the past year?
	3. How often did you have five or more drinks on one occasion in the past year?
CAGE	C: Have you ever felt the need to Cut down on drinking?
	A: Have you ever felt Annoyed by criticism of you drinking?
	G: Have you ever had Guilty feelings about your drinking?
	E: Do you ever take a morning Eye opener?
Patient Health Questionaire-2: PHQ-2	In the last 2 weeks,
	1. Have you often been bothered by feeling down, depressed or hopeless?
	2. Have you often been bothered by little interest or pleasure in doing things?
Generalized Anxiety Disorder-2: GAD-2	Over the last 2 weeks were you bothered by,
	1. Feeling nervous, anxious, or on edge and,
	2. Not being able to stop or control worrying?
Post Traumatic Stress Disorder: PTSD	In your life, have you ever had any experience that was so frightening, horrible, or upsetting that, in the past month, you…
	1. Have had nightmares about it or thought about it when you did not want to?
	2. Tried hard not to think about it or went out of your way to avoid situations that reminded you of it?
	3. Were constantly on guard, watchful, or easily startled?
	4. Felt numb or detached from others, activities, or your surroundings?

(continued)

Table 12.3 (continued)

Woman Abuse Screening Tool: (WAST-SF)	1. In general, how would you describe your relationship? No tension—Some tension—A lot of tension
	2. Do you and your partner work out arguments with… No difficulty—Some difficulty—Great difficulty
Partner Violence Screen: PVS	1. Have you been hit, kicked, punched, or otherwise hurt by someone within the past year? If so, by whom?
	2. Do you feel safe in your current relationship?
	3. Is there a partner from a previous relationship who is making you feel unsafe now?

The USPSTF recommends alcohol abuse screening for all adult patients and especially pregnant women, due to the increased risks to the fetus and pregnancy complications. It also recommends substance screening for patients who have tobacco abuse, frequent trauma-related medical visits, and/or a family history of alcoholism, as they are at a greater risk for substance abuse.

Alcohol Use Disorders Identification Test (AUDIT). This test is the gold standard for detecting alcohol misuse, which has high sensitivity and specificity in English-speaking primary care populations (Saunders, Aasland, Babor, de la Fuente, & Grant, 1993; Smith, Schmidt, Allensworth-Davies, & Saitz, 2009). The scoring profile identifies patients on a continuum from risky drinking behaviors to abuse and dependency. The briefer AUDIT-C version has similar high rates of sensitivity and moderate specificity.

Screening Brief Intervention Referral and Treatment (SBIRT). The Alcohol Screening and Brief Intervention are a combination strategy to screen for alcohol and substance use and for providers to immediately intervene. The screen for risky alcohol use starts with a single question on the number of drinks over a period of time. (See Chap. 13 for a more thorough description of SBIRT) (Babor et al., 2007). The SBIRT model, combining screening with treatment, is now widespread and widely studied (Saunders et al., 1993; Smith et al., 2009). Primary care practices can bill for this combined screening and treatment approach.

CAGE. CAGE a mnemonic acronym for cut down, annoyed, guilt, and eye opener, is a standard clinical interviewing screening protocol in primary care and is integrated into a routine history taking. A positive response indicates further assessment. It targets alcohol abuse and dependence, but is less effective at detecting risky drinking behavior (Fiellin et al., 2000). The screening questions have shown less accuracy in identifying older patients, African Americans, and Latinos with substance abuse symptoms.

CAGE and AUDIT Combination (TWEAK (a mnemonic acronym for tolerance, worried, eye-opener, amnesia, and cut-down), TRACE, Five Shot, RAPS). Combining a few questions from CAGE and AUDIT has created a number of screening tools. For example, TWEAK (Tolerance, Worried, Eye-opener, Amnesia, remember?, K/Cut Down) and TRACE (Tolerance, Annoyance, Cut-down,

Eye-opener) were developed specifically for alcohol screening with women, while the Five Shot and Rapid Alcohol Problems Screen (RAPS) have been validated as screening questions for men and women across diverse ethnic groups (Bischof et al., 2007; Delgadillo et al., 2011).

Mental Health Screening Tools

Mood Disorders: Depression and Bipolar Disorders. Mood disorders are the most prevalent disorders in the general population. Major depression alone has a lifetime prevalence of 20 % in women and 13 % in men, and 20–30 % of these patients experience a re-occurrence of a depressive episode over their lifetime. Consequently, screening adults for depression is recommended by the USPTF (Grade B) when care management processes are in place to assure accurate diagnosis, effective treatment and consistent follow-up care. This recommendation set the standards for integrating a depression screening process into the PCMH (Bauer et al., 2011; Gilbody, Bower, Fletcher, Richards, & Sutton, 2006; Kessler, Sharp, & Lewis, 2005; Solberg, Korsen, Oxman, Fischer, & Bartels, 1999; U.S. Preventive Services Task Force, 2009).

Implementing a depression screening protocol into primary care practices is multifaceted and depression management requires a system of care and a health care team beyond the doctor–patient relationship. The IMPACT model of depression management and the variations on this clinical pathway (e.g., DIAMOND, TIDES) in primary care has set the prototype for an evidence-based approach. Screening the general population of primary care adult patients for signs of depression is an initial step in this clinical protocol (Unutzer & Park, 2012).

The most widely used patient tool for screening depression in primary care is based on the Patient Health Questionnaire (PHQ) (Kroenke, Spitzer, & Williams, 2001; Spitzer, Kroenke, & Williams, 1999). The purpose of the 20-question PHQ tool was to facilitate recognition and diagnosis of depression in all patients establishing care who have not been screened in the previous 12 months, or who are suspected of having a mental health disorder. There is a short PHQ-9 version and an even shorter version PHQ-2, which is used for two initial clinical questions to identify patients who may be flagged at risk for depression (Arroll, Khin, & Kerse, 2003; Kroenke, Spitzer, & Williams, 2003; Kroenke et al., 2011; Lowe, Kroenke, & Grafe, 2005). The PHQ-9 is available free and there are no limitations on the level of training of providers for using this tool. However, results from this screening tool need to be embedded alongside a clinical treatment protocol, with well-defined roles and responsibilities within the health care team and a reliable system for monitoring patients follow-up and their treatment response.

Beck Depression Inventory. BDI-PC is also a well-recognized tool that is less accessible to primary care providers because of its length, the level of advanced training required for interpreting these tools, and the cost (Arnau, Meagher, Norris,

& Bramson, 2001). It may be better suited to primary care settings where behavioral health providers shoulder the responsibility for screening and intervening in depression.

Mood Disorder Questionnaire. While screening for depression is common, screening for the diagnostic differential of bipolar is often missed. The Mood Disorder Questionnaire (MDQ) has been developed as a self-administered, five-question screening tool specifically designed to detect patients who are at risk for the spectrum of bipolar disorders (Hirschfeld et al., 2000). The MDQ more accurately specifies patients who do not show signs of the disorder than detecting patients with the disorder (Hirschfield et al., 2003). Thus, results of the MDQ need to be interpreted within the context of a clinical interview with an experienced clinician. In addition, the MDQ may not be adequate to distinguish between bipolar disorder and personality disorder patients such as Borderline Personality Disorder (Zimmerman et al., 2010). Screening for bipolar disorders is a more complex diagnostic process than screening for a unipolar mood disorder and it may require more sophisticated assessment tools and advanced-level behavioral health providers to accurately identify patients with this disorder.

Specific Patient Populations and Depression Screening

Pregnant and Postpartum Patients and Depression Screening

The prevalence of depression among pregnant and postpartum women is double the rate of matched nonpregnant women, and screening has become a recommended standard of care (USPSTF) (Gavin et al., 2005). The Edinburgh Postnatal Depression Scale (EDPS) is a ten question self-administered tool that can be completed and scored in 3 min. It has been validated across different cultures and languages, with high rates of specificity (80 %) but moderate to low rates of sensitivity (67.7 %). Interestingly, in comparison to other depression diagnostic tools, like BDI, CES-D, and the Postpartum Depression Screening Scale (PDSS), none of these tools performed significantly better or worse in screening for depression among postpartum patients (Gaynes et al., 2005; Olson, Dietrich, Prazar, & Hurley, 2006; Sharp & Lipsky, 2002).

Diabetic Patients and Depression

Given the strong link between mood and self-management in diabetic patients, the American Diabetes Association (ADA) added a standard of psychosocial assessment to its 2005 Clinical Practice Recommendations (McGlynn, Cassel, Leatherman, DeCristofaro, & Smits, 2003). At a minimum, they recommend that providers administer the PHQ-2 at the regular diabetic checkups.

Aging Patients and Depression

Optimal screening for depression in geriatric patients is unknown, but the increased prevalence of depression in patients who are experiencing bereavement, cognitive decline, institutional placement, or chronic medical illnesses is well-established (U.S. Preventive Services Task Force, 2009). In addition, the presence of a chronic painful physical condition increases the likelihood of a positive screen for depression (Ohayon & Schatzberg, 2003).

Geriatric Depression Scale. GDS 30 and GDS 15 are thirty- and fifteen-item self-administered questionnaires that screen for mild to severe ranges of depression in senior patients. The GDS 15 is recommended for late-life depression screening (Heisel, Duberstein, Lyness, & Feldman, 2010; Mitchell, Bird, Rizzo, & Meader, 2010; Unutzer et al., 2002).

Anxiety Disorders

Even though anxiety disorders are prevalent in primary care settings, screening the general adult population is not recommended at this time by the USPSTF or other health organizations (Ebell, 2008). Anxiety disorders, however, are highly prevalent affecting as many as 10 % of the population and 3–20 % of primary care patients seeking care in office visits (Ansseau et al., 2004; Wetherell, Birchler, Ramsdell, & Unutzer, 2007). The variety of anxiety disorders, from Generalized Anxiety, Post-traumatic Stress Disorder, Obsessive Compulsive Disorder or Social Anxiety, significantly overlaps with physiological symptoms and makes the screening and management of anxiety in primary care challenging (Sharp & Lipsky, 2002). Further research into the validity and benefits of screening for anxiety disorders in primary care and the correlations between physiological symptoms continues.

Generalized Anxiety Disorder. The GAD-7 and its shorter version GAD-2 are widely used, self-administered, clinician-scored screening tools developed for use in primary care settings (Donker, van Straten, Marks, & Cuijpers, 2011; Snyder, Stanley, Novy, Averill, & Beck, 2000; Spitzer, Kroenke, Williams, & Lowe, 2006). The psychometric analysis shows these screeners performed well for a range of anxiety disorders such as panic, social phobia, and PTSD.

Post-traumatic Stress Disorder Screener. This tool has been used in primary care military settings to identify personnel who are at risk for PTSD. It has been an effective screening tool for assessing the key characteristics of PTSD in this population but has also been validated within a civilian patient population (Davis, Whitworth, & Rickett, 2009; Freedy & Brock, 2010).

Specific Patient Populations and Behavioral Health Screening

Abuse and Violence

Women, children, and senior patients are targeted patient populations who may be at risk for abuse. The burden of violence toward children, intimate partners, and elders is well documented, yet USPSTF found insufficient evidence to recommend for or against routine screening of parents or guardians for the physical abuse or neglect of children, of women for intimate partner violence, or of older adults or their caregivers for elder abuse. The absence of a screening recommendation is based on the lack of valid measures from the screening process, as well as the absence of data to determine if screening compromises the clinician–patient relationship, especially in low-risk populations, or increases the risk of harm to patients in violent relationships. Some studies suggest that screening for violence without adequate safety and support resources readily available may put the patient at more risk. Nonetheless, many medical organizations, domestic violence coalitions, and child welfare leagues continue to recommend that physicians remain alert to the signs and symptoms of physical and sexual abuse in routine examinations, especially at prenatal visits. The AAFP recommends "being alert" for the presence of family violence in virtually every patient encounter to provide early intervention, even though providers are lacking specific validated tools to detect family violence (American Association of Family Physicians [AAFP], 2012).

Due to the dangers and risks associated with disclosing abuse, there are many nuances that shape the safety and trust between provider and patient in the screening process. Consequently, no single screening tool for violence has well-established psychometric properties. Even the most common tools were evaluated in only a small number of studies. Sensitivities and specificities varied widely within and between screening tools. Further testing and validation are critically needed (Garcia-Esteve et al., 2011; Forgey, Badger, & Krase, 2011; Kapur & Windish, 2011; O'Campo, Kirst, Tsamis, Chambers, & Ahmad, 2011; Snider, Webster, O'Sullivan, & Campbell, 2009). Some of the more common tools are as follows: (1) Hurt, Insult, Threaten, and Scream (HITS) Scale is a self-administered four-item questionnaire that asks how often their partner physically hurt, insulted, threatened with harm, and screamed at them; (2) Woman Abuse Screening Tool (WAST/WAST-Short): WAST and WAST-short forms were developed and validated for use in family medicine clinics; (3) Abuse Assessment Screen (AAS): The AAS is geared toward pregnant women.

Aging Patients: Dementia Screening

Despite the prevalence of dementia increasing, it remains underdiagnosed in the elderly. Still, evidence has been insufficient to recommend for or against screening for dementia in older adults. It remains unclear if screening will result in overall population benefit or risk from introducing drug therapies or other treatments on the course or progression of this disease (Canadian Task Force on the Periodic Health Examination, 1994). Screening can at best identify levels of cognitive dysfunction, but it does not prevent the progression of the disease. Screening for dementia or mild cognitive impairment may be helpful for family members and care givers in preparing to care for a loved one (Prince et al., 2011).

Mini Mental Status Exam. Most dementia screening tools have been derived from the traditional and widely used MMSE, the oldest, most studied, and best known tool for screening for cognitive impairment (Folstein, Folstein, & McHugh, 1975; Howarth, Heath, & Snope, 1999). This provider-administered tool has 11 questions and/or tasks for the patient, and takes 5–10 min to complete. The Modified Mini-Mental State Examination (3MS) is an expanded version that includes items that predict better functional outcome (Teng & Chui, 1987).

Montreal Cognitive Assessment. The MoCA is a 10-min screening tool designed for primary care populations (Nasreddine, Phillips, & Chertkow, 2012). It has high rates of sensitivity and specificity for detecting mild cognitive impairment. It requires provider training and includes tasks such as clock drawing, serial seven's, and orientation, to assess attention, concentration, memory, and executive planning.

General Practitioner Assessment of Cognition. GPCOG was developed for primary care use. It consists of nine interactive tasks—time orientation, clock drawing, and recall, which takes about 4 min to complete and several minutes to review (Brodaty et al., 2002; Brodaty, Kemp, & Low, 2004; Lorentz, Scanlan, & Borson 2002).

Mini-Cog. The Mini-Cog was developed as a tool to assess elderly patients who are multilingual (Borson, Scanlan, Brush, Vitaliano, & Dokmak, 2000). The clinician and patient complete the 3-min three-item recall assessment and clock drawing tool together (Royall, Cordes, & Polk, 1998). It broadly distinguishes patients with or without dementia, but it is not sensitive enough to detect mild cognitive impairment (Borson, Scanlan, Chen, & Ganguli, 2003).

Memory Impairment Screen. The four-item MIS delayed and cued recall test has been used as a quick assessment of dementia, but assesses only memory and not other executive or visual-spacial functioning.

Office Management Practices and Financial Systems

Many barriers stand in the way of consistent screening practices, like inadequate reimbursement, lack of staff time and training, reluctance to label children or adults, limited availability of community resources or specialty treatment centers for when patients in need are identified, and unclear administrative guidelines (Weitzman & Leventhal, 2006). Office management practices, including a clear depiction of the practice office flow of tasks and responsibilities of team members at the beginning, middle, and closure of an office visit, are necessary components for regular screening. The North Carolina Assuring Better Child Health and Development (ABCD), for example, had an increase of more than 70 % in using standardized tools when they implemented practice management strategies, such as conducting staff orientation, sharing data with providers/staff regularly, and identifying key community referral partners into their system (Earls & Hay, 2006; Pinto-Martin et al., 2005).

The sustainability of incorporating screening tools into primary care practices depends not only on well-defined protocols for office staff and provider teams, but also on financial reimbursement, which is currently limited. The 96110 code for a screening tool can be attached to an E/M preventive service code with a modifier (e.g., well-child checkups, well-woman exams). This RVU represents only malpractice and office expense and is allocated primarily for staff administrative responsibilities, but not for physician assessment and discussion with families. While this is a beginning step in building sustainability for using screening tools, this process will need financial support and advocacy from professional organizations, such as the AAP, to extend the financial base for successfully implementing screening tools into primary care (e.g., aapcodinghotline@aap.org).

Practice-Based Data and Quality Improvement Processes Using Screening Tools

The systematic use of screening tools in clinical practice can build a base for effective integrated care initiatives. Screening tools are often used in individual patient encounters depending on the PCP or BH providers' clinical judgment, but aggregate information can be used to enhance population-based patient care and for targeting relevant clinical interventions, to promote healthier outcomes, preventative care, and earlier intervention. Just as mammogram screening provides data on breast cancer prevalence and treatment outcomes, compiling behavioral health screening data from primary care settings gives a broader profile of patient behavioral health characteristics and interventions. Using screening tool information to track individual or group trends in primary care is still in the early stages of development and has not been fully adopted as a standard of care.

There are several examples of how a population-based behavioral health screening initiative can lead to quality improvement processes. The SBIRT screening for alcohol use is an effective, well-researched, and reimbursable activity for the patient-centered medical home and should be routinely implemented for all adult patients (nontargeted adult population). This process of consistent monitoring within the general population has the potential to provide the foundation for quality improvement initiatives in the primary care setting. The IMPACT model, which uses the PHQ-9 to identify patients at risk for depression and also to track patient improvements in depressive symptoms has all of the elements for systems-based use of screening tools for the general adult population. Similarly, the PSC-17 is currently being used in a large public health initiative to increase the identification of psychosocial and behavioral issues with children (Hacker, Williams, Myagmarjav, Cabral, & Murphy, 2009; Murphy et al., 1996). Using standardized screening tools does increase the identification of behavioral health issues, but the challenge of implementing these into standard quality improvement practices remains.

Summary of the Evidence and Essentials

A rich deposit of behavioral health screening tools for use in primary care settings exists. Developmental screening tools for preschoolers, psychosocial concerns for school-age children, depression screening for adolescents, and depression and substance use screening for adults have strong empirical evidence to support screening practice as standard of care. Primary care providers may individually administer behavioral health screening tools depending on their clinical judgment, time, and comfort level. Individual use of these tools in practice, however, is only the first step in setting the context for screening. To reach maximum utility and efficacy, screening needs to be embedded into a system of care, including the identification of team member's roles and expectations for administering, scoring, and reviewing screening results with patients and families, the identification of the population to be screened, selection of the appropriate tool, provision of clinical and office protocols including billing practices, and finally the use of this information for understanding the behavioral characteristics of patients in a community to develop relevant quality improvement interventions.

References

American Academy of Family Physicians. (2012). Retrieved from http://www.aafp.org/online/en/home.html

American Association of Pediatricians. (2001). Retrieved from http://www.aap.org/

Ansseau, M., Dierick, M., Buntinkx, F., Cnockaert, P., De Smedt, J., Van Den Haute, M., et al. (2004). High prevalence of mental disorders in primary care. *Journal of Affective Disorders, 78*(1), 49–55.

Arnau, R. C., Meagher, M. W., Norris, M. P., & Bramson, R. (2001). Psychometric evaluation of the Beck Depression Inventory-II with primary care medical patients. *Health Psychology, 20*(2), 112–119.

Arroll, B., Khin, N., & Kerse, N. (2003). Screening for depression in primary care with two verbally asked questions: Cross sectional study. *British Medical Journal, 327*, 1144–1146. doi:10.1136/bmj.327.7424.1144.

Babor, T. F., McRee, B. G., Kassebaum, P. A., Grimaldi, P. A., Ahmed, K., & Bray, J. (2007). Screening, Brief Intervention, and Referral to Treatment (SBIRT): Toward a public health approach to the management of substance abuse. *Substance Abuse, 28*, 7–30. doi:10.1300/J465v28n03_03.

Badger, L., Robinson, H., & Farley, T. (1999). Management of mental disorders in rural primary care: A proposal for integrated psychosocial services. *The Journal of Family Practice, 48*, 813–818.

Baird, G., Charman, T., Baron-Cohen, S., Cox, A., Swettenham, S., Wheelwright, S., et al. (2000). A screening instrument for autism at 18 months of age: A 6-year follow-up study. *Journal of the American Academy of Child and Adolescent Psychiatry, 39*, 694–702. doi:10.1097/00004583-200006000-00007.

Baron-Cohen, S., Wheelwright, S., Cox, A., Baird, G., Charman, T., Swettenham, J., et al. (2000). Early identification of autism by the Checklist for Autism in Toddlers (CHAT). *Journal of the Royal Society of Medicine, 93*, 521–525.

Bauer, A. M., Azzone, V., Goldman, H., Alexander, L., Unutzer, J., Coleman-Beattie, B., et al. (2011). Implementation of integrated depression management at community-based primary care clinics: An evaluation. *Psychiatric Services, 62*, 1047–1053. doi:10.1176/appi. ps.62.9.1047.

Bischof, G., Reinhardt, S., Grothues, J., Meyer, C., John, U., & Rumpf, H. (2007). Development and evaluation of a screening instrument for alcohol-use disorders and at-risk drinking: The brief alcohol screening instrument for medical care (BASIC). *Journal of Studies on Alcohol and Drugs, 68*, 607–614.

Blanchard, L. T., Gurka, M., & Blackman, J. (2006). Emotional, developmental, and behavioral health of American children and their families: A report from the 2003 National Survey of Children's Health. *Pediatrics, 117*, e1202–e1212. doi:10.1542/peds.2005-2606.

Borner, I., Braunstein, J., St Victor, R., & Pollack, J. (2010). Evaluation of a 2-question screening tool for detecting depression in adolescents in primary care. *Clinical Pediatrics, 49*, 947–953. doi:10.1177/0009922810370203.

Borowsky, I., Mozayeny, S., & Ireland, M. (2003). Brief psychosocial screening at health supervision and acute care visits. *Pediatrics, 112*, 129–133.

Borson, S., Scanlan, J., Brush, M., Vitaliano, P., & Dokmak, A. (2000). The mini-cog: A cognitive 'vital signs' measure for dementia screening in multi-lingual elderly. *International Journal of Geriatric Psychiatry, 15*, 1021–1027.

Borson, S., Scanlan, J., Chen, P., & Ganguli, M. (2003). The mini-cog as a screen for dementia: Validation in a population-based sample. *Journal of the American Geriatrics Society, 51*, 1451–1454.

Brickman, A., Garrity, C., & Shaw, J. (2002). Risk factors for psychosocial dysfunction among enrollees in the State Children's Health Insurance Program. *Psychiatric Services, 53*, 614–619.

Brodaty, H., Kemp, N., & Low, L. (2004). Characteristics of the GPCOG, a screening tool for cognitive impairment. *International Journal of Geriatric Psychiatry, 19*, 870–874. doi:10.1002/ gps.1167.

Center for Disease Control and Prevention. (2011). Retrieved from http://www.cdc.gov

Cook, C., Freedman, J., Freedman, L., Arick, R., & Miller, M. (1996). Screening for social and environmental problems in a VA primary care setting. *Health & Social Work, 21*, 41–47.

Davis, S., Whitworth, J., & Rickett, K. (2009). Clinical inquiries. What are the most practical primary care screens for post-traumatic stress disorder? *The Journal of Family Practice, 58*, 100–101.

Delgadillo, J., Payne, S., Gilbody, S., Godfrey, C., Gore, S., Jessop, D., et al. (2011). How reliable is depression screening in alcohol and drug users? A validation of brief and ultra-brief questionnaires. *Journal of Affective Disorders, 134*, 266–271. doi:10.1016/j.jad.2011.06.017.

Donker, T., van Straten, A., Marks, I., & Cuijpers, P. (2011). Quick and easy self-rating of generalized anxiety disorder: Validity of the Dutch web-based GAD-7, GAD-2 and GAD-SI. *Psychiatry Research, 188*, 58–64. doi:10.1016/j.psychres.2011.01.016.

Drotar, D., Stancin, T., Dworkin, P., Sices, L., & Wood, S. (2008). Selecting developmental surveillance and screening tools. *Pediatrics in Review, 29*, e52–e58. doi:10.1542/pir.29-10-e52.

Earls, M., & Hay, S. (2006). Setting the stage for success: Implementation of developmental and behavioral screening and surveillance in primary care practice–the North Carolina Assuring Better Child Health and Development (ABCD) Project. *Pediatrics, 118*, e183–e188. doi:10.1542/peds.2006-0475.

Ebell, M. H. (2008). Diagnosis of anxiety disorders in primary care. *American Family Physician, 78*, 501–502.

Edlund, M., Unutzer, J., & Wells, K. (2004). Clinician screening and treatment of alcohol, drug, and mental problems in primary care: Results from healthcare for communities. *Medical Care, 42*, 1158–1166.

Engel, C. C., Oxman, T., Yamamoto, C., Gould, D., Barry, S., Stewart, P., et al. (2008). RESPECT-Mil: Feasibility of a systems-level integrated care approach to depression and post-traumatic stress disorder in military primary care. *Military Medicine, 173*, 935–940.

Fiellin, D., Reid, M., & O'Connor, P. (2000). Screening for alcohol problems in primary care: A systematic review. *Archives of Internal Medicine, 160*, 1977–1989.

Filipek, P., Accardo, P., Ashwal, S., Baranek, G., Cook, E., Dawson, G., et al. (2000). Practice parameter: Screening and diagnosis of autism: Report of the Quality Standards Subcommittee of the American Academy of Neurology and the Child Neurology Society. *Neurology, 55*, 468–479.

Folstein, M., Folstein, S., & McHugh, P. (1975). "Mini-mental state": A practical method for grading the cognitive state of patients for the clinician. *Journal of Psychiatric Research, 12*, 189–198.

Forgey, M., Badger, L., & Krase, K. (2011). The development of an evidence based assessment protocol for intimate partner violence in the U.S. Army. *Journal of Evidence-Based Social Work, 8*, 323–348. doi:10.1080/15433714.2011.533946.

Freedy, J., & Brock, C. (2010). Spotting-and treating-PTSD in primary care. *The Journal of Family Practice, 59*, 75–80.

Garcia-Esteve, L., Torres, A., Navarro, P., Ascaso, C., Imaz, M., Herreras, Z., et al. (2011). Validation and comparison of four instruments to detect partner violence in health-care setting. *Medicina Clinica, 137*, 390–397. doi:10.1016/j.medcli.2010.11.038.

Gardner, W., Kelleher, K., & Pajer, K. (2002). Multidimensional adaptive testing for mental health problems in primary care. *Medical Care, 40*, 812–823. doi:10.1097/01.MLR.0000025436.30093.77.

Gardner, W., Kelleher, K., Pajer, K., & Campo, J. (2003). Primary care clinicians' use of standardized tools to assess child psychosocial problems. *Ambulatory Pediatrics, 3*, 191–195.

Gardner, W., Lucas, A., Kolko, D., & Campo, J. (2007). Comparison of the PSC-17 and alternative mental health screens in an at-risk primary care sample. *Journal of the American Academy of Child and Adolescent Psychiatry, 46*, 611–618. doi:10.1097/chi.0b013e318032384b.

Gardner, W., Nutting, P., Kelleher, K., Werner, J., Farley, T., Stewart, L., et al. (2001). Does the family APGAR effectively measure family functioning? *The Journal of Family Practice, 50*, 19–25.

Gavin, N., Gaynes, B., Lohr, K., Meltzer-Brody, S., Gartlehner, G., & Swinson, T. (2005). Perinatal depression: A systematic review of prevalence and incidence. *Obstetrics and Gynecology, 106*, 1071–1083. doi:10.1097/01.AOG.0000183597.31630.db.

Gaynes, B., Gavin, N., Meltzer-Brody, S., Lohr, K., Swinson, T., Gartlehner, G., et al. (2005). Perinatal depression: Prevalence, screening accuracy, and screening outcomes. *Evidence Report/Technology Assessment, 119*, 1–8.

Gilbody, S., Bower, P., Fletcher, J., Richards, D., & Sutton, A. (2006). Integrated care for depression: A cumulative meta-analysis and review of longer-term outcomes. *Archives of Internal Medicine, 166*, 2314–2321. doi:10.1001/archinte.166.21.2314.

Glascoe, F. P. (2005). Screening for developmental and behavioral problems. *Mental Retardation Developmental Disabilities Research Review, 11*, 173–179. doi:10.1002/mrdd.20068.

Hacker, K., Williams, S., Myagmarjav, E., Cabral, H., & Murphy, M. (2009). Persistence and change in pediatric symptom checklist scores over 10 to 18 months. *Academic Pediatrics, 9*, 270–277. doi:10.1016/j.acap. 2009.03.004.

Hamrin, V., Antenucci, M., & Magorno, M. (2012). Evaluation and management of pediatric and adolescent depression. *The Nurse Practitioner, 37*, 22–30.

Hayutin, L., Reed-Knight, B., Blount, R., Lewis, J., & McCormick, M. (2009). Increasing parent-pediatrician communication about children's psychosocial problems. *Journal of Pediatric Psychology, 34*, 1155–1164. doi:10.1093/jpepsy/jsp012.

Heisel, M., Duberstein, P., Lyness, J., & Feldman, M. (2010). Screening for suicide ideation among older primary care patients. *Journal of the American Board of Family Medicine, 23*, 260–269. doi:10.3122/jabfm.2010.02.080163.

Herman-Staab, B. (1994). Screening, management, and appropriate referral for pediatric behavior problems. *The Nurse Practitioner, 19*, 40–49.

Hirschfeld, R., Holzer, C., Calabrese, J., Weissman, M., Reed, M., Davies, M., et al. (2003). Validity of the mood disorder questionnaire: A general population study. *The American Journal of Psychiatry, 160*, 178–180.

Hirschfeld, R., Williams, J., Spitzer, R., Calabrese, J., Flynn, L., Keck, P., et al. (2000). Development and validation of a screening instrument for bipolar spectrum disorder: The mood disorder questionnaire. *The American Journal of Psychiatry, 157*, 1873–1875.

Howarth, D., Heath, J., & Snope, F. (1999). Beyond the Folstein: Dementia in primary care. *Primary Care, 26*, 299–314.

Jellinek, M., Little, M., Murphy, J., & Pagano, M. (1995). The pediatric symptom checklist: Support for a role in a managed care environment. *Archives of Pediatrics & Adolescent Medicine, 149*, 740–746.

Jellinek, M., Murphy, J., Little, M., Pagano, M., Comer, J., & Kelleher, K. (1999). Use of the pediatric symptom checklist to screen for psychosocial problems in pediatric primary care: A national feasibility study. *Archives of Pediatrics & Adolescent Medicine, 153*, 254–260.

Jutte, D., Burgos, A., Mendoza, F., Ford, C., & Huffman, L. (2003). Use of the pediatric symptom checklist in a low-income, Mexican American population. *Archives of Pediatrics & Adolescent Medicine, 157*, 1169–1176. doi:10.1001/archpedi.157.12.1169.

Kapur, N., & Windish, D. (2011). Optimal methods to screen men and women for intimate partner violence: Results from an internal medicine residency continuity clinic. *Journal of Interpersonal Violence, 26*, 2335–2352. doi:10.1177/0886260510383034.

Kessler, D., Sharp, D., & Lewis, G. (2005). Screening for depression in primary care. *British Journal of General Practice, 55*, 659–660.

Kostanecka, A., Power, T., Clarke, A., Watkins, M., Hausman, C., & Blum, N. (2008). Behavioral health screening in urban primary care settings: Construct validity of the PSC-17. *Journal of Developmental and Behavioral Pediatrics, 29*, 124–128. doi:10.1097/DBP.0b013e31816a0d9e.

Kroenke, K., Spitzer, R., & Williams, J. (2001). The PHQ-9: Validity of a brief depression severity measure. *Journal of General Internal Medicine, 16*, 606–613.

Kroenke, K., Spitzer, R. L., & Williams, J. (2003). The patient health questionnaire-2: Validity of a two-item depression screener. *Medical Care, 41*, 1284–1292.

Langberg, J., Froehlich, T., Loren, R., Martin, J., & Epstein, J. (2008). Assessing children with ADHD in primary care settings. *Expert Review of Neurotherapeutics, 8*, 627–641. doi:10.1586/14737175.8.4.627.

Lazarus, A. (1999). Screening for behavioral disorders in primary care. *Managed Care Interface, 12*, 52–55.

Leiner, M., Puertas, H., Caratachea, R., Perez, H., & Jimenez, P. (2010). Sensitivity and specificity of the pictorial pediatric symptom checklist for psychosocial problem detection in a Mexican sample. *Revista de Investigacion Clinica, 62*, 560–567.

Lorentz, W. J., Scanlan, J. M., & Borson, S. (2002). Brief screening tests for dementia. *Canadian Journal of Psychiatry, 47*, 723–733.

Lowe, B., Kroenke, K., & Grafe, K. (2005). Detecting and monitoring depression with a two-item questionnaire (PHQ-2). *Journal of Psychosomatic Research, 58*, 163–171. doi:10.1016/j.jpsychores.2004.09.006.

Mawle, E., & Griffiths, P. (2006). Screening for autism in pre-school children in primary care: Systematic review of English Language tools. *International Journal of Nursing Studies, 43*, 623–636. doi:10.1016/j.ijnurstu.2005.11.011.

McCance-Katz, E., & Satterfield, J. (2012). SBIRT: A key to integrate prevention and treatment of substance abuse in primary care. *The American Journal on Addictions, 21*, 176–177. doi:10.1111/j.1521-0391.2011.00213.x.

McGlynn, E., Cassel, C., Leatherman, S., DeCristofaro, A., & Smits, H. (2003). Establishing national goals for quality improvement. *Medical Care, 41*, 116–129.

McGrady, A., Lynch, D., Nagel, R., & Tamburrino, M. (2010). Coherence between physician diagnosis and patient self reports of anxiety and depression in primary care. *The Journal of Nervous and Mental Disease, 198*, 420–424. doi:10.1097/NMD.0b013e3181e084ce.

Mitchell, A., Bird, V., Rizzo, M., & Meader, N. (2010). Which version of the geriatric depression scale is most useful in medical settings and nursing homes? Diagnostic validity meta-analysis. *The American Journal of Geriatric Psychiatry, 18*, 1066–1077.

Murphy, J., Ichinose, C., Hicks, R., Kingdon, D., Crist-Whitzel, J., Jordan, P., et al. (1996). Utility of the Pediatric Symptom Checklist as a psychosocial screen to meet the federal Early and Periodic Screening, Diagnosis, and Treatment (EPSDT) standards: A pilot study. *Journal of Pediatrics, 129*, 864–869.

Nasreddine, Z., Phillips, N., & Chertkow, H. (2012). Normative data for the Montreal Cognitive Assessment (MoCA) in a population-based sample. *Neurology, 78*, 765–766. doi:10.1212/01. wnl.0000413072.54070.a3.

National Institute of Health and Clinical Excellence. (2012) Retrieved from www.nice.org.uk

Nelson, H., Nygren, P., Walker, M., & Panoscha, R. (2006). Screening for speech and language delay in preschool children: Systematic evidence review for the US preventive services task force. *Pediatrics, 117*, e298–e319. doi:10.1542/peds.2005-1467.

O'Campo, P., Kirst, M., Tsamis, C., Chambers, C., & Ahmad, F. (2011). Implementing successful intimate partner violence screening programs in health care settings: Evidence generated from a realist-informed systematic review. *Social Science & Medicine, 72*, 855–866. doi:10.1016/j. socscimed.2010.12.019.

Ohayon, M., & Schatzberg, A. (2003). Using chronic pain to predict depressive morbidity in the general population. *Archives of General Psychiatry, 60*, 39–47.

Olson, A., Dietrich, A., Prazar, G., & Hurley, J. (2006). Brief maternal depression screening at well-child visits. *Pediatrics, 118*, 207–216. doi:10.1542/peds.2005-2346.

Pagano, M., Cassidy, L., Little, M., Murphy, J., & Jellinek, M. (2000). Identifying psychosocial dysfunction in school-age children: The pediatric symptom checklist as self-report measure. *Journal of School Psychology, 37*, 91–106. doi:10.1002/(sici)1520-6807 (200003)37: 2%3c91::aid-pits1%3e3.0.co;2-3.

Pinto-Martin, J., Dunkle, M., Earls, M., Fliedner, D., & Landes, C. (2005). Developmental stages of developmental screening: Steps to implementation of a successful program. *American Journal of Public Health, 95*, 1928–1932. doi:10.2105/ajph.2004.052167.

Pinto-Martin, J., Souders, M., Giarelli, E., & Levy, S. (2005). The role of nurses in screening for autistic spectrum disorder in pediatric primary care. *Journal of Pediatric Nursing, 20*, 163–169. doi:10.1016/j.pedn.2005.01.004.

Polaha, J., Dalton, W., & Allen, S. (2011). The prevalence of emotional and behavior problems in pediatric primary care serving rural children. *Journal of Pediatric Psychology, 36*, 652–660. doi:10.1093/jpepsy/jsq116.

Prince, M., Acosta, D., Ferri, C., Guerra, M., Huang, Y., Jacob, K., et al. (2011). A brief dementia screener suitable for use by non-specialists in resource poor settings–the cross-cultural derivation and validation of the brief Community Screening Instrument for Dementia. *International Journal of Geriatric Psychiatry, 26*, 899–907. doi:10.1002/gps.2622.

Rausch, J., Hametz, P., Zuckerbrot, R., Rausch, W., & Soren, K. (2012). Screening for depression in Urban Latino adolescents. *Clinical Pediatrics*. doi:10.1177/0009922812441665.

Reijneveld, S., Vogels, A., Hoekstra, F., & Crone, M. (2006). Use of the Pediatric Symptom Checklist for the detection of psychosocial problems in preventive child healthcare. *BMC Public Health, 6*, 197. doi:10.1186/1471-2458-6-197.

Reitman, D., Currier, R., & Stickle, T. (2002). A critical evaluation of the Parenting Stress Index-Short Form (PSI-SF) in a head start population. *Journal of Clinical Child and Adolescent Psychology, 31*, 384–392. doi:10.1207/S15374424JCCP3103_10.

Richardson, L., Keller, A., Selby-Harrington, M., & Parrish, R. (1996). Identification and treatment of children's mental health problems by primary care providers: A critical review of research. *Archives of Psychiatric Nursing, 10*, 293–303.

Richardson, L., McCauley, E., Grossman, D., McCarty, C., Richards, J., Russo, J., et al. (2010). Evaluation of the Patient Health Questionnaire-9 Item for detecting major depression among adolescents. *Pediatrics, 126*, 1117–1123. doi:10.1542/peds.2010-0852.

Robins, D. L. (2008). Screening for autism spectrum disorders in primary care settings. *Autism, 12*, 537–556. doi:10.1177/1362361308094502.

Royall, D., Cordes, J., & Polk, M. (1998). CLOX: An executive clock drawing task. *Journal of Neurology, Neurosurgery & Psychiatry, 64*, 588–594.

Salerno, J., Marshall, V., & Picken, E. (2012). Validity and reliability of the rapid assessment for adolescent preventive services adolescent health risk assessment. *Journal of Adolescent Health, 50*, 595–599. doi:10.1016/j.jadohealth.2011.10.015.

Sanci, L., Lewis, D., & Patton, G. (2010). Detecting emotional disorder in young people in primary care. *Current Opinion in Psychiatry, 23*, 318–323.

Sand, N., Silverstein, M., Glascoe, F., Gupta, V., Tonniges, T., & O'Connor, K. (2005). Pediatricians' reported practices regarding developmental screening: Do guidelines work? Do they help? *Pediatrics, 116*, 174–179. doi:10.1542/peds.2004-1809.

Saunders, J., Aasland, O., Babor, T., de la Fuente, J., & Grant, M. (1993). Development of the Alcohol Use Disorders Identification Test (AUDIT): WHO integrated project on early detection of persons with harmful alcohol consumption–II. *Addiction, 88*, 791–804.

Schonwald, A., Huntington, N., Chan, E., Risko, W., & Bridgemohan, C. (2009). Routine developmental screening implemented in urban primary care settings: More evidence of feasibility and effectiveness. *Pediatrics, 123*, 660–668. doi:10.1542/peds.2007-2798.

Sharp, L. K., & Lipsky, M. (2002). Screening for depression across the lifespan: A review of measures for use in primary care settings. *American Family Physician, 66*, 1001–1008.

Sheldrick, R., Merchant, S., & Perrin, E. (2011). Identification of developmental-behavioral problems in primary care: A systematic review. *Pediatrics, 128*, 356–363. doi:10.1542/peds.2010-3261.

Sices, L., Stancin, T., Kirchner, L., & Bauchner, H. (2009). PEDS and ASQ developmental screening tests may not identify the same children. *Pediatrics, 124*, e640–e647. doi:10.1542/peds.2008-2628.

Simonian, S. J., & Tarnowski, K. (2001). Utility of the pediatric symptom checklist for behavioral screening of disadvantaged children. *Child Psychiatry and Human Development, 31*, 269–278.

Smith, P., Schmidt, S., Allensworth-Davies, D., & Saitz, R. (2009). Primary care validation of a single-question alcohol screening test. *Journal of General Internal Medicine, 24*, 783–788. doi:10.1007/s11606-009-0928-6.

Snider, C., Webster, D., O'Sullivan, C., & Campbell, J. (2009). Intimate partner violence: Development of a brief risk assessment for the emergency department. *Academic Emergency Medicine, 16*, 1208–1216. doi:10.1111/j.1553-2712.2009.00457.x.

Snyder, A., Stanley, M., Novy, D., Averill, P., & Beck, J. (2000). Measures of depression in older adults with generalized anxiety disorder: A psychometric evaluation. *Depression and Anxiety, 11*, 114–120.

Solberg, L., Korsen, N., Oxman, T., Fischer, L., & Bartels, S. (1999). The need for a system in the care of depression. *The Journal of Family Practice, 48*, 973–979.

Spitzer, R., Kroenke, K., & Williams, J. (1999). Validation and utility of a self-report version of PRIME-MD: The PHQ primary care study, primary care evaluation of mental disorders. Patient health questionnaire. *The Journal of the American Medical Association, 282*, 1737–1744.

Spitzer, R., Kroenke, K., Williams, J., & Lowe, B. (2006). A brief measure for assessing generalized anxiety disorder: The GAD-7. *Archives of Internal Medicine, 166*, 1092–1097. doi:10.1001/archinte.166.10.1092.

Stoppelbein, L., Greening, L., Moll, G., Jordan, S., & Suozzi, A. (2012). Factor analyses of the Pediatric Symptom Checklist-17 with African-American and Caucasian pediatric populations. *Journal of Pediatric Psychology, 37*, 348–357. doi:10.1093/jpepsy/jsr103.

Teng, E., & Chui, H. (1987). The Modified Mini-Mental State (3MS) examination. *The Journal of Clinical Psychiatry, 48*, 314–318.

Tolan, P., & Dodge, K. (2005). Children's mental health as a primary care and concern: A system for comprehensive support and service. *American Psychologist, 60*, 601–614. doi:10.1037/0003-066x.60.6.601.

U.S. Preventive Services Task Force. (2008). *USPSTF Grade definitions*. Retrieved from http://www.uspreventiveservicestaskforce.org/uspstf/grades.htm. U.S. Preventive.

U.S. Preventive Services Task Force. (2009). Screening for depression in adults: U.S. preventive services task force recommendation statement. *Annals of Internal Medicine, 151*, 784–792. Retrieved from http://www.annals.org/content/151/11/784.full.pdf+html

U.S. Preventive Services Task Force. (2010). *USPSTF A and B recommendations*. Retrieved from http://www.uspreventiveservicestaskforce.org/uspstf/uspsabrecs.htm

Unutzer, J., Katon, W., Callahan, C., Williams, J., Hunkeler, E., Harpole, L., et al. (2002). Integrated care management of late-life depression in the primary care setting: A randomized controlled trial. *The Journal of the American Medical Association, 288*, 2836–2845.

Unutzer, J., & Park, M. (2012). Strategies to improve the management of depression in primary care. *Primary Care Clinics in Office Practice, 39*, 415–431. doi:10.1016/j.pop.2012.03.010.

Voigt, R., Johnson, S., Mellon, M., Hashikawa, A., Campeau, L., Williams, A., et al. (2009). Relationship between parenting stress and concerns identified by developmental screening and their effects on parental medical care-seeking behavior. *Clinical Pediatrics, 48*, 362–368. doi:10.1177/0009922808327058.

Wallis, K. E., & Pinto-Martin, J. (2008). The challenge of screening for autism spectrum disorder in a culturally diverse society. *Acta Paediatrica, 97*, 539–540. doi:10.1111/j.1651-2227.2008.00720.x.

Wasserman, R., Kelleher, K., Bocian, A., Baker, A., Childs, G., Indacochea, F., et al. (1999). Identification of attentional and hyperactivity problems in primary care: A report from pediatric research in office settings and the ambulatory sentinel practice network. *Pediatrics, 103*, E38.

Weitzman, C., & Leventhal, J. (2006). Screening for behavioral health problems in primary care. *Current Opinion in Pediatrics, 18*, 641–648.

Wetherell, J., Birchler, G., Ramsdell, J., & Unutzer, J. (2007). Screening for generalized anxiety disorder in geriatric primary care patients. *International Journal of Geriatric Psychiatry, 22*, 115–123. doi:10.1002/gps.1701.

Williams, J., Klinepeter, K., Palmes, G., Pulley, A., & Foy, J. (2004). Diagnosis and treatment of behavioral health disorders in pediatric practice. *Pediatrics, 114*, 601–606. doi:10.1542/peds.2004-0090.

Williams, S. B., O'Connor, E. Eder, M., & Whitlock, E. (2009). Screening for child and adolescent depression in primary care settings: a systematic evidence review for the U.S. Preventive Services Task Force. Rockvill, MD. Pediatrics. 2009 Apr;123(4):e716–35

Winter, L., Steer, R., Jones-Hicks, L., & Beck, A. (1999). Screening for major depression disorders in adolescent medical outpatients with the Beck depression inventory for primary care. *Journal of Adolescent Health, 24*, 389–394.

Wren, F., Bridge, J., & Birmaher, B. (2004). Screening for childhood anxiety symptoms in primary care: Integrating child and parent reports. *Journal of the American Academy of Child and Adolescent Psychiatry, 43*, 1364–1371. doi:10.1097/01.chi.0000138350.60487.d3.

Wren, F., Scholle, S., Heo, J., & Comer, D. (2003). Pediatric mood and anxiety syndromes in primary care: Who gets identified? *International Journal of Psychiatry in Medicine, 33*, 1–16.

Zimmerman, M., Galione, J., Ruggero, C., Chelminski, I., Young, D., Dalrymple, K., et al. (2010). Screening for bipolar disorder and finding borderline personality disorder. *The Journal of Clinical Psychiatry, 71*, 1212–1217. doi:10.4088/JCP.09m05161yel.

Zuckerbrot, R., Cheung, A., Jensen, P., Stein, R., & Laraque, D. (2007). Guidelines for Adolescent Depression in Primary Care (GLAD-PC): Identification, assessment, and initial management. *Pediatrics, 120*, e1299–e1312. doi:10.1542/peds.2007-1144.

Zuckerbrot, R. A., & Jensen, P. S. (2006). Improving recognition of adolescent depression in primary care. *Archives of Pediatrics & Adolescent Medicine, 160*, 694–704. doi:10.1001/archpedi.160.7.694.

Zuckerbrot, R., Maxon, L., Pagar, D., Davies, M., Fisher, P., & Shaffer, D. (2007). Adolescent depression screening in primary care: Feasibility and acceptability. *Pediatrics, 119*, 101–108. doi:10.1542/peds.2005-2965.

Chapter 13
Implementing Clinical Interventions in Integrated Behavioral Health Settings: Best Practices and Essential Elements

Daniel J. Mullin and Jennifer S. Funderburk

Abstract The dissemination of Patient-Centered Medical Homes provides an opportunity for primary care practices to attend to the behavioral health and health behavior needs of its patients. This will often include the development of an integrated behavioral health care practice that expands the team membership and develops routines for anticipating and following patients, with a focus on managing a broad range of conditions. Implementation of a successful integrated behavioral health care practice requires attention to building a team, hiring and training that team, developing sustainable workflows, identifying empirically based interventions to include within a clinical pathway, and establishing processes for insuring quality care. This chapter will provide guidance to administrators and review empirical evidence when it exists on all of these topics.

As primary care practices undergo transformation to Patient-Centered Medical Homes (PCMH), it is the ideal time for leadership teams to consider ways to integrate behavioral health services (Hunter & Goodie, 2010). The goal of this chapter is to provide guideposts for heath care providers and administrators in designing organizational systems for incorporating primary care behavioral health services that supports sustainable, evidence-based clinical care. Colocating behavioral health providers within primary care seems intuitively simple. Yet, merely adding behavioral health providers (BHPs) into primary care is not sufficient or adequate for building new approaches that integrate biomedical and psychosocial health care. BHPs are typically hired to provide direct services to primary care patients who

D.J. Mullin, Psy.D. (✉)
Center for Integrated Primary Care, Department of Family Medicine and Community Health, University of Massachusetts Medical School, Worcester, MA, USA
e-mail: Daniel.mullin@umasmemorial.org

J.S. Funderburk, Ph.D.
Center for Integrated Health care, Syracuse VAMC, Syracuse, NY, USA
e-mail: Jennifer.Funderburk@va.gov

M.R. Talen and A. Burke Valeras (eds.), *Integrated Behavioral Health in Primary Care: Evaluating the Evidence, Identifying the Essentials*, DOI 10.1007/978-1-4614-6889-9_13, © Springer Science+Business Media New York 2013

have a range of mental health, behavioral health, or medical needs; however, approaches for incorporating BHPs into primary care are as varied and unique as the setting in which they develop (Katon et al., 2010).

Integrated clinical care is significantly distinct from the traditional referral "specialty" mental health service situated in primary care. The successful integration of behavioral health into practice is a highly complex and multifaceted organizational and clinical process that requires significant planning, resources, and time. This chapter will describe how behavioral health can be embedded within primary care using five parameters of integrated clinical care—(1) defining the clinical team, (2) identifying and focusing on a patient population, (3) using direct clinical interventions or protocols, (4) developing office practices and fiscal sustainability for behavioral health practices, and (5) evaluating quality improvement measures in integrated behavioral health (Peek & Oftedahl, 2010). Table 13.1 provides a clinical case example, and Table 13.2 outlines these five areas delineated, identifying key elements and questions for designing integrated clinical practice. In this chapter, these parameters will be defined and described using examples from clinical practice. The elements of the team will be reviewed, including the team composition along with member roles, responsibilities, training, and communication in direct clinical care. Clinical practices for targeted patients (e.g., depression) and nontargeted patients (e.g., compliance with health regimens) will be reviewed. A review of the evidence for specific integrated clinical care interventions will be described to highlight best-practice approaches and identify areas that need evaluation. The chapter will conclude with a discussion of the role of evaluation and quality improvement measures within the clinical collaborative system of care and how quality improvement is intertwined with clinical practice approaches.

Team Composition: Roles, Responsibilities, Training, and Supervision

Identifying the configuration of an integrated clinical team is a challenging process for health care providers and administrators. In health care centers, providers and staff are often organized within discipline groups rather than in multiprofessional clinical care teams—for example, nurses meet with nurses, physicians with physicians, and support staff with support staff. In contrast, integrated behavioral health begins with multiprofessional teamwork. Multiprofessional teams in primary care vary widely in their composition. Team configurations may range from a structured, well-defined group, such as a primary care provider (PCP), psychiatrist, clinical care manager, and BHP with clear roles, such as the IMPACT model (Unützer et al., 2002) in contrast to the unique, unprescribed, clinical-provider behavioral health patient care approach seen in the Cherokee Health initiatives (Freeman, 2007). Integrated behavioral health and primary care team members may include primary care physicians, psychiatrists, nurses, medical assistants, BHPs (e.g., mental health clinicians), or clinical care managers (CCM). These behavioral health team

Table 13.1 Clinical care case example with parameters (This example portrays a patient who works with the integrated behavioral health team to illustrate specific details incorporated in the chapter)

The patient, Ms. Willard, is a 43-year-old Caucasian female. She lives with her husband of 18 years and two children, aged 16 and 12. She is employed at an elementary school as a Teacher's Aide. Ms. Willard has been a patient of the Fairview Health Center (FHC) for 8 years and her PCP is Dr. Bergman. She has been diagnosed with hypertension and elevated cholesterol. Ms. Willard's weight gradually increased over the years, and her BMI is currently 34. She suffers from chronic pain in her left knee and left ankle from an injury sustained in a motor vehicle accident a decade before. Ms. Willard has a history of major depressive disorder, which has been treated intermittently with an antidepressant medication.

As a patient at FHC, she has attended appointments when she has had acute health concerns. For example, she has suffered from occasional sinus infections and has had flu three times in the past 10 years. She has attended annual physical exams some years, but not every year. Her appointment frequency recently increased to address concerns about her knee and ankle pain. Most of these appointments have been with Dr. Bergman, but on occasion she saw one of his practice partners.

Team Composition and Communication

Within the past 2 years the FHC hired a part-time Clinical Care Manager (CCM), Ms. Martin, who is a Registered Nurse, and a Behavioral Health Provider (BHP), Ms. Donner, who is a Licensed Clinical Social Worker. Ms. Martin received training in approaches to CCM through a statewide learning collaborative, which was developed to help practices with the transformation to the Patient-Centered Medical Home. Ms. Donner completed clinical training rotations in medical settings, but she has never worked in a primary care setting. She has training in Cognitive-Behavioral Therapy and an introduction to brief interventions, such as Solution-Focused Therapy.

The team members communicate about patients through electronic communications in the health center's Electronic Health Record. They meet formally every 2 weeks for an hour over lunch. They also discuss shared patients informally in hallway consultations.

Shared Identified Patient

Ms. Willard was first identified by her nurse and PCP at an appointment for acute sinusitis after completing a Patient Health Questionnaire-9 (Kroenke, Spitzer, & Williams, 2001), with positive screening results for depressive symptoms. A medical assistant on the team administered the written questionnaire when she noticed that Ms. Willard had not been screened in the past 12 months. The positive screen activated a targeted consultation process within the FHC, through which the patient was referred to the CCM. The CCM was responsible for monitoring her progress. The PCP assessed Ms. Willard's depressive symptoms and invited the CCM to meet with the patient.

Prior to entering the exam room, the PCP told the CCM about Ms. Willard's intermittent episodes of depression and her reluctance to engage in psychotherapy. The CCM then met with Ms. Willard and answered her questions, confirming that she understood the importance of taking her antidepressant medication regularly. During this discussion, the CCM presented the possibility of meeting again to discuss different skills that might help her feel better. Using Motivational Interviewing skills, she asked Ms. Willard about her readiness to make some behavioral changes to help improve her mood. Ms. Willard indicated a low readiness to change when asked about her depressed mood, but a high readiness to change regarding her difficulties with sleeping. She expressed an interest in figuring out ways to help improve her sleep without using sleep medications, as she believed that those medications would leave her feeling groggy all day. The CCM asked Ms. Willard if she would be willing to meet with the BHP to discuss some potential ways she might be able to improve her sleep. The CCM also described her role and prepared her for a phone call in 2 weeks to check up on her symptoms and provide support.

(continued)

Table 13.1 (continued)

Clinical Intervention: Sleep Stimulus Control and Motivational Interviewing
Ms. Willard and the BHP, Ms. Donner, met in another exam room. Ms. Donner assessed
Ms. Willard's current sleep schedule, her current difficulties with sleep using the
Insomnia Severity Index (Morin, Belleville, Bélanger, & Ivers, 2011), and identified
several areas for improvement. The BHP explained the importance of a regular sleep
schedule and associating Ms. Willard's bed with sleep. Using MI skills, the BHP asks
Ms. Willard to identify on a 1–10 scale her confidence in being able to make the
changes they have discussed and the importance of these changes to her. Using that
information, they continued to discuss potential barriers and the BHP provided
additional relevant information.

Quality Improvement: Patient Level
Each time Ms. Willard met with the CCM or BHP, they assessed her depressive symptoms
using the Patient Health Questionnaire-9 (PHQ-9) and her level of sleep disturbance
using the Insomnia Severity Index. After meeting with the BHP two times, Ms.
Willard's score on the ISI significantly decreased and she reported greater satisfaction
with her sleep. The CCM noted that Ms. Willard's PHQ-9 score also decreased as she
has maintained medication compliance. Ms. Willard continued to be reluctant to
engage in cognitive-behavioral treatment for depression, but she stated that she will
consider it if she does not feel better soon.

Table 13.2 Clinical case example understood through parameters

Integrated behavioral health parameters		Clinical case example
Team	1. Team composition and roles	• PCP: initial assessment, medication and evaluation and referrals
		• CCM: follow-up with patient, track progress
		• BHP: provide CBT and MI, document patient-centered goals and progress
	2. Level of collaboration or integration	• Integrated—shared space, EHR systems, shared care plans, shared culture
		• Biweekly team meetings to review patient care
Identification of population	3. Nontarget or targeted population screening	• Identification of an adult patient during an acute care visit using the PHQ-9
		• PCP identifies patient behavioral/emotional factors interfering with chronic illness care, chronic pain, sleep, and fatigue
Clinical system	4. Population identification and screening	• Clinical protocol initiated for individual with positive PHQ-9 scores
		• Referral to CCM at time of visit (warm hand-off)
		• Follow-up session(s) scheduled with BHP after patient meets with CCM
	5. Clinical interventions	• Standard Chronic Care model of clinical pathways: PCP identification, referral to CCM and BHP
		• BHP incorporates evidence-based interventions: Sleep Stimulus Control treatment and MI
		• CCM monitors patient care, routine f/u phone calls
	6. Level of patient engagement	• Explicit shared decision-making between BHP and patient
		• Chronic Care Model is clinic team driven

(continued)

Table 13.2 (continued)

Integrated behavioral health parameters		Clinical case example
Office practice and financial system	7. Level of practice reliability/ standardization	• Standard practice of MA and PCP screening adult patients for depression at all visits • Consistent referral process to CCM and BHP • Shared—transparent documentation of treatment plans between providers
	8. Business model/ billing system	• Billing for screening process • CCM is supported through grant funds • BHP services are billed with Health and Behavioral codes
QI and effectiveness measurement	9. Practice-based data collection, analysis, and actual use	• PHQ-9 and Insomnia Screening tool are used to monitor individual progress • PHQ-9 data for adult patients is compiled • No routine team review of population-based data

members may have a variety of roles and responsibilities ranging from coordinating patient care and follow-up, educating patients regarding their health, improving patient engagement in their health care, prescribing medications, or providing behavioral health coaching via phone or face-to-face. There is no research that specifically evaluates or compares the benefits or limitations between different composition of integrated clinical care teams and standard primary care so there are no set guidelines for key elements in a collaborative team other than the inclusion of a team member who is skilled at implementing behavioral health interventions. However, there are some general principles that can guide administrators and providers in building teams that support integrated behavioral health and primary care practices. These principles are: (1) defining roles and expectations of each team member, (2) educational/training experiences necessary, including specialized training in integrated behavioral health and/or knowledge, clinical skills, and professional attitude, and (3) team communication—all of which will help build a successful integrated behavioral health practice.

Defining Expectations and Responsibilities

Successful integrated teams need to delineate clear expectations and responsibilities between the team members. For example, team members need to define who is responsible for clinical tasks from screening to referrals to follow-up visits, and follow-up monitoring and reassessing. For example, the nurse may be designated to administer a screening tool, the PCP's role is to review the screening tool and make a referral to behavioral health, the BHP has a follow-up assessment and treatment and flag PCP with progress and recommendations, and the CCM has the task of scheduling monthly follow-up phones for monitoring. Organizing and clarifying these communication practices are critical. These practices typically include routines for follow-up care and ensure that the practice's patients are not lost to follow-up.

Educational/Training Experiences

The educational foundation for BHPs in primary care is an emerging area for workforce development in health care. Individuals with diverse educational backgrounds, such as social work, nursing, psychology, counseling, marriage and family counseling, and psychiatry, may function as BHPs in primary care settings. Their educational background typically includes Master and Doctoral degrees, or medical degrees. Even some primary care physicians have fellowship training in psychiatry and are doubled boarded or are licensed marriage and family therapists. However, it is *not* common for these different disciplines to have specific training in the foundations of primary care behavioral health. Currently, there is no states licensure specifically for behavioral health providers. Typically, individuals may focus on areas (e.g., clinical health psychology, medical social work, etc.) that mesh with the knowledge and skills for primary care clinical practice (Alexopoulos, Reynolds, Bruce, et al., 2009; Hunter, Goodie, Oordt, & Dobmeyer, 2009; Robinson, 2005). The advantage of incorporating advanced degree BHPs (e.g., Ph.D., MD) is that they usually have training and knowledge of psychiatric assessment and empirically supported clinical interventions, such as Motivational Interviewing or Cognitive-Behavioral Therapies. They are also able to help patients with complex mental health issues, as well as help to train and supervise other team members on behavioral health issues/interventions.

CCMs are typically providers with medical assistant or nursing backgrounds. In PCMHs there is renewed interest in including CCMs with advanced behavioral health skills. There is a growing recognition that many primary care patients have chronic co-occurring medical and behavioral health needs that can be managed by CCMs with behavioral health expertise. This role has been supported by the research on depression in primary care (Unützer et al., 2002). CCMs may function as the coordinators of behavioral health after a referral from the PCP or screening assessment for behavioral health care has been initiated. CCMs may provide continuity of care in a variety of ways. They support patients' medication regimens, monitor patients' follow-up appointments with a PCP or psychiatrist, provide phone contact and assess patients for risk factors, and refer patients into more intensive clinical care options when necessary. The CCMs serve the crucial role of connecting patients with other members of the primary care team and with specialty services as needed. Typically, these team members have a Bachelor's or Master's degree that may include specific behavioral health training (Alexopoulos et al., 2009; Rubenstein et al., 2010). However, CCMs may have limited prior experience in caring for patients with complex comorbid medical and behavioral needs. Often times they will have expertise in one of these areas, but require support in developing confidence and expertise in the others.

Medical providers—physicians, psychiatrists, advanced nurse practitioners—provide another function within the integrated behavioral health and primary care approach. These team members have the expertise to assess and treat patients with medications and help monitor other health risks with medically complex patients (e.g., hypertension, drug interactions, diabetes). When caring for patients with complex comorbid medical and behavioral health needs, the perspective offered by this continuity is often critical for engaging patients and improving outcomes.

Specialized Training in Integrated Behavioral Health

Many different mental health disciplines offer foundational behavioral health skills, but few programs offer specific training for the knowledge, skills, and professionalism that is specifically applicative to integrated behavioral health. There are only a small percentage of graduate programs, clinical practicums, internships, or fellowships specifically designed to train providers in the unique knowledge and skill set for primary care. For psychologists, social workers, and marriage and family therapists, most of this training tends to occur within internship and postdoctoral programs (Garcia-Shelton & Vogel, 2002; McDaniel, et al., 2004). For instance, Malcolm Grow Medical Center's Primary Care Training internship program at Andrews Air Force base offers doctoral psychology students a chance to gain experience in behavioral health consultation in primary care through a required 6-month rotation for 1 day per week (Dobmeyer, Rowan, Etherage, & Wilson, 2003). The Collaborative Family Healthcare Association maintains a helpful website that lists current internship programs (see http://cfha.net//pages/Clinical-Internships/).

There are few graduate programs that are being designed to address the need for specialized training in medical family therapy, behavioral health, or clinical health psychology. For instance, the Doctorate of Behavioral Health program at Arizona State University provides specialized coursework and practicum experiences focused on developing a new brand of providers capable of working effectively within integrated health care systems (see http://sls.asu.edu/dbh/about.html). This 18-month program, while not governed by an accrediting body, does require a prerequisite of a clinical master's degree.

There are also certificate programs in Primary Care Behavioral Health. The University of Massachusetts Medical School's Center for Integrated Primary Care hosts a certificate program that consists of 36 hours of didactic and interactive training, delivered in 6 full-day workshops. Behavioral health professionals enrolled in this program can choose from two tracks: one for those who work as generalist behavioral health professionals in primary care settings and one for those who work with patients with severe and persistent mental illnesses (see http://www.umassmed.edu/cipc). Fairleigh Dickinson University also hosts a certificate program in Integrated Primary Care, delivered through a distance format, utilizing the Internet and email to deliver 20 interactive modules (see http://integratedcare.fdu.edu). Both certificate programs cost around $1,500. While continuing education credits are provided through discipline-specific organizations, there is no accrediting body that oversees such certificate programs and it is not recognized formally within specific disciplines. Also, these are knowledge-base programs do not require direct clinical supervision experiences within primary care settings for the certificate. Psychologists can also obtain a board certification from the American Board of Professional Psychologists in clinical health psychology. Individuals with this certification have a significant level of training in clinical health psychology; however, they may not have had specific training in primary care (see http://www.abpp.org/i4a/pages/index.cfm?pageid=3353).

All team members, including CMC, PCP, and BHPs, will benefit from continuing professional development opportunities as this field takes shape. Workshops and conferences, such as those offered during the Collaborative Family Healthcare Association Annual Conference (see www.cfha.net) and the web-based training program offered by the University of Massachusetts Medical School (Blount & Miller, 2009) (see http://www.umassmed.edu/cipc) or by the National Council of Community Behavioral Health Care (see http://www.thenationalcouncil.org), offer opportunities to provide continuing education opportunities.

Knowledge, Clinical Skills, and Professional Attitudes

There are a range of clinical competencies that are important for providers to function effectively within an integrated behavioral health team (see Table 13.3 for a summary). The various team members may need to develop competencies in different areas for effective clinical care.

First, BHPs need to have a foundational knowledge in behavioral medicine and health psychology. Specifically, it is important that they have a solid foundation in common medications, especially psychotropic medications, and basic knowledge of medical terminology and chronic diseases (Hunter et al., 2009; Robinson & Reiter, 2007). BHPs must have conceptual and scientific knowledge of the interrelationship between biomedical and psychosocial factors in health risks and health promotion. Other members of the team must have an awareness of when and how BHPs can add to effective patient care and health outcomes.

Second, BHPs and PCPs must develop strong relationship and communication skills, as well as assessment, consultation, and brief intervention skills. Assessment skills must be relevant to the primary care setting. For example, BHPs often administer and interpret behavioral health assessments such as the Patient Health Questionnaire-9 and share this information with their clinical team. BHPs should be comfortable administering the various types of mental health assessments, such as screening tools or brief cognitive assessment within an integrated behavioral health practice. Assessing a patient's risk for suicide, violence, or significant mental disorder is another critical BHP skill. PCPs often care for patients reporting serious mental health symptoms and rely on the BHPs to provide an assessment, support, coaching, and crisis intervention or referrals for these patients.

Table 13.3 Summary of the clinical competencies to consider prior to hiring a BHP/CM

Knowledge base
- Strong background in behavioral medicine and healthy psychology needed to collaborate with primary care providers
  - Solid foundation in common psychotropic medications
  - Basic knowledge of medical terminology and disease
  - Understanding of biopsychosocial relationships involved in symptom presentation

Patient communication
- Ability to translate medical terminology into everyday language
- Provision of a clear explanation of the biopsychosocial relationships related to patient's symptom presentation

Mental health assessments
- Selection of reliable and valid assessment tools for specific presenting problems
- Administration of assessment tools
- Scoring and interpretation of measures
- Selection of evidence-based practices based on assessment results
- Use of results to monitor reduction/escalation of symptom presentation

Risk assessment
- Comfort with risk assessments with patients reporting suicidal ideation
- Knowledge of risk management protocols and available resources

Solid foundation in motivational interviewing
- Prior training (involving feedback and coaching) aids in the effective delivery of Motivational Interviewing techniques, used to motivate patients towards changing their behaviors ranging from alcohol use to medication adherence
- Members of the Motivational Interviewing Network of Trainers (MINT) can train others

Other essential clinical skills for all members of the integrated team, especially the BHP, include brief Cognitive-Behavioral Therapy and brief Problem Solving interventions in addition to a solid foundation in health behavior change approaches such as Motivational Interviewing (MI). MI is a method of communication that has been found to be effective in helping to motivate patients to change behaviors ranging from alcohol use to medication adherence (Burke, Arkowitz, & Menchola, 2003; Lundahl, Kunz, Brownell, Tollefson, & Burke, 2010; Rubak, Sandboek, Lauritzen, & Christensen, 2005; Vasilaki, Hosier, & Cox, 2006). Research has shown that attendance at a MI workshop alone (without feedback or additional coaching) does not yield individuals who will be able to maintain proficiency at implementing MI (Miller, Yahne, Moyers, Martinez, & Pirritano, 2004). Rather, it is important to find candidates who have had additional feedback and coaching in the implementation of MI.

Third, all of the team members must demonstrate the professional attitudes and awareness of each other's professional cultural-climate to bridge the communication between biomedical and psychosocial worlds. Developing the professional sensitivity to communicate with a diverse professional team is crucial for integrated behavioral health. BHPs are often cultural brokers and translators between patient's understanding and values and the medical provider's perspective and goals (Hunter et al., 2009; Robinson & Reiter, 2007). A fundamental component of every integrated behavioral health model is the ability of all of the team members to demonstrate respect and acknowledge the value of behavioral health issues to whole-person care. Without being able to demonstrate these professional attitudes of respect and shared vision of patient care, the team members will function in silo, parallel practice modes.

BHPs are also behavioral health ambassadors at the frontline of primary care, helping to close the gap between biomedical and psychosocial worlds. BHPs may help defuse the stigma that PCPs or patients have towards behavioral health. In addition, BHPs help bridge the services and communication between the specialty mental health services and primary care centers. This coordination can happen when the BHP providers have confidence, assertiveness, and flexibility, and especially when they are a trusted member of the primary care team.

HOW: Team Communication

Defining who is part of the collaborative team and the knowledge and skills of team members is only one aspect of integrated behavioral health. Collaborative teams need to define the method of communication (e.g., Electronic Health Record (EHR), team meetings, huddles) and how often team members communicate about patient care. Daily team huddles before clinic or monthly team meetings are some common methods for team interactions, but teams may also communicate through EHR system sharing assessment and patient treatment plans. The shared EHR also makes it possible for team members to post follow-up messages to each other. No single approach to coordinating care or communicating between team members has been demonstrated to be superior to other approaches, but the advantage of integrated behavioral health is the accessibility between team members and the ease of "impromptu" hallway consultations.

Building a high functioning integrated behavioral health team requires intentional planning. Members must be recruited with the appropriate skills, and knowledge gaps must be addressed with additional training. Encouraging patterns of regular communication is also essential. This section highlights the different knowledge, skills, and professional team factors that are critical for effective team communication. Chapter 10 describes in more detail the variety of team roles and communication processes with integrated behavioral health systems.

Clinical Care for Targeted and Nontargeted Patient Populations

Integrated behavioral health and primary care programs will vary based on which populations they serve. As a result, successful integrated behavioral health and primary care teams are intentional in identifying protocols that focus team members to work with a defined patient population as well as provide specific clinical pathways for treatment. It is possible to develop these protocols and pathways by first distinguishing between targeted and nontargeted patients. Targeted patients are those who have been identified through screening or medical exam to have a specific symptom or condition that may benefit from behavioral health interventions. These conditions may be either psychiatric conditions (e.g., depression, anxiety, substance abuse) or medical conditions with behavioral components (e.g., tobacco use, diabetes, obesity). Nontargeted primary care patients are those patients who may benefit from a wide range of behavioral health clinical strategies to improve patient health outcomes, healthy choices, self-management, or goal setting.

Patients identified through targeted or nontargeted screening are connected with the appropriate members of the primary care team. Typically, these team members may be BHPs or CCMs. It is the responsibility of the BHP or the CCM to provide the patient with an evidence-based intervention suitable to the patient's needs. The decisions about what intervention(s) should be provided are typically made through a collaborative process that includes the integrated behavioral health team, the patient, and the best evidence-based approaches.

Evidence-Based Clinical Approaches for Targeted Populations

For integrated behavioral health programs that have identified targeted consultation pathways to be used by CCMs or BHPs (e.g., all patients with Major Depressive Disorder), the delivery of evidence-based clinical interventions can be relatively straightforward. A variety of resources are available summarizing evidence-based interventions for a wide variety of populations. These assessments and interventions can be developed into well-defined paths for patients in the targeted population. Detailed descriptions of pathways for select populations are already available (Collaborative Care for Depression in the Primary Care Setting: A Primer on VA's TIDES Project, 2008). Based on the USPTF findings, there are only a handful of targeted patient populations that have empirical support within the primary care setting (www.USPTF.org). This section provides an overview of those clinical interventions/pathways that have significant evidence supporting their usefulness in primary care or are evidence-based and would be feasible within the constraints of an integrated primary care setting.

Alcohol misuse. Screening, Brief Intervention, and Referral to Treatment (SBIRT) is a population-based approach that incorporates universal screening, interventions, and treatment strategies that target substance use disorders and at-risk substance use (Babor et al., 2007) within primary care at the point of care (Saitz, 2010). The United States Preventive Services Task Force (USPSTF) identifies alcohol screening and intervention as having sufficient evidence (e.g., level B) to recommend this as a standard of clinical care. The international wealth of literature supporting the efficacy of brief alcohol interventions in reducing alcohol use within the primary care setting for patients reporting at-risk drinking (e.g., often defined as drinking that involves repeated consequences or drinking greater than 14 (7 for women or men ≥65 years old) standard drinks per week or greater than 5 (4 for women or men ≥65) on any given occasion) (US Department of Health and Human Services. National Institute on Alcohol Abuse and Alcoholism, 2005) is quite extensive (Funderburk, Maisto, Sugarman, Smucny, & Epling, 2008). This literature has found that these interventions can help reduce alcohol use by an average of 38 g per week (Bertholet, Daeppen, Wietlisbach, Fleming, & Burnand, 2005) and help reduce the number of at-risk drinkers by 12 % compared to no intervention (Beich, Thorsen, & Rollnick, 2003). Evidence supporting the efficacy of brief alcohol interventions for reducing alcohol consumption in those patients meeting criteria for alcohol dependence is not available to date (Saitz, 2010). It remains unclear whether brief alcohol interventions are useful within that population.

Although descriptions of brief alcohol interventions vary in content and format (e.g., ranging from one 5-min intervention to 45-min with two telephone booster sessions), six core elements that are provided during effective brief alcohol interventions are identified: (1) Feedback on personal risk, (2) Responsibility resides within the person for change, (3) Advice about changing, (4) Menu of change options, (5) Expression of empathy by the clinician, and (6) Increase self-efficacy (otherwise known as FRAMES)[28]. A majority of the research programs used primary care providers as the main interventionists, while several used research staff that varied in educational backgrounds (Funderburk et al., 2008).

The World Health Organization (see http://www.who.int/substance_abuse/activities/sbi/en/index.html#content) and the National Institute of Alcohol Abuse and Alcoholism (see http://pubs.niaaa.nih.gov/publications/practitioner/pocketguide/pocket_guide.htm) have helpful information including brief alcohol intervention materials and trainings.

Tobacco use. U.S. Preventive Services Task Force (2008) conducted a thorough literature review and concluded that there was enough evidence to support the effectiveness of brief and intensive counseling in reducing tobacco use (Fiore et al., 2008). This is the only behavioral health intervention that has a strong level A recommendation from the USPSTF. Brief counseling usually employs the 5 A's (e.g., Ask, Advise, Assess, Assist, Arrange) (Whitlock, Orleans, Pender, & Allan, 2002) and occurs within 3 min during the primary care visit. Intensive treatment, which consists of approximately four or more follow-up sessions that are more than 10 min and focuses on problem solving and skills training, is more effective than brief counseling (Fiore et al., 2008). Similar to alcohol use, there are many online resources for patients and providers (e.g., see http://www.smokefree.gov/).

Sleep disorders. The Academy of Sleep Medicine has recommended the following behavioral interventions due to empirical support of their effectiveness in treating chronic insomnia: (1) cognitive-behavioral treatment (e.g., help patient change his/her beliefs about sleeping while also teaching behavioral strategies, such as stimulus control, relaxation, or sleep restriction) (Morgenthaler et al., 2006), (2) stimulus control therapy (e.g., help patient learn how to reassociate the bed/bedroom with sleep (Bootzin, Epstein, & Wood, 1991)), (3) relaxation training (e.g., help patient to reduce tension and intrusive thoughts prior to bed using progressive muscle relaxation or autogenic training (Morgenthaler et al., 2006)), (4) sleep restriction (e.g., help patient maximize his/her sleep efficiency by curtailing the amount of time in bed to approximate the time spent sleeping (Spielman, Saskin, & Thorpy, 1987)), and (5) multicomponent therapy (e.g., combine sleep restriction and stimulus control (Morgenthaler et al., 2006)). However, few research studies have examined these interventions within the primary care setting, even though rates of chronic insomnia in primary care are high [e.g., 19 % (Shochat, Umphress, Israel, & Acoli-Israel, 1999)]. Two randomized controlled studies have evaluated abbreviated forms of cognitive-behavioral treatment (CBT) of insomnia within a primary care setting, which were delivered by members of the research staff. These studies found CBT outperformed a sleep hygiene intervention (e.g., education about good sleep practices) across several study outcome measures (Edinger & Sampson, 2003; Edinger et al., 2009). The CBT format ranged from two sessions to four biweekly sessions. McCrae, McGovern, Lukefahr, and Stripling (2007) found that brief multicomponent treatment (two 50-min individual sessions and two 25-min phone sessions) delivered by behavioral health providers (e.g., social worker, counselor) outperforms sleep hygiene. This initial research within the primary care setting is promising. In addition, stimulus control and sleep restriction can be easily adapted to a primary care setting. However, research has not addressed all the complexities of implementing interventions for sleep within the primary care setting.

Depression and Anxiety

Problem solving treatment tailored for primary care. PST-PC has been tailored for primary care and has been found to be effective at reducing depressive symptoms (Wolf & Hopko, 2008). Many studies focused on patients with Major Depressive Disorder and compared PST-PC to pharmacological interventions (Mynors-Wallis, Gath, Day, & Baker, 2000). The treatment consists of six sessions (e.g., initial 60 min session followed by five 30-min sessions) led by a research staffed medical provider or nurse that focus on teaching the patient effective problem solving skills by focusing on a problem they are currently experiencing in an effort to increase psychosocial functioning (see http://impact-uw.org/tools/pst_manual.html for treatment manuals). To date, there is no consensus about the effectiveness of PST-PC for dysthymia and minor depression (Alexander, Amkoff, & Glass, 2010). Several studies have also reported that PST-PC can be effectively delivered by various medical professionals, including nurses (Katon, Unutzer, & Simon, 2004; Mynors-Wallis, Davies, Gray, Barbour, & Gath, 1997).

Interpersonal Process Therapy. IPT has been identified as an empirically valid treatment for depression outside of primary care, which focuses on helping patients improve interpersonal relationships in an effort to reduce depressive symptomatology (DeRubeis & Crits-Christoph, 1998). Several research studies have examined an abbreviated version of IPT, which has been implemented in either six or ten sessions, within the primary care setting. These studies have found this abbreviated version of IPT to be effective in reducing depressive symptoms compared to a control condition (Klerman et al., 1987) and usual care, which typically is medication (Mossey, Knott, Higgins, & Talerico, 1996). This abbreviated form of IPT was also incorporated as the treatment when patients did not want medication within the studies examining a care management intervention (e.g., PROSPECT). IPT was delivered by clinical care managers with various educational backgrounds from nurses to psychologists (Alexopoulos et al., 2009).

Cognitive-Behavioral Therapy Tailored for Primary Care. This is another treatment that, due to its efficacy in treating depression and anxiety outside of primary care (Olatunji, Cisler, & Deacon, 2010; Powell, Abreu, de Oliveira, & Sudak, 2008), several studies have evaluated within the primary care setting targeting depressive and anxiety symptoms. Scott, Tacchi, Jones, and Scott (1997) conducted a preliminary study examining if six sessions of CBT enhanced PCP's usual care for patients with depression. They found that there was some evidence that adding CBT with a behavioral health provider may result in decreased depressive symptoms and increased recovery rates at 7 weeks. Miranda and Munoz (1994) examined whether participation in an 8-week CBT course would result in a reduction of depressive symptoms in primary care patients reporting minor depression. They found the CBT course to significantly lower depressive symptoms as compared to a control condition. Although future research needs to expand the size and scope of these research studies, these findings provide initial evidence that brief-CBT may be of value to depressed patients who are seen within the primary care setting.

Two studies have examined CBT for treatment of anxiety disorders in primary care. Roy-Byrne et al. (2005) demonstrated that six sessions of CBT delivered by a BHP combined with psychopharmacology within a primary care setting yielded sustained improvements of anxiety symptoms in individuals with Panic Disorder. Stanley et al. (2009) found ten sessions of CBT to reduce worry severity and depressive symptoms compared to usual care in patients with Generalized Anxiety Disorder. However, they did not find any differences in their measure of generalized anxiety severity.

Obesity

Due to the devastating effects and significant prevalence of obesity within the USA, the US Preventive Services Task Force recommended regular height and weight measurements in primary care in an effort to screen for obesity (US Preventive Services Task Force, 1996) and to begin to intervene using intensive behavioral counseling. Unfortunately, the small amount of research on behavioral interventions conducive to the primary care setting is still very limited. One review of the literature revealed that low-to-moderate intensity PCP counseling yielded no clinically significant weight loss (Tsai & Wadden, 2009). A few research studies have examined collaborative interventions conducted by the primary care team (e.g., nurse, dietician) typically resulting in an additional 8–28 in-person or telephone visits, but demonstrating mixed results when it came to weight loss ranging from −0.2 to −4.3 kg (Ashley et al., 2001; Ely et al., 2008; Logue et al., 2005). Therefore, the research is still limited on interventions that can be useful in targeting obesity.

Diabetes and Hypertension

"Disease self-management" is a term applied to any formalized patient education program aimed at teaching skills needed to carry out medical regiments specific to the disease, guide health behavior change, and provide emotional support for patients to control their disease and live functional lives (Bourbeau et al., 2003). Several literature reviews have concluded that disease self-management techniques improve health status (e.g., reduce systolic blood pressure) and reduce health care utilization when the self-management programs focus on diabetes and hypertension. The evidence is less clear for diseases, such as arthritis, asthma, and COPD (Bodenheimer, Lorig, Holman, & Grumbach, 2002; Bourbeau et al., 2003; Chodosh et al., 2005; Dennis et al., 2008; Warsi, Wang, LaValley, Avorn, & Solomon, 2004). Research still needs to be conducted to identify the essential elements of self-management programs, as they remain unknown (Chodosh et al., 2005).

Evidence-Based Clinical Interventions for Nontargeted Patient Population

Working with nontargeted patients, meaning, "whoever comes through the clinic doors today," is a common experience for BH providers in primary care. Yet, there are few specific clinical pathways for knowing the best strategies to manage the vast array of concerns that patients share during a medical visit. Patients who come into the health center may or may not have a specific mental health or substance abuse disorder, but may have a general behavioral health concern related to their physical condition such as diabetes, hypertension, or asthma. Patients may, for example, express concern about their long history of failures with trying to walk more. PCPs, at the time of the office visit, may identify that the patient could benefit from behavioral interventions to improve their health outcome, enhance the patient's engagement within the medical home, or curtail inappropriate use of medical services. These patients are often not part of a disease registry or systematic screening process for an age group (e.g., developmental screening for children) in the clinic system. Therefore, consultation pathways for the nontargeted patients may entail generic referral processes and "on call consultations" during the clinic hours. Office managers, referral coordinators, and supervisors may be instrumental in outlining standard protocols for health providers to refer to the BHP or CM services when a patient needs behavioral health coaching with a grab-bag of health issues. The development of these pathways is often influenced by the type of integrated behavioral health model implemented within a clinic and the types of patients the PCP tends to encounter. Typically, a nontargeted patient begins with a PCP provider on the integrated behavioral health and primary care team identifying a patient who may need support in goal setting, for example, and the provider may use a "warm hand-off" to introduce the patient to the BHP or CCM at the time of the medical visit (Strosahl, 2000). Initial research has shown an introduction to a BHP or CCM will likely increase attendance at subsequent appointments (Cummings, O'Donohue, & Cummings, 2009; Guck, Guck, Brack, & Frey, 2007). The culture, economic status, or gender of patients, however, may influence the follow-through of patients who are introduced to a BHP at their medical visit. The other potential benefits to health care outcomes and follow-up care following a "warm hand-off" are yet to be examined.

When a collaborative contact is initiated, the CCM or BHP may employ evidence-based interventions appropriately, following the "warm hand-off." Due to the population approach of primary care, interventions are typically delivered in a brief solution-focused format [e.g., 15–30 min, 1–3 sessions (O'Donohue, Byrd, Cummings, & Henderson, 2005)] allowing the providers to address the patient's unique needs and encouraging patient's to identify the focus of their care. Many of the evidence-based interventions that have been developed within mental health context can be adapted to patients who are seen in primary care. Specific interventions that have been used with targeted patient groups (e.g., depression and anxiety) along with general techniques, such as Motivational Interviewing, have anecdotally been adapted to this nontargeted group of patients with diverse health care concerns. However, the nature of key components of these behavioral health interventions in relationship to the primary care context have not yet been well articulated, developed, or evaluated.

SUPPORTED BY: Practice Management and Office Systems

Operations and Payment

It is difficult to provide explicit guidance regarding the financial and operational details of integrated behavioral health practices. The type of organization (e.g., FQHC, CHC, nonprofit), the local health care environment and state regulations will greatly impact financial and operational decisions. This section will review some of the common decisions that need to be addressed and offer general guidance on payment and operational decisions that are relevant to delivering evidence-based integrated behavioral health interventions.

Operations. Integrated behavioral health and primary care organizations that rely on integrated scheduling, billing, and registration systems will have a distinct advantage over practices that manage these practice management routines separately. A unified system allows patients to call one number to schedule an appointment and complete one registration and checkout process. A unified registration process will allow them to schedule and check in for their visits with both providers through a single interaction with a support staff member. This unity of scheduling and registration allows for a more seamless patient experience. It also conveys the message that integration of behavioral and medical services are valued and supported in the everyday operations of the health center.

Payment. In some states there are barriers to billing and payment that present significant challenges to building integrated care practices. For example, in many states the Medicaid regulations do not allow for same day billing of behavioral health and medical encounters. Those interested in integrated behavioral health need to understand and address these policies (see Chap. 4 for a discussion on policy).

Some integrated behavioral health practices have been successful in using the Health and Behavior CPT codes (CPT 96150-4), which allow BHPs to be reimbursed for care targeting patient's medical conditions. These codes are most often approved for licensed psychologists, but BHPs with other credentials (e.g., LICSW, LPCC) have also reported success in using these codes (Kessler, 2008). Medicare has approved the use of these codes, as have some private insurers such as BC/BS and Cigna. Unfortunately, in a majority of states, Medicaid programs do not reimburse for these service codes.

There is optimism that the national movement to implement medical home models will bring with it payment reform, which will allow for new financial models of care that will make it easier to develop integrated behavioral health practices. As payment shifts to capitated payments, whereby practices are paid fees to care for a population of patients rather than for being reimbursed for each visit with a patient, the opportunities for integrated behavioral health to demonstrate financial value will be increased. Much of the care in a capitated system will shift to preventive care and targeting patients with complex comorbid medical and behavioral health needs. BHPs and CCMs are positioned to contribute to this preventive care and to attend to the needs of a smaller number of complex patients who account for a disproportionate level of health care resources and cost.

Practice-Based Data and Quality Improvement Processes

This final section is devoted to describing a quality improvement process that will facilitate the ongoing management and improvement of clinically integrated behavioral health practices. Due to an ever-changing health care environment and significant financial pressures that require constant demonstration of the value and outcomes associated with a program, it is impossible to ignore the value of assessing quality outcomes associated with an integrated behavioral health program. In addition, these outcomes may be a required component for primary care practices that are pursuing recognition as a PCMH. For example, the development of processes and workflows for screening patients for unmet behavioral health needs is an essential component of the PCMH, as described by the NCQA. The documentation of such screening and the communication between BHP/CCMs and PCPs will support a practice's application for recognition as a PCMH. For these reasons, it is essential that administrators develop systematic processes for practice-based quality improvement. Three different levels of quality improvement can be considered when creating an integrated behavioral health program: patient, provider, and system. Each level is important in evaluating a program and requires different strategies for implementing, collecting data, evaluating the results, and building quality improvement initiatives within a health care setting.

Patient Level

There are two basic areas for evaluating the impact of integration on patient care—patient satisfaction and health outcomes. The evaluation of patients' perceptions of care in an integrated behavioral health service is critical, especially within a health care environment that is increasingly focused on providing patient-centered care. Patient satisfaction is a key indicator of quality. Typically, patient satisfaction is assessed via self-report questionnaires. It is important to remember there are many aspects of patient satisfaction with a primary care behavioral service, including: access to appointments, coordination of care, ease of referral process between medical and behavioral health, wait times and length and frequency of encounters, etc. Therefore, it is important to design questionnaires to describe the potential strengths and weaknesses of integrated behavioral health, while recognizing that the patients may not have a clear understanding of the underlying integration between biomedical and psychosocial care.

Patient health outcomes are another factor often included in quality improvement processes. These outcomes can include physical, social, or emotional indicators. However, defining the health outcome to be measured can be complex depending on the breadth of the behavioral health needs of a targeted integrated behavioral health service. The more diverse the integrated behavioral health service, the more difficult it will be to assess patient outcomes. For instance, care management programs that target patients with Major Depressive Disorder can focus on reduced depressive symptoms and improved functioning. However, those nontargeted patient groups who receive behavioral health interventions for a range of health concerns (e.g., chronic pain, fatigue, insomnia) may have other medical or biologically based health outcomes that can be used to assess and evaluate integrated behavioral health initiatives. Typically, patient outcomes are assessed via simple metrics, such as the percentage of patients reporting a decrease in negative symptoms or an increase in healthy behaviors (e.g., social support, activity levels). The level of symptom change is often measured using validated self-report questionnaires (Kroenke et al., 2001; Kroenke, Spitzer, Williams, Monahan, & Löwe, 2007; Morin et al., 2011; Parkerson, Broadhead, & Tse, 1990; Saunders, Aasland, Babor, & de la Fuente, 1993). Many of the screening tools described in Chap. 12 used to identify cases of behavioral health problems (e.g., AUDIT-C, PHQ-9, and the GAD-7) have also been used to monitor clinical progress and outcomes. It is important to decide what patient outcomes to measure and what empirically validated self-report questionnaire can be used to monitor changes. Most importantly, integrated behavioral health addresses how behavioral health changes physical health, such as diabetic management (e.g., HgA1c, BMI, Hypertension). These are important areas to monitor along with mental or behavioral health indicators.

Provider Level

Evaluating the quality of work conducted by the BHP/CCM provides information on the quality of the primary behavioral health service from the provider level. Satisfaction between the BHP/CCMs and the PCPs is an essential evaluation process, especially within an organization that has recently reorganized. Evidence suggests that BHP/CCMs and PCPs are typically satisfied with integrated behavioral health services (Chomienne et al., 2010; Farrar, Kates, Crustolo, & Nikolaou, 2001; Funderburk et al., 2010). However, poor satisfaction with behavioral health service can have significant impact on the collaboration between team members. PCPs and other health providers can provide significant feedback on the clinical performance of the BHP/CCM, since many of their responsibilities are difficult to assess directly. For example, the BHP/CCMs responsiveness to PCPs, nurses, and MAs requests for assistance, or timely consultation may impact the health providers' perceptions of the importance of behavioral health services. Gathering systematic feedback from providers and staff will assist in the identification of opportunities for improvement in the integrated behavioral health care service. Likewise, feedback from BH on health care providers' level of collaboration is an important yet underinvestigated area for quality improvement. The bidirectional nature of communication and professional shared investment can add to identifying the essential ingredients for quality care.

Another way to evaluate the quality of integrated behavioral health and primary care is via chart review. However, this is rarely accomplished in health care settings because it depends on a systematic approach to documenting behavioral health interventions and assessments. One of the obstacles centers on obtaining reliable and consistent data. This is often complicated when BHP/CCMs documentation is inconsistent or in a free text format. It is important to evaluate whether the BHP/CCMs are following established protocols for predetermined patient populations or providing appropriate assessment/treatment based on the patient's presenting problem. In addition, it is important to ensure that the BHP/CCM is following payer and state/federal law regulations. Often, this can be accomplished through regular peer/supervisor review of progress notes. Because the documentation is significantly different than those notes typically found in specialty mental health clinics, it is important to have individuals knowledgeable about the requirements for peer review. For example, comprehensive psychiatric evaluations are often not conducted within most models of integrated behavioral health (Strosahl, 1998). In order to facilitate the evaluation of quality clinical care, clinicians must be encouraged to clearly document the problem they are treating and the interventions they provide. Health records that have standard categories for treatment approaches, progress notes, and patient factors may help organize this information for the clinical tracking and descriptive data.

A third approach to evaluating clinician/provider quality improvement is through periodic live observation of BHP/CCMs or audio review of patient encounters. This intensive review process can provide increased confidence in the BH providers' fidelity to the evidence-based interventions discussed above. Regular case reviews and review of critical incidents may also contribute to improvements in care. Whenever possible these discussions of patient care should include all members of the primary care team to further emphasize collaboration within team-based care approach.

System Level

There are programmatic evaluations that administrators may complete to evaluate the quality of the program at a system level. This level of assessment is essential if the integrated behavioral health service is newly implemented because it focuses on the overall system's ability to provide behavioral health services within primary care and identifies the essential qualities of the integrated behavioral health service being implemented. This evaluation can be further separated into process and outcome measures. Some systems-based evaluations have used surveys to assess a site's level of integration to track the integration of behavioral health within primary care.

Process measures focus on a variety of indicators of how the integrated behavioral health service is functioning. These indicators are derived from the model of integrated behavioral health being implemented and the goals of that program. For example, a program that is implementing a Primary Care Behavioral Health model (Strosahl, 1998) may choose measures such as: mean number of sessions provided by BHP (e.g., expected 2–3 based on model), mean length of sessions provided by BHP (e.g., expected 15–30 min), time between a patient's appointments (e.g., expected 2–3 weeks), time between referral and first appointment (e.g., close to zero because model endorses walk downs), number of same day appointments available per day, etc. A program that has committed itself to implement universal screening for depression may consider monitoring how often this routine screening is being completed in practice. These process measures can provide administrators with an understanding of how a program of integrated behavioral health and primary care is functioning.

Programs may also be assessed by outcome measures; however, this is dependent on the model chosen and the goals identified. Examples include: percentage of patients with BHP/CCM contact who discontinue use of tobacco or percentage of patients with BHP/CCM who recover from a major depressive episode. These outcome measures can provide data on the functioning of the entire program of integrated behavioral health and primary care, or the performance of individual clinicians.

A robust system of quality improvement is an essential element of a high functioning integrated behavioral health service. Patient, provider, and service level data can provide assurances that a program is actually functioning as intended. In addition, opportunities for improvement can be identified. Both measures of process and outcome should be monitored as part of health center's routine quality improvement process. That is, a truly integrated program will use the same quality improvement resources to evaluate both its "medical" and "behavioral" health services.

Summary

This chapter has highlighted several areas such as team interactions, training, and clinical improvement that need to be delineated prior to implementation of direct clinical integrated behavioral health and primary care. The success of the direct clinical integrated behavioral health services depends on several factors: team roles and composition, structured evidence-based clinical pathways, and quality improvement methods. Currently, there is evidence on clinical guidelines that support the treatment of mental health conditions such as depression in primary care using a team of PCP and CCM. BH is usually reserved for those patients who would benefit from intensive individual brief treatments such as CBT or PST. However, the clinical protocols for behavioral health interventions for patients with chronic diseases (e.g., diabetes, hypertension) or other health conditions (e.g., sleep, obesity, headaches), otherwise known as "whoever steps through door," are not well defined or researched and need our attention. And, the quality improvement strategies to evaluate the strengths and limitations of these integrated behavioral health approaches need to be built into our systematic review processes from the patient, provider, and health care system levels. This chapter highlights the beginning foundation to build on evidence-based approaches in clinical practice. This overview also depicts how team composition, population-based models, clinical protocols, and quality improvement factors are important ingredients for future clinical care initiatives in the years to come.

References

Alexander, C. L., Amkoff, D. B., & Glass, C. R. (2010). Bringing psychotherapy to primary care: Innovations and challenges. *Clinical Psychology: Science and Practice, 17*, 191–214.

Alexopoulos, G. S., Reynolds, C. F., Bruce, M. L., et al. (2009). Reducing suicidal ideation and depression in older primary care patients: 24-month outcomes of the PROSPECT study. *The American Journal of Psychiatry, 166*, 882–890.

Ashley, J. M., St Jeor, S. T., Schrage, J. P., Perumean-Chaney, S. E., Gilbertson, M. C., McCall, N. L., et al. (2001). Weight control in the physician's office. *Archives of Internal Medicine, 161*, 1599–1604.

Babor, T. F., McRee, B. G., Kassebaum, P. A., Grimaldi, P. L., Ahmed, K., & Bray, J. (2007). Screening, brief intervention, and referral to treatment (SBIRT): Toward a public health approach to the management of substance abuse. *Substance Abuse, 28*, 7–30.

Beich, A., Thorsen, T., & Rollnick, S. (2003). Screening in brief intervention trials targeting excessive drinkers in general practice: Systematic review and meta-analysis. *British Medical Journal, 327*, 536–542.

Bertholet, N., Daeppen, J. B., Wietlisbach, V., Fleming, M., & Burnand, B. (2005). Reduction of alcohol consumption by brief alcohol intervention in primary care: Systematic review and meta-analysis. *Archives of Internal Medicine, 165*, 986–995.

Blount, F. A., & Miller, B. F. (2009). Addressing the workforce crisis in integrated primary care. *Journal of Clinical Psychology in Medical Settings, 16*, 113–119.

Bodenheimer, T., Lorig, K., Holman, H., & Grumbach, K. (2002). Patient self-management of chronic disease in primary care. *Journal of the American Medical Association, 288*, 2469–2475.

Bootzin, R. R., Epstein, D., & Wood, J. M. (1991). Stimulus control instructions. In P. Hauri (Ed.), *Case studies in insomnia* (pp. 19–28). New York: Plenum Publishing Corp.

Bourbeau, J., Julien, M., Maltais, F., Rouleau, M., Beaupre, A., Begin, R., et al. (2003). Reduction of hospital utilization in patients with chronic obstructive pulmonary disease: A disease-specific self-management intervention. *Archives of Internal Medicine, 163*, 585–591.

Burke, B. L., Arkowitz, H., & Menchola, M. (2003). The efficacy of motivational interviewing: A meta-analysis of controlled clinical trials. *Journal of Consulting and Clinical Psychology, 71*, 843–861.

Chodosh, J., Morton, S. C., Mojica, W., Maglione, M., Suttorp, M. J., Hilton, L., et al. (2005). Meta-analysis: Chronic disease self-management programs for older adults. *Annals of Internal Medicine, 143*, 427–438.

Chomienne, M., Grenier, J., Gaboury, I., Hogg, W., Ritchie, P., & Farmanova-Haynes, E. (2010). Family doctors and psychologists working together: Doctors' and patients' perspectives. *Journal of Evaluation in Clinical Practice, 17*, 282–287.

Cummings, N. A., O'Donohue, W. T., & Cummings, J. L. (2009). The financial dimension of integrated behavioral/primary care. *Journal of Clinical Psychology in Medical Settings, 16*, 31–39.

Dennis, S. M., Zwar, N., Griffiths, R., Roland, M., Hasan, I., Powell Davies, A., et al. (2008). Chronic disease management in primary care: From evidence to policy. *Medical Journal of Australia, 188*, S53–S56.

DeRubeis, R. J., & Crits-Christoph, P. (1998). Empirically supported individual and group psychological treatments for adult mental disorders. *Journal of Consulting and Clinical Psychology, 66*, 37–52.

Dobmeyer, A. C., Rowan, A. B., Etherage, J. R., & Wilson, R. J. (2003). Training psychology interns in primary behavioral health care. *Professional Psychology: Research and Practice, 34*, 586–594.

Edinger, J. D., Olsen, M. K., Stechuchak, K. M., Means, M. K., Lineberger, M. D., Kirby, A., et al. (2009). Cognitive behavioral therapy for patients with primary insomnia or insomnia associated predominately with mixed psychiatric disorders: A randomized clinical trial. *Sleep, 32*, 499–510.

Edinger, J. D., & Sampson, W. S. (2003). A primary care "friendly" cognitive behavioral insomnia therapy. *Sleep, 26*, 117–182.

Ely, A. C., Banitt, A., Befort, C., Hou, Q., Rhode, P. C., Grund, C., et al. (2008). Kansas primary care weighs in: A pilot randomized trial of chronic care model program for obesity in three rural Kansas primary care practices. *The Journal of Rural Health, 24*, 125–132.

Farrar, S., Kates, N., Crustolo, A. M., & Nikolaou, L. (2001). Integrated model for mental health care: Are providers satisfied with it? *Canadian Family Physician, 47*, 2483–2488.

Fiore, M., Jaen, C. R., Baker, T. B., Bailey, B. C., Benowitz, N. L., Curry, S. L., et al. (2008). A clinical practice guideline for treating tobacco use and dependence: 2008 update a U.S. public health service report. *American Journal of Preventive Medicine, 35*, 158–176.

Freeman, D. (2007). Blending behavioral health into primary care at Cherokee Health Systems. *The register report*. Retrieved June 1, 2012, from http://www.nationalregister.org/trr_fall07_ freeman.html

Funderburk, J. S., Maisto, S. A., Sugarman, D. E., Smucny, J., & Epling, J. (2008). How do alcohol brief interventions fit with models of integrated primary care? *Families, Systems & Health, 26*, 1–5.

Funderburk, J. S., Sugarman, D. E., Maisto, S. A., Ouimette, P., Schohn, M., Lantinga, L. J., et al. (2010). The description and evaluation of an integrated healthcare model. *Families, Systems & Health, 28*(2), 130–145.

Garcia-Shelton, L., & Vogel, M. E. (2002). Primary care health psychology training: A collaborative model with family practice. *Professional Psychology: Research and Practice, 33*, 546–556.

Guck, T. P., Guck, A. J., Brack, A., & Frey, D. R. (2007). No-show rates in partially integrated models of behavioral health care in a primary care setting. *Families, Systems & Health, 25*, 137–146.

Hunter, C. L., & Goodie, J. L. (2010). Operational and clinical components for integrated-collaborative behavioral healthcare in the patient-centered medical home. *Families, Systems & Health, 28*, 308–321.

Hunter, C. L., Goodie, J. L., Oordt, M. S., & Dobmeyer, A. (2009). *Integrated behavioral health in primary care: Step-by-step guidance for assessment and intervention*. Washington, DC: American Psychological Association.

Integrated behavioral health for Depression in the Primary Care Setting: A Primer on VA's TIDES Project. (2008). *VHA, Office of Research and Development*. http://www.hsrd.research.va.gov/ publications/internal/depression_primer.pdf

Katon, W. J., Lin, E. H. B., Von Korff, M., Ciechanowski, P., Ludman, E. J., Young, B., et al. (2010). Integrated behavioral health for patients with depression and chronic illnesses. *The New England Journal of Medicine, 363*, 2611–2620.

Katon, W., Unutzer, J., & Simon, G. (2004). Treatment of depression in primary care: Where we are, where we can go. *Medical Care, 42*, 1153–1157.

Kessler, R. (2008). Integration of care is about money too: The health and behavior codes as an element of a new financial paradigm. *Families, Systems & Health, 26*, 207–216.

Klerman, G. K., Budman, S., Berwick, D., Weissman, M. W., Damico-White, J., Demby, A., et al. (1987). Efficacy of a brief psychosocial intervention for symptoms of stress and distress among patients in primary care. *Medical Care, 25*, 1078–1088.

Kroenke, K., Spitzer, R. L., & Williams, J. B. W. (2001). The PHQ-9. Validity of a brief depression severity measure. *Journal of General Internal Medicine, 16*, 606–613.

Kroenke, K., Spitzer, R. L., Williams, J. B. W., Monahan, P. O., & Löwe, B. (2007). Anxiety disorders in primary care: Prevalence, impairment, comorbidity, and detection. *Annals of Internal Medicine, 146*, 317–325.

Logue, E., Sutton, K., Jarjoura, D., Smucker, W., Baughman, K., Capers, C., et al. (2005). Transtheoretical model-chronic disease care for obesity in primary care: A randomized trial. *Obesity Research, 13*, 917–927.

Lundahl, B. W., Kunz, C., Brownell, C., Tollefson, D., & Burke, B. L. (2010). A meta-analysis of motivational interviewing: Twenty-five years of empirical studies. *Research on Social Work Practice, 20*, 137–160.

McCrae, C. S., McGovern, R., Lukefahr, R., & Stripling, A. M. (2007). Research evaluating brief behavioral sleep treatments for rural elderly (RESTORE): A preliminary examination of effectiveness. *The American Journal of Geriatric Psychiatry, 15*, 979–982.

McDaniel, S. H., Hargrove, D. S., Belar, C. D., Schroeder, C. S., & Freeman, E. L. (2004). Recommendations for education and training in primary care psychology. In R. G. Frank, S. H. McDaniel, J. H. Bray, & M. Heldring, (Eds.), *Primary care psychology* (pp. 63–92). Washington, DC: American Psychological Association.

Miller, W. R., Yahne, C. E., Moyers, T. B., Martinez, J., & Pirritano, M. (2004). A randomized trial of methods to help clinicians learn motivational interviewing. *Journal of Consulting and Clinical Psychology, 72*, 1050–1062.

Miranda, J., & Munoz, R. (1994). Intervention for minor depression in primary care patients. *Psychosomatic Medicine, 56,* 136–142.

Morgenthaler, T., Kramer, M., Alessi, C., Friedman, L., Boehlecke, B., Brown, T., et al. (2006). Practice parameters for the psychological and behavioral treatment of insomnia: An update. An American Academy of Sleep Medicine report. *Sleep: Journal of Sleep and Sleep Disorders Research, 29,* 1415–1419.

Morin, C. M., Belleville, G., Bélanger, L., & Ivers, H. (2011). The Insomnia Severity Index: Psychometric indicators to detect insomnia cases and evaluate treatment response. *Sleep: Journal of Sleep and Sleep Disorders Research, 34,* 601–608.

Mossey, J. M., Knott, K. A., Higgins, M., & Talerico, K. (1996). Effectiveness of a psychosocial intervention, interpersonal counseling, for subdysthymic depression in the medically ill elderly. *Journals of Gerontology, 51,* 172–178.

Mynors-Wallis, L., Davies, I., Gray, A., Barbour, F., & Gath, D. (1997). A randomized controlled trial and cost analysis of problem-solving treatment for emotional disorders given by community nurses in primary care. *The British Journal of Psychiatry, 170,* 113–119.

Mynors-Wallis, L., Gath, D., Day, A., & Baker, F. (2000). Randomized controlled trial of problem solving treatment, antidepressant medication, and combined treatment for major depression in primary care. *British Medical Journal, 320,* 26–30.

O'Donohue, W., Byrd, M., Cummings, N., & Henderson, D. (2005). *Behavioral integrative care: Treatments that work in the primary care setting.* New York: Brunner-Routledge.

Olatunji, B. O., Cisler, J. M., & Deacon, B. J. (2010). Efficacy of cognitive behavioral therapy for anxiety disorders: A review of meta-analytic findings. *Psychiatric Clinics of North America, 33,* 557–577.

Parkerson, G. R., Broadhead, W. E., & Tse, C. K. (1990). The Duke health profile. A 17-item measure of health and dysfunction. *Medical Care, 28,* 1056–1072.

Peek, C. J., & Oftedahl, G. (2010). A consensus operational definition of Patient-Centered Medical Home (PCMH) also known as Health Care Home. *University of Minnesota and Institute for Clinical Systems Improvement,* 1–17

Powell, V., Abreu, N., de Oliveira, I., & Sudak, D. (2008). Cognitive-behavioral therapy for depression. *Revista Brasileira de Psiquiatria, 30,* S73–S80.

Robinson, P. (2005). Adapting empirically supported treatments to the primary care setting: A template for success. In W. T. O'Donohue, M. R. Byrd, N. A. Cummings, & D. A. Henderson (Eds.), *Behavioral integrative care: Treatments that work in the primary care setting.* New York: Brunner-Rutledge.

Robinson, P. J., & Reiter, J. T. (2007). *Behavioral consultation and primary care: A guide to integrating services.* New York: Springer.

Roy-Byrne, P. P., Craske, M. G., Stein, M. B., Sullivan, G., Bystritsky, A., Katon, W., et al. (2005). A randomized effectiveness trial of cognitive-behavioral therapy and medication for primary care panic disorder. *Archives of General Psychiatry, 62,* 290–298.

Rubak, S., Sandboek, A., Lauritzen, T., & Christensen, B. (2005). Motivational interviewing: A systematic review and meta-analysis. *British Journal of General Practice, 55,* 305–312.

Rubenstein, L. V., Chaney, E. F., Ober, S., Felker, B., Sherman, S. E., Lanto, A., et al. (2010). Using evidence-based quality improvement methods for translating depression integrated behavioral health research into practice. *Families, Systems & Health, 28,* 91–113.

Saitz, R. (2010). Alcohol screening and brief intervention in primary care: Absence of evidence for efficacy in people with dependence or very heavy drinking. *Drug and Alcohol Review, 29,* 631–640.

Saunders, J., Aasland, O., Babor, T., & de la Fuente, J. (1993). Development of the Alcohol Use Disorders Identification Test (AUDIT): WHO collaborative project on early detection of persons with harmful alcohol consumption: II. *Addiction, 88,* 791–804.

Scott, C., Tacchi, M. J., Jones, R., & Scott, J. (1997). Acute and one-year outcome of a randomised controlled trial of brief cognitive therapy for major depressive disorder in primary care. *The British Journal of Psychiatry, 171,* 131–134.

Shochat, T., Umphress, J., Israel, A. G., & Acoli-Israel, S. (1999). Insomnia in primary care patients. *Sleep, 22*(2), S359–S365.

Spielman, A. J., Saskin, P., & Thorpy, M. J. (1987). Treatment of chronic insomnia by restriction of time in bed. *Sleep: Journal of Sleep Research and Sleep Medicine, 10*, 45–56.

Stanley, M. A., Wilson, N. L., Novy, D. M., Rhoades, H. M., Wagener, P., Greisinger, A., et al. (2009). Cognitive behavior therapy for generalized anxiety disorder among older adults in primary care: A randomized clinical trial. *Journal of the American Medical Association, 301*(14), 1460–1467.

Strosahl, K. (1998). Integrating behavioral health and primary care services: The primary mental health care model. In A. Blount (Ed.), *Integrated primary care: The future of medical and mental health collaboration* (pp. 139–166). New York: Norton & Co.

Strosahl, K. (2000). The psychologist in primary health care. In A. J. Kent, M. Hersen, A. J. Kent, & M. Hersen (Eds.), *A psychologist's proactive guide to managed mental health care* (pp. 87–112). Mahwah, NJ: Lawrence Erlbaum Associates.

Tsai, A. G., & Wadden, T. A. (2009). Treatment of obesity in primary care practice in the United States: A systematic review. *Journal of General Internal Medicine, 24*, 1073–1079.

Unützer, J., Katon, W., Callahan, C. M., Williams, J., Hunkeler, E., Harpole, L., et al. (2002). Collaborative care management of late-life depression in the primary care setting: A randomized controlled trial. *Journal of the American Medical Association, 288*, 2836–2845.

U.S. Preventive Services Task Force. (1996). *Guide to clinical preventive services* (2nd ed., pp. 219–229). Washington, DC: Office of Disease Prevention and Health Promotion.

U.S. Preventive Services Task Force (2003). Counseling to prevent tobacco use and tobacco-caused disease: recommendation statement. Rockville, MD: Agency for Healthcare Research and Quality. Accessed at http://www.uspreventiveservicestaskforce.org on 24 September 2008.

US Department of Health and Human Services. National Institute on Alcohol Abuse and Alcoholism. (2005). *Helping patients who drink too much: A clinician's guide*. Bethesda, MD: National Institute of Health.

Vasilaki, E. I., Hosier, S. G., & Cox, W. M. (2006). The efficacy of motivational interviewing as a brief intervention for excessive drinking: A meta-analytic review. *Alcohol and Alcoholism, 41*, 328–335.

Warsi, A., Wang, P. S., LaValley, M. P., Avorn, J., & Solomon, D. H. (2004). Self-management education programs in chronic disease: A systematic review and methodological critique of the literature. *Archives of Internal Medicine, 164*, 1641–1649.

Whitlock, E. P., Orleans, C. T., Pender, N., & Allan, J. (2002). Evaluating primary care behavioral counseling interventions: An evidence-based approach. *American Journal of Preventive Medicine, 22*, 267–284.

Wolf, N. J., & Hopko, D. R. (2008). Psychosocial and pharmacological interventions for depressed adults in primary care: A critical review. *Clinical Psychology Review, 28*, 131–161.

Chapter 14
Working with Complexity in Integrated Behavioral Health Settings

Macaran A. Baird, C.J. Peek, William B. Gunn, and Andrew Valeras

Abstract This chapter provides a practical approach for understanding and dealing with patient "complexity" in a health care context. Complexity is defined as the interaction of patient, provider, and care delivery variables, which intermingle to create situations where usual treatments are not working—or not working as well as patients and clinicians are expecting. These situations can only be understood by looking at the complex interaction of those variables and adopting new models of understanding and implementing new care-giving strategies. The chapter begins with a review of different approaches to dealing with complexity within the USA and in Europe. A particular method and clinical checklist is described in detail. A "real world" application, the Complex Continuity Clinic, using this and other methods of engaging patients in complex situations, is outlined, with clinical examples. Finally, the important implications of a complexity approach to emerging health care reform is described, shedding light on how effective approaches that embrace complex biopsychosocial health issues can result in greater quality and reduced costs.

M.A. Baird, MD, MS (✉) • C.J. Peek, PhD
Department of Family Medicine and Community Health, University of Minnesota
Medical School, 6-240 Phillips-Wangensteen Building, MMC 381,
420 Delaware Street SE, Minneapolis 55455, MN, USA
e-mail: baird005@umn.edu; cjpeek@unm.edu

W.B. Gunn, PhD
NH/Dartmouth FPR Program, 250 Pleasant St., Concord 03301, NH, USA
e-mail: wgunn@crhc.org

A. Valeras, DO, MPH
New Hampshire Dartmouth Family Medicine Residency, 250 Pleasant St.,
Concord 03301, NH, USA
e-mail: Andrewvaleras@gmail.com

M.R. Talen and A. Burke Valeras (eds.), *Integrated Behavioral Health in Primary Care:*
Evaluating the Evidence, Identifying the Essentials, DOI 10.1007/978-1-4614-6889-9_14,
© Springer Science+Business Media New York 2013

Introduction

As we enter the second decade of the twenty-first century, efforts to integrate behavioral/mental health into primary care practices face many challenges. Among the most influential issues for the long run is the need to redirect our model of assessing patients with emotional distress. Some of that distress is from diagnosable mental conditions and some of it is from situational or social distress that is more like "the human condition" than "mental illness." Our diagnostic and treatment efforts are heavily influenced by the current model of naming psychiatric conditions/illnesses via the Diagnostic and Statistical Manual of Mental Disorders (DSM) now in its 5th Edition. But there is more to the story than discovering and treating diagnosable mental conditions.

The focus of this chapter is to define and explore the concept of a patient's social complexity including his or her interactions with a complex medical environment, which may complicate diagnosis and treatment for any condition the patient may have. We will briefly outline (1) what is meant by *patient social and health system complexity* versus the more general field of complexity science and (2) how to recognize when and how to evaluate a patient's social or care complexity in addition to medical complexity—the latter being more commonly the focus for medical clinicians.

The renewed interest in complexity science has stimulated more discussion about this concept as we enter the second decade of the twenty-first century. In that context, "complexity" refers to the nature of "complex adaptive systems." Such systems have several characteristics that often confound the ability to predict the impact of an intervention in one part of the system. Those core features are:

1. Multiplicity: the number of interacting elements
2. Interdependency: how connected are the elements
3. Diversity: the degree of heterogeneity of the elements

These features interact in patterns, but precise prediction of the behavior of a complex adaptive system is relatively difficult compared to noncomplex systems. For example, adding a payment incentive in a complex human system might yield counter-intuitive results instead of yielding a predicable increase in a desired behavior. Or, adding a site to improve access to care in one place might yield additional parallel services and an overall increase in local demand rather than meet predicted needs based upon prior volume estimates for a local population. As one thing changes in a complex adaptive system that change interacts with all other elements and there may be random, unexpected ripple effects throughout the system of care. System changes are rarely linear, sequential, and predictable (Sargut & McGrath, 2011). This broad field of endeavor or new science of complexity is beyond the scope of this chapter. However, this definition of complexity in complex adaptive systems exists as an important background for our more focused and grounded discussion of patient and care system complexity.

Another background recognition is that medical complexity (the interaction of several or many medical conditions or diagnoses) has a combined and complex impact upon the patient and providers who care for medically complex patients. Grant et al. (2011) report their findings from interviews with primary care physicians regarding their sense of patient complexity being more than the simply additive nature of multiple comorbidities. They found that their sample of physicians estimated that over 25 % of their patients were complex, but those complexities included such factors as medical, social, and behavioral factors that did not correlate well with prior comorbidity or strictly medically defined complexity. In this model of quantitatively defined complexity, there was poor concordance or poor predictability of complexity as perceived by the physicians compared to comorbidity-defined complexity. "Complexity is multidimensional and is not adequately captured in measures that focus only on comorbid conditions" (p. 798). This paper did not describe further the social variables within the perceived complexity. However, it was clear that physician perception of "complexity" tapped something beyond the number of medical conditions for a specific patient.

In this chapter we will explore past and current efforts to improve care by identifying patients with social or care complexity that cuts across current description-based diagnoses based on symptoms. A new language is evolving for being clear about what an "illness" is and what a complicating social or environmental factor is, with new attempts at identifying clusters of patients with common identifying characteristics beyond the familiar disease- or diagnostic-oriented clusters. This approach works to identify and alter traditional care patterns when routine care options do not yield positive outcomes for such "complex" patients (Peek, Baird, & Coleman, 2009; Safford, Allison, & Kiefe, 2007; Weiss, 2007). This expanded concept of complexity is based upon social and care system variables rather than just a longer list of medical and mental health diagnoses. In other words, "patient complexity" goes beyond "medical complexity," encompassing social and/or care system complexity that interferes with care or with a patient's ability to engage in care.

Medical Complexity and Social or Care Complexity

It is especially important to consider this two-dimensional approach to "patient complexity" in the USA where we may overuse mental health diagnoses, especially depression, to describe patients who face these other social and care system obstacles. This has reached the popular as well as academic press (Carlat, 2010a, 2010b; Kirsch, 2010; Waters, 2010a, 2010b). The rise in the use of antidepressants to help patients (and the increasing questions about their effectiveness, especially with mild to moderate severity) is well-known (Fournier et al., 2010; Pigott, Leventhal, Alter, & Boren, 2010). This may be a result of treating symptoms that are well-documented in the DSM but do not systematically describe and understand that proportion of patients' despair, demoralization, discouragement, and withdrawal that is related to "complexity" derived from nonmedical factors that inhibit quality of life and can block improvement from routine medical or mental health care. If our current model for mental health diagnoses and treatment is not working well enough in this area, we must consider a systematic change in our approach. This chapter will briefly explore this alternative model for addressing these challenges to improve patient outcomes.

The "biopsychosocial model," introduced by Engel (1977, 1980), calls for shifts gradually being operationalized in a practical way (Borrell-Carrio, Suchman, & Epstein, 2004). One example comes from Amundson (2001), who created a model that reached beyond medical and psychiatric diagnoses and used interprofessional teams to implement care plans for complex patients beginning in the early 1990s. He consulted with primarily smaller hospitals in the USA to help them better manage their own small populations of expensive patients who often had little or no insurance, but significant medical problems and complex social and mental health issues. These patients were frequent visitors to emergency rooms and hospitals. His model offered hospitals the opportunity to identify the top 20–50 patients with these characteristics and with whom the hospitals often lost several million dollars. Interprofessional teams that included social workers created care plans at the cost of a few hundred thousand dollars to prevent the loss of millions of dollars in undercompensated or entirely uncompensated care. Therefore, the hospitals gained an economic benefit by losing less money while providing better care.

Baird worked with a team in a large Midwestern integrated group practice to create a "reflective interview" for a select group of complex patients who had been seen in the primary care practices more than ten times in a year while having no concrete medical problem that would predict frequent visits to the clinic. These one-time consultations with a mental health provider interviewing both the patient and the primary care provider were shown to reduce hospital costs in this small study (Rasmussen et al., 2006).

A similar approach has been used with different names for this activity, such as a "reflecting team" approach (Lebensohn-Chialvo, Crago, & Shisslak, 2000), in which the team participates in the patient interview, sometimes behind a one-way mirror with the patient's full permission and gives feedback to both the clinician and the patient about what is observed. However, these have been created in academic teaching practices and have not been tested in a community practice in a scientific manner. Others have used mathematical models to identify these socially complex patients (Safford, Allison, & Kiefe, 2007) by creating weighted values for a variety of medical and social variables that might impact patients. The model was then tested for its ability to predict which patients would face issues that might impair their care. These approaches are all attempts to understand social variables or what is sometimes called the "social determinants of health" (Institute of Medicine, 2002; Kottke & Pronk, 2009; Pronk, Peek, & Goldstein, 2004).

Efforts continue in this direction. In 2010 a new term, "Hot Spotters," has been used to describe those clinical and social support teams that are identifying patients who have combined medical, mental health, and social conditions that result in poorly coordinated and very expensive care (Gawande, 2011). By simultaneously addressing whatever problems these patients face from housing to safety to needing better coordinated or integrated medical and mental health care, patients' health has improved and the annual cost of care has been reduced, sometimes dramatically. Hot Spotters is a new and positive trend in approaching complex patients who often fail to connect well with traditionally organized medical, mental health, and social systems.

We have learned about a set of concepts for complexity assessment within a tool called INTERMED from clinicians in the Netherlands through a collection of papers including de Jonge, Huyse, & Stiefel (2006); Huyse, Stiefel & de Jonge (2006) and Stiefel, et al (2006). This tool systematically assesses patient and health care system complexity in a template designed for the European specialty or hospital-based settings. With permission from the Dutch group, a team from Minnesota (Peek, Baird, & Coleman, 2009) adapted that model for use in the fast-paced US outpatient care systems. This primary care version is called the Minnesota Complexity Assessment Method (MCAM) (See Fig. 14.1), which is being tested and modified further in Scotland as MECAM, the Minnesota Edinburgh Complexity Assessment Method (Maxwell et al., 2011).

The term "complexity" has many applications and shadings within the domain of health and health care. Medical clinicians commonly use the word "complex" to mean complicated or difficult, particularly as shorthand for a difficult patient-clinician relationship. Complexity may also refer to multiple interacting medical conditions, such as those frequently encountered in care of chronic illness—sometimes termed "medical complexity." In nursing, "complexity" can be a property of particular roles (and a staffing issue), referred to as "work complexity" or as social or mental health factors that elevate the risk to patients and staff in hospitals (Weydt, 2009). Similarly, "complexity" has also been discussed as a property of ambulatory care visits (Katerndahl, Wood, & Jaen, 2010). Others, especially those studying health care as a system and the applications of complexity science to health care, use "complexity" to mean the many possible ways that interconnected components of a health care system and its patients and communities can interact or adapt for successful fit in the environment (Zimmerman, Lindberg, & Plsek, 2008). A specific example is a model of "Complex Adaptive Chronic Care" for addressing chronicity in chronic care models that goes beyond disease-oriented thinking (Martin & Sturmberg, 2009; Peek, 2009). All these meanings and shadings of the versatile term "complexity" are important, but this chapter focuses on complexity as factors that interfere with standard care and decision-making (Peek, Baird, & Coleman, 2009).

While all clinicians instinctively relate to the concept of "complex patient," there has been little shared definition in the field for what that means. For example, when encountering a patient they believe is "complex," they may react with, "Oh my gosh!" or "Things aren't going as I expected," or "I don't feel so good about this," or "With these conditions, the patient should be getting better." Recall that Grant et al. (2011) said that physician attribution of "complex" goes beyond what would be predicted by medical comorbidity alone. The field needs a more standard definition and vocabulary that allow clinicians to say more clearly for a given patient situation exactly what is complex and what to do about it—and then to incorporate complexity-linked interventions into the care plans already geared to diseases and conditions. The following paragraphs regarding definitions and domains of complexity are paraphrased or quoted from Peek, Baird, & Coleman, (2009).

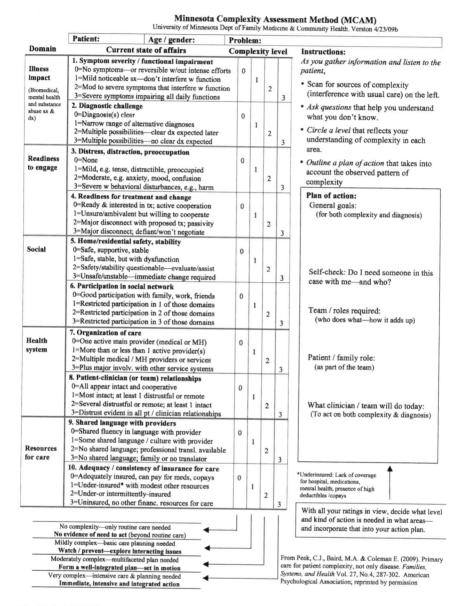

Fig. 14.1 MCAM scoring page

One definition of patient complexity:

[A complex patient] is one for whom clinical decision-making and required care processes are not routine or standard. For complex patients, many recommendations from evidence-based medicine are unlikely to apply in a straightforward manner because of "exceptions" such as: multiple interacting chronic conditions, other comorbid conditions and socioeconomic factors such as homelessness or absence of adequate family caregivers or other support systems. (Weiss, 2007, p. 375)

A series of papers on "Managing Complexity in Chronic Care" based on this definition appears as a special issue of the *Journal of General Internal Medicine* (Kupersmith, 2007; Safford, Allison & Kiefe, 2007; Weiss, 2007). The Dutch authors cited above also think of patient complexity as interference with standard care and offer an important distinction with a set of domains and a tool that were first designed for use in inpatient settings.

> It is appealing to distinguish between complexity that arises from characteristics of a patient—such has having multiple interacting diseases that may complicate each other ... and complexity of care delivery, such as involvement of multiple systems and specialties that require interdisciplinary communication to be effective .... (de Jonge, Huyse, & Stiefel, 2006, p. 680)

This foundational Dutch work is the basis for a US outpatient adaptation that employs similar but modified concepts and domains:

1. An illness domain that includes diagnostic uncertainty and functional impairment due to symptom severity
2. A readiness domain that includes distress, distraction, and readiness to engage in treatment
3. A social domain that includes participation in the social network and home safety and stability
4. A health system domain that includes organization of care and patient-clinician relationships
5. A resources for care domain that includes the degree of shared language with providers and the adequacy and consistency of insurance for care

These domains, each with two areas of inquiry and definitions of increasing levels of complexity, are illustrated in Fig. 14.1 as the Minnesota Complexity Assessment Method, an outpatient adaptation of the original INTERMED domains and questions (Stiefel et al., 2006). Each item in Fig. 14.1 represents a separate source of potential complexity, which if high, flags an area to potentially address as an interference with standard care.

The goal of these assessment models is to more usefully understand the nature of the obstacles that are keeping usual care from yielding the expected positive outcomes. By noting these barriers and sorting them into specific categories or domains, the team can more accurately understand the specific context of patients who are not making the expected progress toward health. The goal then becomes helping the patient deal more successfully with those specific barriers. If the barriers are not at a high level, then no action is needed beyond routine medical care. But if the specific area of challenge or "domain" is noted to be a large barrier for a specific patient, the primary care clinician and/or care manager on the primary care team can enlist other team members or community services to more constructively address the barrier. This enlarged team is only fully engaged when the patient assessment suggests it is necessary. However, more detailed understanding of the targeted domain needing attention can determine who else should be involved in the team-based care and which community resources and/or patient resources may be needed. For example, if the patient has never trusted a health care professional, the first step can be to

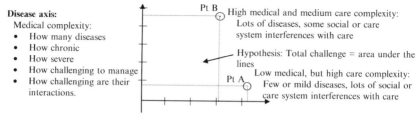

Disease axis:
Medical complexity:
- How many diseases
- How chronic
- How severe
- How challenging to manage
- How challenging are their
  interactions.

Pt B   High medical and medium care complexity:
       Lots of diseases, some social or care
       system interferences with care

       Hypothesis: Total challenge = area under the
       lines
Pt A   Low medical, but high care complexity:
       Few or mild diseases, lots of social or
       care system interferences with care

Social/care delivery axis: (as per Peek et al. 2009)
    Non-medical complexity—Domains:
- *Illness impact*—levels of impairment and diagnostic
  uncertainty
- *Readiness*—distress, distraction and readiness to engage
- *Social*—social safety, support, and participation
- *Health system*—organization of care and relationships
- *Resources for care*—common language, adequate insurance

Fig. 14.2 Axes of patient complexity (From Peek 2010. Building a medical home around the patient: what it means for behavior. *Families, Systems, & Health*, Vol. 28, No. 4, p. 331. Published by American Psychological Association; reprinted with permission)

arrange for more focused contact and trust-building time with the primary care provider or someone else the patient recognizes as part of the team. In other instances, the patient may need someone from community social services to facilitate a connection to a nearby community group such as YWCA or other social group to overcome social isolation.

A patient may have a list of medical diagnoses suggesting medical complexity. That same patient may also face interfering factors (social or care complexity) in the domains of social and health systems. The combination of high medical and high social/health system complexity makes usual care and care planning much less likely to yield the desired outcome. This patient faces the dilemma of dealing with both medical and social/care system complexity or must manage the "area under the line" as noted in Fig. 14.2 (Peek, 2010).

A hypothesis (or way of thinking) is that the net challenge for care of a particular patient may be a product of both axes (medical complexity and care complexity), not just the more familiar medical complexity. To address both, the clinic should have both these axes in mind. Providers and patients getting together not only to plan care but to create strategies to reduce predictable interferences with that care is shown in Fig. 14.1. The investment in medical care plans is not protected unless patients and providers together ask themselves what person-specific factors will predictably interfere with those care plans and with usual or customized care for the patient's conditions. On the patient side, patients can often be confused by their own illnesses, complicating life factors, and stresses. Whether articulated or not, these undermine confidence in their ability to do carry out their own self-care and patient engagement behaviors. Patients can begin to feel like a failure, "difficult," or that no one wants to see them anymore. But this is often not due to lack of motivation or "noncompliance," but to very real interferences with care from social or care delivery sources (Peek, Baird, & Coleman, 2009; Peek, 2010).

High levels of complexity on the social/care delivery axis can point clinicians and care teams toward broader or supplementary interventions or connections than their medical care plans might do alone. For example, here are some aspects of care planning that might be included for high levels of social or care complexity:

1. *Illness impact—levels of impairment and diagnostic uncertainty.* If diagnostic uncertainty or disagreement with the patient on diagnosis is an issue, it may be helpful to revisit diagnosis or reopen the conversation about "what's really wrong" with the patient. Functional impairment that exceeds what would be expected from the condition also points to further inquiry rather than just labeling the patient "overreacting."
2. *Readiness—distress, distraction, and readiness to engage.* High levels here calls for understanding the patient's current life situation and what else is competing for attention. There may be things going on that seem much more urgent than a complicated care plan for diabetes, for example.
3. *Social—social safety, support, and participation.* If the patient is isolated—with few if any friends, work life, or family connections, there is likely no one to understand and support the patient's role in their care plan. This form of discouragement affects "adherence" as well. What social supports may help the person become better integrated into their social world?
4. *Health system—organization of care and relationships.* If there are many providers, especially if they are not communicating or communicating conflicting information and advice, care coordination, and organizing the care plan may be necessary. If the patient has no providers, especially no PCP, finding one may be high on the list of priorities. If the patient does not trust providers or has a history of disappointments, building one safe relationship may be the first order of business.
5. *Resources for care—common language, adequate insurance.* If the patient does not speak the same language as the provider, it may be important to arrange for a professional interpreter who understands the culture as well as the language. If the patient has insufficient insurance to pay for copayments, transportation, or other expenses for care, it may be helpful to involve a financial planner to help the person find a public health plan or other way to pay for necessary care.

In Minnesota (and possibly other states) medical practices with state "health care home" certification are now paid a small care management fee based upon the medical complexity of each patient. This fee has been augmented modestly to encourage care teams to address two domains of social complexity: having language barriers and a mental health diagnosis. The last factor is a known risk for increased cost for patients needing medical care but can be a blended factor with despair, isolation, and an overwhelmed emotional state for patients. Being overwhelmed is not a medical diagnosis, but the despairing symptoms can result in a diagnosis of depression, not otherwise specified (NOS). This intellectual dilemma was discussed in the first part of this chapter. In fact, that diagnosis, Depression NOS, is common in primary care and can yield increased attention to help the patient. Unfortunately, if that assistance consists only of medication, it does not assist the patient in dealing with their domains of social and care system complexity that are overwhelming them such as lack of trust in health professionals, a disengaged stance toward their illness, lack of social support, lack of resources/insurance, and uncoordinated care from a variety of providers.

However, increased payment for some dimensions of social complexity is an early sign that some reimbursement systems are seeking ways to fund care systems that seek to assist patients in the reality of their complex lives. These increased payments for social complexity are a beginning of efforts to find sustainable payment models to support primary care practices as they try to improve outcomes for patients when usual care does not succeed.

The gradual emergence of payment models to address some dimensions of social complexity serves as a reminder that not all "complexity" is from a mental health condition. This reminds us to go beyond the familiar mental health taxonomy into a new vocabulary for what makes patients complex—including the predictable interferences with care. The DSM-based model rests upon a descriptive taxonomy rather than underlying etiology (Althoff & Waterman, 2011). We diminish our positive clinical impact on patients when our assessment methods are descriptive of symptoms but less sophisticated about clarifying the nature of their distress. Psychiatric training changes are needed, as recommended by Althoff & Waterman, to improve the understanding of patients' entire situations beyond psychiatric diagnosis and medication tolerance. In primary care, we also need to gain more insight into patient's total dilemma rather than base our clinical insights primarily upon the diagnosis as defined in the DSM. We need to go beyond treating with medications alone or medications supported by mere encouragement, "pep talk," or other positive messages that do not necessarily get at the specific factors that are distressing people (Salazar-Fraile, Sempere-Verdu, Mossakowski, & Bryan, 2010). Our approach to mental health diagnosis has been compared to the "field guide" approach of a bird-watching book—identifying mental disorders with checklists of characteristics similar to those used by birdwatchers (Lane, 2007). This indeed describes what we see, but leaves us without tools that improve our understanding of why we see different symptoms or patterns of distress in our patients. A new model of care that deals with patient complexity is possible, does not depend upon the DSM diagnostic model, and can address very real issues that confound patients and providers and interferes with usual care based upon diagnosis alone.

State of the Art in Evaluating Social or Care Complexity

Assessment of social and care system complexity beyond the usual medical complexity is early and rudimentary. Studies underway now seek to validate the idea that we can reliably identify social and care system variables that impede the positive impact of usual care. Also studies are underway to validate the domains themselves to ensure they are reasonably discrete from one another.

Early and informal feasibility testing shows the MCAM to be reasonably time efficient. Nurses, care coordinators, and physicians report they can do an assessment in 3 min or less when they already know the patient. Of course, when clinicians realize they do not know the answer to certain questions, it alerts them to take the additional time to find out. Team training is needed to create a shared understanding among clinicians about the use of the assessment tool, when to use it, and how to engage the patient in the process of assessment. We have found that physicians often relate more easily to the first several domains that connect more closely to medical concerns while nurses and social workers often engage more readily on three through five. However, a team discussion is enriched by the overall team assessment and can lead to more specific action steps than previous global assessments, such as "the patient is stuck and not making progress."

Scottish collaborators are testing a patient version of MCAM and an Edinburgh version (MECAM) using slightly different language patterns fitting each culture (Maxwell et al., 2011). Adaptation of language for describing and assessing social or care complexity should be tailored to the language actually in use for these concepts in particular communities (Lyons, 2006).

MCAM and MECAM capture information that sometimes was collected via a genogram or annotated family history in the clinical setting (Doherty & Baird, 1983). This method got at some but not all domains of patient complexity. However, even during the 1980s and 1990s, which was the high point of enthusiasm for using genograms or a "family tree," relatively few physicians used them in actual practice. By sorting the social and care system complexity into domains with gradations of severity or importance to improving health, MCAM/ MECAM have gathered information that is more easily transferable to other team members. Rather than leaving clinicians with an undifferentiated, often pejorative "assessment" of a challenging patient ("Ugh!" or "The patient is stuck," or "The patient is nonadherent,") these methods provide an action-oriented language for pointing at the reasons to engage a larger team or seek support from family or a community agency and create a more targeted action plan. In summary, these concepts and tools create ways to talk about the patient's complexity that reaches beyond the medical diagnoses (medical complexity) into the many individual factors that may affect care and the patient's ability to engage in it.

Care systems across the USA are testing various methods that are parallel to MCAM and INTERMED for use by primary care physicians, care managers, and care coordinators. Drs. Gunn and Valeras implemented the following examples in a family medicine residency clinic that serves many patients with complex social situations.

Practical Application of Complexity Thinking

Problem of Primary Care and Complex Patient Needs

The setting. The primary care setting, as we usually know it, is designed for acute care visits and uncomplicated chronic disease management with engaged patients who are partners in their health care plans (a well-supported patient, a straightforward protocol, things proceeding as expected). Many primary care clinic settings are, however, ill-equipped for patients who have multiple and complex medical and social situations or when usual care is not working, leaving an individual provider to address multiple needs in short visits. This can lead to frustrated providers and patients, reduced quality, and higher costs. These costs are often in the form of increased testing, emergency room visits, and unnecessary hospitalizations. Addressing this "disconnect" quickly and effectively with complex patients will require a "special" program or arrangement in most primary care practices.

The Concord Hospital Family Health Center in Concord, New Hampshire, is a "safety net" primary care clinic, which also houses the Dartmouth Family Medicine Residency and a primary care behavioral health-training program. Fifteen thousand patients, many who are uninsured or have government insurance, are served in the clinic. Social workers, psychologists, and marriage and family therapists train alongside family physicians and mid-level providers (physician assistants and nurse practitioners). Together, we continually design practice processes and educational experiences which address the needs of patients with complex biopsychosocial-spiritual issues.

The health care team. The clinic administrators and faculty/clinicians recognized the need for greater continuity and resources for developing health care teams that could consistently manage the needs of our population, particularly around complex patient situations. The position of "integrated behavioral health clinician" (IBHCs) was established. The IBHCs are licensed social workers, psychologists or marriage and family therapists who partner with each of the four small clinical teams within the clinic. The IBHCs, the faculty physician, and the supervising nurse are a triad of team leaders in each clinical pod and are given responsibility for helping their team design effective care protocols and processes. These leaders are in frequent consultation with the clinical director of nursing, the manager of behavioral health services, and the medical director to discuss broader population-based issues. The physician-nurse-behavioral health leadership triads meet weekly prior to their pod meetings to discuss logistical and clinical issues. Sustainable quality and effectiveness occurs when structure, governance, and leadership roles are clear and highly functional.

Complex Continuity Clinic: A Patient-Centered and Learner-Centered Experience

One clinical initiative all pods have established is the Complex Continuity Clinic (CCC). The overall objective of this clinic is to implement patient-centered medical home concepts into practice by integrating biomedical and psychosocial care providers through high functioning teams. This care is provided to patients and their families who have at least a moderate degree of complexity. "Complex" is defined as: "when usual care is not working."

In the CCC, there are three goals: (1) to provide clinical care for our complex patient group, (2) to educate our medical residents, behavioral health trainees, and allied health care staff about team-based care for challenging patients, and (3) to provide a professional development opportunity and have an educational strategy to help residents identify complex patients within their patient panel for whom they are responsible. All individual providers, regardless of their position or years of experience, have some situations that are more uniquely challenging for them in particular. The individual history, the experience of the provider, and their unique attitude toward patients with complex situations are variables in complexity and are frequent topics of conversation.

CCC began in 2008 as a half-day clinic with two "complex patients" scheduled. Residents were scheduled to do 10–12 of these clinics during six months of their third year. Prior to seeing patients, residents meet with their precepting team (faculty physician and behavioral health clinician) to discuss general concepts relating to what makes a situation complex, as well as specific goals for the upcoming appointments and strategies to accomplish the goals. Following the session, the team discusses how the plan went and what the next steps are. This dialog provides an opportunity to identify the resident's needs and patient-related themes. The IBHCs and nurses contribute significantly as well, based on their knowledge of the patient. At times, community members from other agencies involved in the case are also present.

It was quickly discovered that, with a two-patient CCC session, the efficacy of time, provision of service, and the learning was limited if one or both of those patients canceled or did not show. CCC was transformed into a schedule that had two longer slots and three or four acute visits. This format still allowed for discussion of the complexity involved in the cases, but also offered a more sustainable model that could be replicated after training.

Each CCC patient encounter involved the creation or addition to a patient-centered care plan (PCCP), which lives in the electronic medical record, and contains life goals established with the team, instead of solely disease-oriented medical goals. (See Chap. 10 for a more thorough description of PCCPs.) CCC is specifically designed to enable a longer visit with the patient, allowing for the entire team (physician, nurse, behavioral health member, patient, and family members) to participate in the development of an individualized care plan. This is a strength not typically built into primary care clinics.

Following the CCC visits, the health care team manages this subgroup of patients through phone calls or appointments to ensure connection and adherence to plan. Key to success is the use of face-to-face conversation between providers or communication capabilities within the EHR.

Key components. Patient complexity concepts based on the MCAM have been useful for understanding the difference between social or care complexity and the more familiar "medical complexity." The incorporation of IBHCs as leaders on the primary care teams moved these concepts into practice, in that these teams are accustomed to working together on the expanded scope of problems and in developing care plans formed in CCC, as well as enhancing the community linkages in follow-up activity.

Financial. CCC services have been billed using Level IV time codes, which is used when a provider spends at least 25 minutes of face-to-face counseling. However, it would be difficult to sustain CCC this way in a busy practice on a routine basis given the fee-for-service environment. However, many of the cost savings will come from better planning at the beginning of illness episodes and less cost shifting to more expensive settings, such as the emergency room or hospital. The tremendous advantage of CCC is that it provides more time at crucial junctures, like when the treatment plan is not working, when the patient is hospitalized or visits the emergency room frequently, or when behavioral or social issues are clouding the picture and need to be addressed. The weaknesses of CCC include the amount of clinician time and the financial support provided by the traditional fee-for-service payment system. In an ACO environment, having sessions scheduled in this way could result in tremendous advantages, with highly satisfying results for clinicians, patients, families, and third party payers.

Outcomes. Over three years, 24 residents have experienced CCC. They have seen an average of 11 different patients, with some of these patients returning two or three times for follow-up visits. Ninety-five percent of patients surveyed about their satisfaction with the CCC format feel that having the time to tell their story and work through the issues has been extremely beneficial. Providers have been able to identify particular insightful themes for themselves in working with complex patients and this greater clarity is itself a benefit to clinicians. The ability of a provider to know what his or her own "blind spots" are in working with complexity is critical to success. The following questions are routinely pondered by the interdisciplinary team and, in particular, the resident:

1. What is my role in maintaining the problem?
2. How do I open up the symptoms to reveal the patterns and the bigger picture?
3. What should be the major "theme" at this time? (Support, trust, adherence, etc.)
4. How do I not try to do everything myself and use my team?

5. How do I negotiate or help others to negotiate effectively when there is disagreement between providers, between patient and provider, between family and patient, between family and provider?
6. How do I soften up, listen, be curious, and open? *OR*
7. How do I take a harder, more assertive approach, and be more focused and clear?

We have not kept clinical outcome data on all patients seen, but we have anecdotal stories of patients that have substantially reduced ER utilization and decreased frantic phone calls to the pod for emergent issues. We now have a team-based post-hospital visit where many of these same concepts can be applied.

Applications to practice. Some resident graduates have told us they now schedule one complex patient team visit once or twice a week in their practice, either at the beginning or the end of a session. They also create and maintain complex care plans with selected patients to fill out and bring to the visits, or discuss during annual physicals. Clinicians discuss complex cases at team meetings so all members can reinforce a high leverage goal, such as understanding context or building trust with the team or working together toward better patient and family care.

CCC Case Examples

C.L.

CL is a 52-year-old white female who was new to the patient panel and to the state of the resident author (AV) a few months into his third year of residency. She moved to live with her youngest sister after her elder sister (and roommate) died unexpectedly. It was through a CCC visit that the complexity in CL's life was realized, as well as the impact of this model for providing integrated team care.

Medical complexity. CL's past medical history was complicated by multiple medical and psychological comorbidities. CL's paper chart from her previous provider listed nine different chronic diseases, including Diabetes Mellitus type 2, COPD, fibromyalgia, benign essential hypertension, hyperlipidemia, chronic back pain status post-surgical lumber discectomy and subsequent vertebral fusion, coupled with a history of drug abuse and opiate addiction. The significant disease interaction proved especially challenging for medical management in the setting of minimal interaction with the patient in her initial 12 months in the state.

Non-medical complexity: Illness impact. As a result of her previous trauma history, CL's resiliency was compromised and minimal stressors would lead to exaggerated perception of medical need and a perceived urgency to all physical symptoms. As a result of her perceived medical crisis, CL presented to the local Emergency Department (ED) repeatedly for months on end with an array of symptoms ranging from back pain, chest pain, anxiety, groin pain, abdominal pain, GI bleeding, shortness of breath, suicidal ideation, and depression. This was extremely frustrating to the resident provider because his specialist colleagues and emergency room physicians developed assumptions about his lack of ability to "control" CL's behavior. He felt responsible and somehow accountable to a patient that he had never met.

Readiness. During an extended CCC visit, CL revealed that her sister (her current roommate) would often take advantage of her because of her disease and medical treatment. CL described once being locked in the closet for hours while her sister foraged through her belongings looking for her prescription pain medication, which she finally found and stole. CL responded by avoiding regular medical care and treatment to prevent her sister's exploitation.

Social. CL, being new to the state, had no local social connections other than this abusive sister. She reported feeling isolated, which contributed to worsening symptoms of depression and suicidal ideation.

Health system. Within one year, CL had 19 separate ED visits. In that timeframe, she underwent 4 abdominal CT scans, 1 head CT, 8 chest x-rays, 11 abdomen and pelvis x-rays, 6 lumbar x-rays, and she gave 108 independent blood and urine samples for laboratory studies. Twelve different providers in the ED cared for CL during that period of time.

In this same one-year period, CL kept only two appointments with her PCP; one of which was immediately followed by an ED visit. The disposition of all of CL's ED visits was "discharge to home," with the exception of one, for which she was admitted for rule-out chest pain, but she signed out against medical advice so was therefore never admitted to the hospital. The charges billed to Medicaid in this same time period were upwards of $32,000.

Resources for care. Soon after arriving to the state, CL acquired Medicaid, allowing her to overcome access barriers to care; however, in this case access to care does not guarantee receiving appropriate care, especially when considering complex medical and social needs.

CL is described here, not because her level of complexity is severe or insurmountable, but because she is an example of success and the potential capacity of the system and of the health care team's perspective to change, when complexity is considered. Nine months after meeting CL for the first time, she was invited to a CCC visit during her PCP's third year of residency. The interaction was precepted (supervised) by an attending physician, a behavioral health faculty, an IBHC, and a nurse.

This type of visit also provides an opportunity to introduce the concept of a health care team to a patient. It was during this appointment that CL's true medical and social complexity was realized and understood by the team, and as a result, could be incorporated into her care plan. The most compelling outcome of this visit with CL was the pattern change in where she chose to access the health care system, and her subsequent decreased ED utilization. Since that time, she has been to the ED only once, when she was directed there by clinic staff due to lack of appointments and triage guideline protocol.

Her PCP interviewed CL recently about her experience and inquired about this sudden and dramatic change in her utilization of the ED. CL pointed to her CCC visit, explaining, "After that visit, I felt I had a team at the Family Health Center and even if you are not there, or you go away, I know that there is someone else at FHC that will help me. Now I don't have to go to the ER anymore." CL's ability to change her perception of when and by whom her urgent care needs will be met speaks to the importance of feeling "known" by a health care team. CCC provided a venue through which to "know" the patient in a way that embraced CL's complexity, rather than trying to ignore it, and allowed for its incorporation into the patient's plan of care.

For learners of family medicine, third year of residency provides the early feelings that competence in the provision of medicine is achievable on some level. That is, however, when the patient's presentation and interaction is straightforward. In these situations, it is easy to rely on medical school and residency experience to provide a viable path forward in negotiating the patient's best plan of care under the established medical model. CCC provided a framework of care that could be utilized when some perceived barrier (either the patient's, the practitioner's, the team's, or all) stands in the way of providing the best care possible. Often times, however, the barrier is not recognized and it manifests in the patient's, provider's, or team's frustration. It was in these instances that CCC became useful for CL's provider, as a learner, in developing strategies and skills to explore personal frustration in a safe and supportive environment. Exploring patients' frustrations with the care they received, when the medical model did not suffice to meet their needs, often led to the conclusion that only team-based integrated care would allow for everyone to progress toward their predefined goals.

C.G.

CG is a 62-year-old male asked to come to CCC because of a personal sense of the resident provider's frustration in relation to the care that he was receiving.

Medical complexity. As part of residency training, CG was cared for by his PCP both in and out of the hospital, throughout his frequent admissions for abdominal pain related to chronic pancreatitis, hepatitis C, and stage-four liver cirrhosis. CG carried these diagnoses stoically behind a graying handle bar mustache and heavily monochrome tattooed skin. CG attended the majority of his scheduled outpatient visits, which were primarily focused on how to keep him out of the hospital. At the end of these visits, however, it did not feel to the provider that anything had been accomplished. CG would be rehospitalized a few weeks later and this cycle repeated itself over and over again for two years. CG was always pleasant and respectful, but over more than two years, he never gave any confirmation or acknowledgement of the existence of this endless cycle that had no gains in either the doctor-patient relationship or the treatment plan to relieve his chronic abdominal pain. Throughout this time CG was also reluctant to see any subspecialist regarding his care. The patient was stuck, and the provider was stuck with him.

Nonmedical complexity: Illness impact. CG gastrointestinal pathology was "real" from the medical model perspective, but its impact on CG was discordant with his frequent presentation to ED. It became apparent that his abdominal pain was spurred by stress, which he was reluctant to share the source of.

Readiness. Each CCC is prefaced with a team discussion surrounding the resident's reasons for asking the patient to come to this type of appointment. What makes this patient complex? It was in exploring CG's reluctance to engage with his health care team, beyond his physical symptoms, that unlocked CG's greater plight. During the pre-visit huddle, the team voiced an unanswered question. CG had been incarcerated for 12 years prior to coming to FHC, and out of genuine curiosity, they asked "What was he in prison for?" With their prodding and encouragement, the visit began with this question, explaining that better understanding his history and the context of his current life situation would help his health care team treat his needs. After a long moment of awkward silence, CG replied "I've been wanting to tell you for two years but I didn't know how." He began to cry, as he explained that he was the victim of childhood physical and sexual abuse, and later in life, he completed the cycle of abuse and became a sexual offender.

Social. As a result of CG's incarceration and specific offense, CG was isolated from mainstream society, was unable to find work, was cut off from his family, and only interaction was with his parole office and health care team.

Health system. CG's experience thus far with the health care system had instilled distrust. He feared that when his "story" was known he would be treated differently or worse, he would be refused care. His past experiences reinforced this; he had been scorned and treated with pure contempt and hatred when revealing his "sex offender" status in other situations.

Resources for care. Due to social isolation and hesitancy to engage the system due to fear of humiliation and dishonor, CG had limited access to resources.

CG reported during a follow-up visit, "Since that visit I feel a wall that existed between us has been broken down." It became clear that prior to this visit, the provider frustration was reciprocated, reinforcing a barrier between doctor and patient, both uncertain how to overcome it, until the opportunity was provided. CCC provided that opportunity for the resident, and for the health care team as a whole. The greatest gift of CCC was the time to explore his story through genuine curiosity, with the support of the team. The next challenge for residents is not how to manage a complex patient, but how to incorporate this understanding of the value of that time in a future practice that is not necessarily structured to allow such opportunities.

Practical Application of Complexity Concepts

HOW: Care Coordination in the Medical Home

Care coordination is a key function of the patient-centered medical home (McDonald et al., 2012; NCQA, 2011; Peek & Oftedahl, 2010). Though the concept is broadly defined and interpreted, the main functions are summarized in a consensus operational definition of patient-centered medical home (Peek & Oftedahl):

(A) Practice-based care coordination or care management within and between times of acute care, preventive care, and chronic care, including:

- Patient engagement (patient and family actions are also part of the picture)
- Transition management—integration of care from one setting to the next
- Tracking information to facilitate clinical communication, access, and patient safety

(B) Coordinating with the "health care neighborhood" of other teams, practices, and community resources shaped around the needs of specific patients, including:

- Specialists (including behavioral health), hospitals, other facilities
- Social services and community resources
- Patients and families themselves who move across this "health care neighborhood"

Sources of patient complexity described in this chapter (and with examples from the Complex Continuity Clinic) affect the kind and level of care coordination required for a given patient. Care coordinators often play a role in medical home settings—often keeping track of information on registries, bringing providers together, acting as a contact point for patients, and helping the care team accomplish those care coordination functions. Specific care coordinator functions vary from setting to setting, but they all witness "complexity" and need to take it into account.

Incorporating complexity concepts and questions into workflows. The authors (Peek and Baird) have noticed in family medicine practices at the University of Minnesota that care coordinators are aware of complexity concepts and in some cases, the MCAM checklist shown in Fig. 14.1. But rather than having "another piece of paper" or a disconnected screen on an electronic health record, care coordinators have indicated a wish to incorporate the complexity questions into their existing care coordinator workflows—so the information naturally falls into place rather than being experienced as "extra questions and forms" to somehow fit into what they mainly do. This is one of the challenges of incorporating complexity concepts into daily work—integrating the questions seamlessly into workflows and information tools. One approach proposed to a small group of family medicine clinic care coordinators is described here. It is offered only as *an example of a way of thinking* about incorporating complexity into workflows, because it has been only the subject of experimentation, not full implementation and testing.

Level of care coordination needed (Peek & Van Riper, 2011). Not everyone needs the same level of care coordination. All the clinic's patients may be in the medical home. But not all of them require intensive care coordination. Even those who do require care coordination will differ in how extensive and what the focus of coordination should be. Care coordinators will need a practical way to determine the level and focus for care coordination required for each patient

Medical complexity and level of coordination needed. The patient's medical complexity is oriented primarily to the number and severity of illnesses as in the medical complexity axis shown in Fig. 14.2. For example, Minnesota certified health care homes employ a tier system for medical complexity that care coordinators can use to help determine the level of care coordination needed. This tier also affects the size of bundled care management fees. But this does not completely determine the level of care coordination needed. For example, a person with significant chronic illnesses but strong social and personal supports (and few interferences with care) may not present high care coordination needs. On the other hand, a patient with relatively fewer or simpler illnesses but significant social or other interferences with care and activation may require a high level of care coordination. This social or care complexity axis is also illustrated in Fig. 14.2.

Dimensions for assessing level of care coordination needed for each patient. Building off AHRQ care coordination work (citation), the level of care coordination needed could be assessed using three dimensions:

1. Medical complexity: Number, severity, ambiguity, and impairments related to illnesses.
2. Risk of fragmentation: Likelihood of care plan being incomplete, poorly understood, or poorly coordinated.
3. Interference with patient capacity: Distress, distraction, social realities likely to interfere with care or participation in it.

In this way of thinking, each patient is assigned a level of low, medium, or high need on each dimension. This results in an individualized patient profile (check the box that applies for each dimension):

Individual Care Coordination Profile

	Low	Med	High
Medical complexity			
Risk of fragmentation			
Interference w patient capacity			

Using individual care coordination profile to determine level of care coordination needed. Some profiles call for minimal care coordination and others call for intensive care coordination—and with different foci. For other patients a more moderate level of care coordination is needed—with the specific care coordination tasks and intensity related to which "cells" in the profile are grayed out. For example, a patient with high medical complexity and risk of fragmentation might require care coordination more focused on integrating treatments and specialists and health system communication. A patient with a simpler medical picture but with significant life stresses or situations that tend to interfere with care might require care coordination focused more on enhancing patient capacity to cope with illness and carry out treatments. In all cases, the level of care coordination and its main foci will depend on the patient's particular profile. The care coordinator would have a visual reminder of what kinds and level of intensity of care coordination tasks are likely most relevant for that particular patient.

Information to arrive at an individual care coordination profile. A care coordinator has, or can probably find, information that helps assign "low-medium-high" to each dimension (rows in the table above) using a combination of the familiar medical information produced by the primary care providers and team and the complexity assessment questions that appear in Fig. 14.1 (Minnesota Complexity Assessment Method). Without showing all the details of Fig. 14.1 or a real worksheet, the information to arrive at "high, medium, low" for the three dimensions of the individual care coordination profile dimensions could be gathered using the areas of inquiry below:

Areas of inquiry for establishing "high-medium-low" on the three dimensions of care coordination profile:

(A) Medical complexity:

1. Medical complexity "tier": How many and what diseases or conditions at what level of severity and interaction[1]
2. Functional impairments that interfere with daily life
3. Diagnostic challenge or uncertainty: not being sure about or disagreeing on diagnoses

(B) Risk of fragmentation:

4. Organization of care: How many providers, services, service systems—how well coordinated
5. Patient-clinician (or team) relationships: intact, cooperative or more distrustful, remote
6. Shared language (or cultural understandings) with clinicians and care team
7. Adequacy or consistency of insurance for care

(C) Interference with patient capacity:

8. Distress, distraction, preoccupation with other things going on in life
9. Readiness for treatment and change—agreement and interest in proposed care plan
10. Home or residential safety and stability
11. Participation in social network (family, work, friends, other)

---

[1]In Minnesota, the medical complexity "tier" is provided by a state system based in "Ambulatory Diagnostic Groups" (ACG or ADGs), a system for predicting the utilization of ambulatory health services within a patient group – based on the person's age, gender, and broad clusters of diagnoses and conditions (Starfield, Weiner, Mumford, & Steinwachs, 1991; Weiner, Starfield, Steinwachs, & Mumford, 1991).

This care coordination profile now exists only as a concept on an experimental paper worksheet. But a basic pattern of incorporating complexity concepts in an electronic care coordinator workflow could be done—thus avoiding "extraneous" papers and forms floating around outside it. If complexity concepts are to become mainstream in care planning, they have to be embedded in workflows—electronic and otherwise.

Patient participation in providing or confirming complexity-related information. The form on Fig. 14.1 and the areas of inquiry above are written in clinician language in the form of a clinician checklist. But patients could be involved in supplying or confirming information on those areas. A care coordinator or nurse who is rooming a patient could interview the patient to fill out the team's understanding of things that might influence the care. For example, a nurse or care coordinator could preface such a conversation with, "Your providers would like to be sure they are aware of anything in your situation that might affect or interfere with care for your conditions—and identify any concerns you have about your conditions or treatments." Taking this step helps patients themselves understand complexity concepts (what might interfere with my care), hence helping to mainstream these concepts from the patient point of view as well.

Taking this a step further, a patient version of a complexity assessment checklist might be used to get the patients thinking about these ideas as they wait for their provider visit or care coordinator phone call. For example, authors (Peek and Baird) have written (but not tested) a simplified patient version of the questions in Fig. 14.1 called "Concerns with Care Checklist" with the stem question, "Do you have any concerns about...." followed by those ten areas put into simple patient-friendly language. If the patient says "yes" or "maybe" to any of the questions, it signals the nurse or care coordinator to find out more—and address these concerns in the care plan.

Conclusion

Health care clinicians, administrators, payers, and policymakers will all have to work with social and care complexity in a practical way in today's environment. It is not sufficient for care systems and payment systems to become increasingly sophisticated about diagnosis and treatment of medical conditions and diseases (medical complexity) but remain distant or vague about the social complexities that will predictably interfere with those sophisticated medical care plans. At present, mastery of diagnostic and disease-oriented assessment and treatment greatly exceeds mastery of all those other factors that will interfere with care. Yet mastery of this area is necessary to protect the investment in disease-oriented care plans and treatments.

Clinicians, clinics, health plans, and patients themselves will need enough concrete assistance in the area of "complexity" to make a difference. This starts at a minimum with developing a practical and more widely used vocabulary for what kinds of factors predictably interfere with care and make for "patient complexity." The Dutch, Scottish, and Minnesota work on complexity assessment takes a step in that direction through establishing domains of complexity and assessment questions that can be asked of any patient. Beyond developing and adopting such a practical vocabulary, practice routines are needed—simple enough procedures that can be consistently built into practice to reveal the individual patient factors that are likely to interfere with care so that the investment in medical care plans and treatments is protected and a practical balance between medical and social factors is maintained for each patient. The author's (Gunn's) work with "Complex Continuity Clinic," the work on "Reflective Interviews" (Rasmussen et al., 2006) and other even more systematic applications of complexity assessment concepts (Kathol, Perez, Cohen, & Huyse, 2010) will be needed.

Complexity concepts such as social factors or deprivations that interfere with care often produce discouragement or demoralization. These need to be distinguished from mental health conditions and not automatically "medicalized" in a way that prematurely stops the conversation about what is going on. Not all situational discouragement is depression in the diagnostic sense, though often enough in ordinary language is felt to be "depressing." Complexity concepts offer additional vocabulary for evaluating and caring for discouraged patients who are distracted by other things in their lives or in their relationships with health care.

Attention to social and care complexity as intertwined with medical complexity is critical. This is especially true as we move toward an "accountable care organization" (ACO) environment when the kinds of teams described in this chapter are responsible for a population of patients—along with their colleagues in specialty care and hospitals. We must be strategic in how we rebalance care toward inclusion of social and care complexity factors, rather than just pile it on the growing list of obligations that health care clinics are supposed to do on their own. The main strategy is to build practical connections between primary care clinics and community resources—the "patient-centered medical home" with appropriate division of labor between health care settings and the community with patients, families, and neighborhoods also doing their own parts in addressing the problem.

However, this message is not to be understood as a pejorative recommendation to "turn primary care clinics into social service agencies" or to consider such community connections merely as "social services" as "less than." The era of medical home, ACO, and the Triple Aim calls for (1) integration of care between clinics, specialists, hospitals, and community resources; and (2) differentiation of roles for each of these players of the "health neighborhood." All these roles are needed, there is no room for pejorative stereotyping or a "pecking order," and each must be enabled to do its own work—the part that it does best. The gaps and sources of fragmentation between them are what need attention, for example, communication between health care professionals and each other, gaps between these professionals and the patients and families they serve, gaps between systems of care in the "health neighborhood," and gaps between the professional system and the community and individual resources that exist apart from the health care system. This vision of integrated care goes beyond the primary care practice and beyond the larger professional system of health care delivery to include all the players including citizens and patients themselves. This is teamwork *writ large* ("embodied in greater, more prominent magnitude") with complexity concepts embedded that include but are not limited to medical complexity.

Ultimately, communities will be making decisions on how to use their limited resources for health. Some of this can be for ever-more sophisticated disease care and some of it can be to address the sources of social complexity and distress that interferes with care and can mimic health care conditions, such as mild to moderate depression. In a world of limited of resources, there are choices for communities to make, such as whether it is better to build up schools, families, or other social institutions or to build more and more clinics as if all health problems can be taken care of in health care settings.

References

Althoff, R. R., & Waterman, G. S. (2011). Commentary: Psychiatric training for physicians: A call to modernize. *Academic Medicine, 86*, 285–287.

Amundson, B. (2001). America's rural communities as crucibles for clinical reform: Establishing collaborative care teams in rural communities. *Families, Systems & Health, 19*, 13–23.

Borrell-Carrio, F., Suchman, A. L., & Epstein, R. M. (2004). The biopsychosocial model 25 years later: Principles, practice, and scientific inquiry. *Annals of Family Medicine, 2*, 576–582.

Carlat, D. (2010a). *The trouble with psychiatry: A doctor's revelations about a profession in crisis.* New York: Free Press.

Carlat, D. (2010b). Mind over meds. *The New York Times.* Retrieved April 29, 2013, from http://www.nytimes.com/2010/04/25/magazine/25Memoir-t.html?pagewanted=all&_r=0

de Jonge, P., Huyse, F. J., & Stiefel, F. C. (2006). Case and care complexity in the medically ill. *Medical Clinics of North America, 90*, 679–692.

Doherty, W. J., & Baird, M. A. (1983). *Family therapy and family medicine: Toward the primary care of families.* New York: Guilford Press.

Engel, G. L. (1977). The need for a new medical model: A challenge for biomedicine. *Science, 196*, 129–136.

Engel, G. L. (1980). The clinical application of the biopsychosocial model. *The American Journal of Psychiatry, 137*, 535–544.

Fournier, J. C., DeRubeis, R. J., Hollon, S. D., Dimidjian, S., Amsterdam, J. D., Shelton, R. C., et al. (2010). Antidepressant drug effects and depression severity: A patient-level meta-analysis. *Journal of the American Medical Association, 303*, 47–53.

Gawande, A. (2011). The hot spotters: Can we lower medical costs by giving the neediest patients better care? *The New Yorker.* Retrieved April 29, 2013, from http://www.newyorker.com/reporting/2011/01/24/110124fa_fact_gawande

Grant, R. W., Ashburner, J. M., Hong, C. C., Chang, Y., Barry, M. J., & Atlas, S. J. (2011). Defining patient complexity from the primary care physician's perspective: A cohort study. *Annals of Internal Medicine, 155*, 797–804.

Huyse, F., Stiefel, F., & deJonge, P. (2006). Identifiers or "red flags" of complexity and need for integrated care. Medical Clinics of North America 90 (2006) 703–712.

Institute of Medicine. (2002). Confronting racial and ethnic disparities in health care. *National Academy of Sciences.* Retrieved April 29, 2013, from http://www.iom.edu/Reports/2002/Unequal-Treatment-Confronting-Racial-and-Ethnic-Disparities-in-Health-Care.aspx

Katerndahl, D. A., Wood, R., & Jaen, C. R. (2010). A method for estimating relative complexity of ambulatory care. *Annals of Family Medicine, 8*, 341–347.

Kathol, R., Perez, R., Cohen, J., & Huyse, F. (2010). *The integrated case management manual: Assisting complex patients regain physical and mental health*. New York: Springer.

Kirsch, I. (2010). *The emperor's new drugs: Exploding the antidepressant myth*. New York: Basic Books.

Kottke, T. E., & Pronk, N. P. (2009). Taking on the social determinants of health: A framework for action. *Minnesota Medicine, 92*, 36–39.

Kupersmith, J. (2007). Managing patient and system complexities to improve the quality and outcomes of chronic care: papers from VA's state-of-the-art conference: Managing complexity in chronic care. *Journal of General Internal Medicine, 22*, 373–444.

Lane, C. (2007). *How normal behavior became a sickness*. Binghamton, NY: Vail-Ballou Press.

Lebensohn-Chialvo, P., Crago, M., & Shisslak, C. M. (2000). The reflecting team: An innovative approach for teaching clinical skills to family practice residents. *Family Medicine, 32*, 556–560.

Lyons, J. S. (2006). *Communimetrics: A communication theory of measurement in human service settings*. New York: Springer.

Martin, C. M., & Sturmberg, J. P. (2009). Perturbing ongoing conversations about systems and complexity in health services and systems. *Journal of Evaluation in Clinical Practice, 15*, 549–552.

Maxwell, M., Hibberd, C., Pratt, R., Cameron, I., & Mercer, S. (2011). Development and initial validation of the Minnesota Edinburgh complexity assessment method (MECAM) for use within the Keep Well Health Check. 2011, Healthier Scotland: Edinburgh.

McDonald, K. M., Schultz, E., Pineda, N., Lonhart, J., Chapman, T., & Davies, S. (2012). *Care coordination accountability measures for primary care practice* Prepared by Stanford University under subcontract to Battelle on Contract No. 290-04-0020 (AHRQ Publication No. 12-0019-EF). Agency for Healthcare Research and Quality. Retrieved April 29, 2013, from http://www.ahrq.gov/research/findings/final-reports/pcpaccountability/index.html

National Committee for Quality Assurance. (2011). *2011 PCMH standards and guidelines*. National Committee for Quality Assurance. Retrieved April 29, 2013, from http://www.iafp.com/pcmh/ncqa2011.pdf

Peek, C. J. (2009). Integrating care for persons, not only diseases. *Journal of Clinical Psychology in Medical Settings, 16*, 13–20.

Peek, C. J. (2010). Building a medical home around the patient: What it means for behavior. *Families, Systems & Health, 28*, 322–333.

Peek, C. J., Baird, M. A., & Coleman, E. (2009). Primary care for patient complexity, not only disease. *Families, Systems & Health, 27*, 287–302.

Peek, C. J., & Oftedahl, G. (2010). *A consensus operational definition of Patient-Centered Medical Home (PCMH) also known as health care home*. Minneapolis, MN: University of Minnesota and Institute for Clinical Systems Improvement.

Peek, C. J., & Van Riper, K. (2011). *Level of care coordination needed*. Unpublished instructional draft, Department of Family Medicine and Community Health, University of Minnesota Medical School, Minneapolis, MN.

Pigott, H. E., Leventhal, H. M., Alter, G. S., & Boren, J. J. (2010). Efficacy and effectiveness of antidepressants: Current status of research. *Psychotherapy and Psychosomatics, 79*, 267–279.

Pronk, N. P., Peek, C. J., & Goldstein, M. G. (2004). Addressing multiple behavioral risk factors in primary care. A synthesis of current knowledge and stakeholder dialogue sessions. *American Journal of Preventive Medicine, 27*, 4–17.

Rasmussen, N. H., Furst, J. W., Swenson-Davis, D. M., Agerter, D. C., Smith, A. J., Baird, M. A., et al. (2006). Innovative reflecting interview: Effect on high-utilizing patients with medically unexplained symptoms. *Disease Management, 9*, 349–359.

Safford, M. M., Allison, J. J., & Kiefe, C. I. (2007). Patient complexity: More than comorbidity. The vector model of complexity. *Journal of General Internal Medicine, 22*(Suppl 3), 382–390.

Salazar-Fraile, J., Sempere-Verdu, E., Mossakowski, K., & Bryan, J. (2010). "Doctor, I just can't go on." Cultural constructions of depression and the prescription of antidepressants to users who are not clinically depressed. *International Journal of Mental Health, 39,* 29–67.

Sargut, G., & McGrath, R. G. (2011). Learning to live with complexity. *Harvard Business Review, 89*(68–76), 136.

Starfield, B., Weiner, J., Mumford, L., & Steinwachs, D. (1991). Ambulatory care groups: A categorization of diagnoses for research and management. *Health Services Research, 26,* 53–74.

Stiefel, F. C., Huyse, F. J., Sollner, W., Slaets, J. P. J., Lyons, J. S., Latour, C. H. M., et al. (2006). Operationalizing integrated care on a clinical level: The INTERMED project. *Medical Clinics of North America, 90,* 713–758.

Trangle, M., Dieperink, B., Gabert, T., Haight, B., Lindvall, B., Mitchell, J. et al. (2012). Institute for Clinical Systems Improvement. Major depression in adults in primary care. http://bit.ly/Depr0512. Updated May 2012.

Waters, E. (2010a). *Crazy like us: The globalization of the American psyche.* New York: Free Press.

Waters, E. (2010b). The Americanization of mental illness. *The New York Times.* Retrieved April 29, 2013, from http://www.nytimes.com/2010/01/10/magazine/10psyche-t.html?_r=1&pagewanted=all

Weiner, J. P., Starfield, B. H., Steinwachs, D. M., & Mumford, L. M. (1991). Development and application of a population-oriented measure of ambulatory care case-mix. *Medical Care, 29,* 452–472.

Weiss, K. B. (2007). Managing complexity in chronic care: An overview of the VA state-of-the-art (SOTA) conference. *Journal of General Internal Medicine, 22*(Suppl 3), 374–378.

Weydt, A. P. (2009). Defining, analyzing, and quantifying work complexity. *Creative Nursing, 15,* 7–13.

Zimmerman, B., Lindberg, C., & Plsek, P. (2008). *Edgeware: Lessons from complexity science for health care leaders.* Irving, TX: Plexus Institute.

Zwarenstein, M., Treweek, S., Gagnier, J. J., Altman, D. G., Tunis, S., Haynes, B. et al. (2008). Improving the reporting of pragmatic trials: An extension of the CONSORT statement. British Medical Journal, 337, a2390. doi: 10.1136/bmj.a2390.

Part IV
Connecting Concepts, Research and Practice

Chapter 15
Integrated Behavioral Health in Primary Care: Summarizing the Lay of the Land, Marking the Best Practices, Identifying Barriers, and Mapping New Territory

Mary R. Talen, Aimee Burke Valeras, and Larry A. Cesare

Abstract This concluding chapter pulls together the evidence and essential elements on the macro, meso, and micro levels of integrated behavioral health care. The research base for what is known and what is unknown in integrated behavioral health care practices has been thoroughly assessed; the process of which has helped identify common key ingredients for integration, based on the organizing template and lexicon of integrated behavioral health care. Even with strong vision and mission for integrated behavioral health, even with evidence-based clinical protocols for population-based care, even with sustainable funding mechanisms and quality improvement measures—the obstacles and barriers are formidable. This chapter outlines these challenges and unintended consequences of team-based care. Through surveying the landscape of integrated behavioral health care, we delineate the opportunities for advancing the field, highlighting anchor points for behavioral health practices and a variety of methods for placing behavioral health into the mix of primary care. Future directions and recommendations for research initiatives, clinical practices, team-based care, and advocacy in policy are discussed for future opportunities for growth, cultural shift, and potential for transforming health care.

M.R. Talen, Ph.D. (✉)
Northwestern Family Medicine Residency, Erie Family Health Center,
2570 W. North Ave. Chicago, IL 60647, USA
e-mail: mary.talen@gmail.com

A.B. Valeras, Ph.D., MSW
NH Dartmouth Family Medicine Residency, Concord Hospital Family Health Center,
250 Pleasant St., 03301, Concord, NH, USA
e-mail: aimeevaleras@gmail.com

L.A. Cesare, Psy.D.
Human Capital Specialists of San Diego,
877 Greensview Drive, Wooster, OH 44691, USA
e-mail: lacesare@ymail.com

M.R. Talen and A. Burke Valeras (eds.), *Integrated Behavioral Health in Primary Care:* *Evaluating the Evidence, Identifying the Essentials*, DOI 10.1007/978-1-4614-6889-9_15, © Springer Science+Business Media New York 2013

Organizing the State of Integrated Behavioral Health Care

The purpose of this book has been to help organize our descriptions of integrated behavioral health care, compare a host of initiatives using a common filter, and propel the field of integrated behavioral health care toward a coordinated future. The field has been inundated with a cacophony of initiatives that makes it difficult to decipher the essential message and key components of behavioral health in primary care. These chapters have helped us review the landscape of integrated behavioral health using a common template and terms to describe and evaluate an array of integrated behavioral health perspectives.

Part I: Essentials of Integrated Behavioral Health

Our guiding conceptual principles for these chapters have been anchored in the newly developed lexicon for integrated behavioral health care (Peek, 2011). In Chap. 2 (*Integrated Behavioral Health and Primary Care: A Common Language*), Dr. Peek (2011) provides a community-building lexicon as a promising foundation to bring robust organizing principles to integrated behavioral health care research and clinical practices. This conceptual model has grown out of discussions with the community of stakeholders. We are at a crossroads where the larger integrated behavioral health community needs to adopt, utilize, and maintain this language to engage in effective dialogues and comparative studies. The lexicon can become our "go to" reference to help administrators, policy makers, researchers, and clinicians communicate among each other about what integrated behavioral health means. This lexicon provides operational definitions of integrated care: **how** it functions with teams; **what** it entails for patients and providers; and the ways that behavioral health care is **supported by** in systems of care. This chapter outlines the parameters for describing what constitutes integrated care, how it functions within teams, identified populations, clinical protocols, and how it is supported by sites, financial-practice management, and quality improvement. The authors of the subsequent chapters used these principles to evaluate and compare a range of integrated behavioral health approaches. These processes helped us corral our different voices and begin to bring some movement and harmony between initiatives on the macro, meso, and micro levels of integrated behavioral health care.

The Patient-Centered Medical Home (PCMH) and Accountable Care Organizations (ACO) are the macro levels of health care that have a global vision of offering whole person-centered care, providing ample opportunity for integrated behavioral health care to become embedded. In Chap. 3 (*Integrated Behavioral Health and the Patient-Centered Medical Home*), Drs. Auxier, Miller, and Rogers delineated the potential for behavioral health in PCMH, as well as the risk of continued marginalization of behavioral health that are evident in the details of the design. Although NCQA added the integration of behaviors affecting health, mental health, and substance abuse to its 2011 standards, none of the "must-pass" elements for PCMH certification requires behavioral health. Behavioral health is addressed in six of the non-must-pass elements for PCMH certification (out of 152 factors listed to gain certification) and continues to have a minority voice in the larger health care redesign dialogue. While a health care center can be certified as a PCMH using behavioral health elements such as screening and treatment for depression or substance abuse, these elements are not required to get certified. The adoption of PCMH offers unique opportunities for behavioral health but adopting this vision for behavioral health needs strong advocates and empirical support to gain a stronger foothold.

The health care reform initiatives through the Patient Affordable Care Act provide an impetus to place primary care that focuses on the whole person at the front and center of community health care-related conversations. Drs. Miller, Talen, and Patel, in Chap. 4 (*Advancing Integrated Behavioral Health and Primary Care: The Critical Importance of Behavioral Health in Health Care Policy*), describe how the ACA and PCMH fit into our current political climate and provide a unique opportunity to integrate behavioral health in a more coordinated and comprehensive way. While there are several ways to measure the PCMH, they all remain consistent in their recognition that a more tightly coordinated primary care system, including mental health, is needed. These initiatives have all of the elements to make the cultural shift to promoting and integrating biopsychosocial health care. However, behavioral health advocates and leaders have the responsibility to be at the national, state, and local levels table to reinforce, promote, and define this vision.

Part II: Meso Levels of Care

Chapters (2, 3, and 4) that address the macro level of current integrated behavioral health systems illustrate that we are still incubating and forming the structural anatomy of integrated behavioral health care. Drs. Kwan and Nease conclude in Chap. 5 (*The State of Evidence for Integrated Behavioral Health Care*) that, in general, meta-analyses show that integrated behavioral health care can lead to better health outcomes for certain patients. The majority of studies have focused on outcomes in patients with a mental health diagnosis and on integrated behavioral health care approaches that were based on variations of the chronic care model (Wagner, 2000). These studies have several common key elements: (1) standardized screening standards for identification of patients, (2) clinical care management services and consistent follow-up, (3) medical monitoring and medications, and (4) brief behavioral health treatment. Screening and treatment for depression and substance abuse have received the most consistent evaluation through RCT and are thus backed by the strongest empirical support.

Our current evidence-based foundation, however, is hindered by several limitations posed by narrow definitions of quality empirical research. Newer research initiatives are less amenable to classic randomized trial designs and rely upon less rigorous but more organic evaluation methods that allow for the exploration of a host of interrelated processes from teamwork to identifying the patients that are the "best fit" for a range of behavioral health strategies. As potentially more sustainable health care delivery systems evolve, contemporary, translational research approaches are needed to accommodate comprehensive and complex primary care questions about essential elements, effective interventions, and implementation strategies for behavioral health. In response, researchers in integrated behavioral health care are in the throes of redefining these research paradigms to make room for evaluative efforts that can expand to meet the complex and multilayered issues in integrated behavioral health care.

Kwan and Nease call for the community of researchers to go beyond the traditional randomized trial and implement creative, yet rigorous methods to fill these evidence gaps. Forthcoming pioneering researchers would benefit from using the integrated behavioral health care lexicon to help organize the foundational concepts and essential components that constitute an integrated behavioral health care model. Real-world and translational studies that build on broader and more robust behavioral health strategies in the context of primary care are only recently incubating and consequently the outcomes of these newer studies are limited. Innovative techniques such as mixed quantitative and qualitative methods, pragmatic trials, and other process-observational approaches have the potential to define more comprehensively what constitutes behavioral health care, translate key components of integrated behavioral health care within local health care centers, and determine the effectiveness of such approaches.

Drs. Mendenhall, Doherty, Burge, Fauth, and Tremblay offer one such novel example of how newer paradigms for integrated behavioral health care practices and research can come together in Community-Based Participatory Research (CBPR) in Chap. 6 (*Community-Based Participatory Research: Advancing Integrated Behavioral Health Care Through Novel Partnerships*). This approach focuses on partnering professionals with community members to create health initiatives that thrive on the interactions and synergy between group members. The core tenets and processes of CBPR include on-going relationship building between interested and invested professional and community members around a shared health concern.

A key piece of CBPR is the process of conducting qualitative interviews with key community stakeholders around the dimensions of the health issues, as developing an action plan sets the stage for trusted relationships for shared investigation processes and ownership of the initiative. Democratic planning and decision-making are core principles that help build shared leadership to propel communities toward improved health. This model selectively uses the resources of process-oriented researchers and quality improvement approaches to evaluate the impact of action plans on the health of the community. Projects are sustainable, too, by nature of being owned-and-operated by the communities, rather than relying on grant-driven initiatives.

Integrated behavioral health care providers who are interested in this approach to community-based research initiatives need a flexible temperament, an ability to be culturally responsive, hold the characteristics to exercise curious humility, and demonstrate the personal commitment to be full participants with community members over several years. Participants in CBPR believe in what they are doing and are energized by the collective energy they share to promote broad and meaningful change. Overall, this approach builds on strengths and resources within the community, promotes co-learning and capacity-building between partners, and focuses on the cyclical process in which problems are identified and solved. In this manner, solutions are developed within the context of the community's resources and interventions are modified based on responsive community feedback. CBPR projects deserve the full attention of integrated behavioral health care stakeholders, but this trail-blazing pathway is not for those with short attention spans, as it can be a slow and messy process that requires a long-term engagement, trusted working relationships, and a commitment to the work of the shared community vision.

Funding has been a nemesis for sustaining integrated behavioral health care initiatives. Drs. Hodgson and Reitz, in Chap. 8 (*The Financial History and Near Future of Integrated Behavioral Health Care*), describe how financial support for integrated behavioral health care has been subject to limited fixed resources and has fluctuated based on the ebb and flow of grant funding, the complexities of reimbursement within public and private sources, and inconsistent payment policies between local, state, and national levels. The vast majority of programs that integrate medical and behavioral health struggle with financial sustainability. Funding integrated behavioral health care as a reimbursable behavioral health fee-for-service in primary care has not been sustainable. The growth and development of mechanisms that support grass roots integration highlights the creativity and sheer will of communities, states, and health care systems that have implemented these services in primary care over time.

Dr. Chris Hunter describes the Department of Defense's unique perspective on the key elements for integrated care (Chap. 9, *Department of Defense Integrated Behavioral Health in the Patient-Centered Medical Home*). Even with their single-payer financial base, advancing integrated care is challenging. Developing and initiating an integrated behavioral health care service is a long developmental process. This chapter outlines the essential elements for weaving behavioral health into a single-payer, specified primary care service. These six elements are strong, sustained leadership, a evidence-based rationale for integrated behavioral health care, inclusion of stakeholders in the "game," using a common language, develop structured protocols and measures for quality control and improvement.

In contrast to the government fund DoD system, public, private, or public-private collaborative sector initiatives have many more faces. Because there is so much variety, these behavioral health initiatives in primary care require a shared vision and mission to hold the many pieces together. Many health centers are struggling to incubate a variety of approaches to support best practices in integrated behavioral health care. Integrated behavioral health care has been more commonly implemented in safety net settings, such as FQHCs and CHCs, as described by Drs. Mauch and Bartlett in Chap. 7 (*Integrated Behavioral Health in Public Health Care Contexts: Community Health and Mental Health Safety Net Systems*). These authors describe the historically divergent funding streams between medical and mental health for underserved patients, which has contributed to the great divide between these two unequal systems of care. The expansion of FQHCs has created a climate where these two worlds can merge. Reverse location—primary care services in CMHCs—has gained traction and holds promising opportunities for integrating behavioral health and primary care services. The Cherokee system in Tennessee has been the flagship enterprise for merging primary care into community mental health systems. Successful systems of integrated care have had tenacious leaders who have sustained the mission and vision from the clinical and policy levels over decades. In systems where they have sustained a level of integration, programs still face challenges in financial solvency, billing complexities, and obstacles in going beyond treating the patient with the mental health diagnosis. Medical residency programs have also been an incubator for innovative integrated behavioral health projects. But even in these settings, services are widely written off or sustained by time-limited grant funding or support for behavioral health faculty positions from graduate medical education funds. Integrated behavioral health care has made little penetration in health care systems with a substantive population of privately insured patients. Even when organizations, leaders, and providers have a shared vision of providing integrated care between medical and behavioral health, funding mechanisms hinder their sustainability.

From a financial perspective, integrated behavioral health care initiatives are primarily pilot projects funded by private foundations, while some are sustained through state or local funds, but few are mainstream service lines (e.g., Tennessee's Cherokee System). Local CHC and CMHC organizations seeking private foundation support have been the quintessential mechanism for getting started in integrated behavioral health care. Few pilot projects, however, have evolved into larger-scale integrated behavioral health care programs with financial support from NIMH, NIH, or CMS. In order for integrated behavioral health care to advance beyond grant-supported initiatives, pilot projects, or locally funded projects, a system-wide and sustainable source of revenue will need to be adopted. The financial ingredients for sustaining behavioral health services in primary care are promising, given the Affordable Care Act and PCMH initiatives, though there are many uncharted issues that need time, evaluation, and continued leadership for progress toward the integrated behavioral health care vision.

Part III: Micro Levels of Care

In the integrated behavioral health care approach, the doctor-patient relationship is emerging as a team-patient relationship. In Chap. 10 (*Collaborative Partnerships Within Integrated Behavioral Health and Primary Care*), Drs. Hern, Valeras, Banker, and Riebe describe some of the various ways that teams have formulated, depending on their setting and mission. The role of the primary care physician has been pushed, in recent years, into allowing or cajoling team members to help manage the vastness of the scope of primary care. This chapter confronts the reality that patients' health care needs and requests, at any given moment, have an impact on interactions not just with their physician, but also a number of other professionals. There are obvious members that have a clear place in the medical team, like nurses, medical assistants, physician assistants, registrars, office managers, and an array of medical specialists and health educators, like diabetic educators and nutritionists. A more novel member to this amorphous team is the behavioral health clinician. Team-based care has been proceeding without strong evidence that identifies the best, most effective ways to integrate behavioral health clinicians into the team. This is a virgin area where the role, responsibilities, and communication skills of behavioral health providers can be maximized and their indispensable skill set can be capitalized.

Even the most in-sync teams benefit from guidelines around how, when, and which patients should work with the multidisciplinary approach, and then how much of which type of intervention is necessary. Drs. Talen and Valeras, in Chap. 11 (*Identification of Behavioral Health Needs in Integrated Behavioral and Primary Care Settings*), describe the variety of ways that patients who might benefit from interacting with a behavioral health clinician are targeted in primary care. These patients can be identified for a range of concerns such as promoting or encouraging healthy habits or health behavior change, or to identifying areas of stress across the biopsychosocial spectrum of functioning, or shedding light on underlying mental health or substance use risk factors. The more systematic processes of screening groups of patients for behavioral health and mental health issues is reviewed by Drs. Talen, Baumer, and Mann in Chap. 12 (*Screening Measures in Integrated Behavioral Health and Primary Care Settings*). There is no shortage of validated and reliable screening tools, and selecting tools is the least complicated part of population-based approach to screening. However, the systematic processes for implementing screening are complex and require a concerted team approach. Using the lexicon and parameters, these two chapters highlight the differences between targeted and non-targeted patient screening techniques and emphasize that the process for screening is dependent more on the health care team's intentions and consistent protocols rather than finding the "right" standardized tools for screening a range of behavioral health concerns for a specific group of patients (e.g., children, men, women, or seniors).

The vast majority of screening is focused on mental health disorders such as depression, anxiety, or substance abuse. Indeed, initiatives that systematically screen patients in primary care for a mental health concern has provided an important foundation for building evidence to identify and treat mental health in primary care. There are, however, several cautionary notes to this practice. First, screening has often been confused with diagnosis, instead of prompting follow-up assessment and treatment with behavioral health providers. Second, screening for mental health, rather than more generous concepts of behavioral health, is limiting. Rarely are quality of life, self-efficacy, or patient engagement status—factors that influence health risks and status—the focus of behavioral health identification or screening. The next generation of health care teams could benefit from expanding their concepts of screening from traditional mental health concerns to more encompassing life style behaviors that impact health outcomes.

Drs. Mullin and Funderburk, in Chap. 13 (*Implementing Clinical Interventions in Integrated Behavioral Health Settings: Best Practices and Essential Elements*) delve into the specific clinical interventions that may transpire after patients are identified as having the potential to benefit from interacting with a behavioral health clinician. This chapter also touches upon the importance of fit in choosing a behavioral health clinician based on a variety of professional training and clinical competence. Behavioral health professionals must find ways to appreciate the biomedical aspects of clinical presentations in their case formulations and to become better prepared to function effectively in the world of primary care by (a) being immediately available for "warm handoff" referrals, (b) conducting rapid, targeted assessments, (c) developing expertise in brief, solution-focused, and evidence-based interventions, (d) delivering succinct, practical consultative information and recommendations, and (e) developing the capacity for initiating and following-up with linkages to external services when necessary. Currently, there is evidence on clinical guidelines that support the treatment of mental health conditions, specifically, depression and substance abuse in primary care using a team of PCP and CCM. BH is usually reserved for those patients who would benefit from intensive individual brief treatments such as CBT or PST. However, the clinical protocols for behavioral health interventions for patients with chronic diseases (e.g., diabetes, hypertension) or other health conditions (e.g., sleep, obesity, headaches), otherwise known as "whoever steps through door," are not well defined or researched and needs our attention. And, the quality improvement strategies to evaluate the strengths and limitations of these integrated behavioral health approaches are rarely built into our systematic review processes from the patient, provider, and health care system levels.

Moving a level beyond screening and intervention, Drs. Macaran, Peek, Gunn, and Valeras describe in Chap. 14 (*Working with Complexity in Integrated Behavioral Health Settings*) the presence of complexity in primary care. A complex pattern can develop when psychosocial factors, fragmentation within the health care system, and diverse medical symptoms combine to result in patient-provider interactions that have the potential to drain and exhaust an entire system. The authors recognize, however, that a patient does not possess complexity alone; complexity does not exist in a vacuum, but rather within a relationship. The ideas, beliefs, experiences, ideologies, personality, fears, emotions, and approach of each member of the health care team can clash with the presentation of the patient in such a way that both parties feel unheard, unvalidated, and discouraged. This chapter offers a progressive tool—the MCAM—to assess patient complexity, but also offers a teaching tool—the Complex Continuity Clinic—that provides the space and support for providers and entire teams to voice their own role in a dysfunctional relationship and to brainstorm ways to experiment with approaches that are less comfortable or traditional to repair the healing relationship.

The concept of complexity is presented at the micro-level in Chap. 14—how to assess it and work with it in patient-team interactions. Applying this concept of working with complexity—finding innovative solutions to multifaceted problems—to a macro-level approach may be a parallel process for how to integrate behavioral health into primary care. Complexity care initiatives may need to move from individual-case-based approaches to more systematic assessment and structured protocols to address the diverse needs of patients.

Barriers and Unintended Consequences

Given the economic downturn, states' budget deficits, and the astronomical cost of health care in the USA, constituents across all political lines agree on the necessity to eliminate waste in health care and reduce cost of health care, while maintaining and enhancing the quality of health care provision. Recognizing and embracing the overlap between psychological health, social determinants of health, and physical health is an obvious step in conceptualizing a economically feasible and coordinated quality model of health care. If the health care system is to adapt to embrace a integrated behavioral health care model, the systemic mental models upholding our current health care industry must be confronted head-on.

The conflicting agendas of the multiple entities that make up the health care world (public and private insurance companies, government agencies, policy makers, hospitals and clinics, medical and nonmedical providers, and patients) serve to uphold an entrenched system. This system is embedded in the medical model and the scientific method, the frameworks under which Western medicine has primarily progressed, which has resulted in pharmaceutical discoveries, diagnostic clarification and treatment, increased life expectancy, and decreased maternal and infant mortality, among other advancements. It has also simultaneously generated a generation that is living with chronic disease, rather than dying from it. The focus on identifying and treating disease has resulted in massive tertiary care centers, state of the art emergency departments, and a subspecialty approach to disease management.

The present vehement dialogue about health care reform is the evidence of the public acknowledgement of the need to visualize a system that allows for embracing the successes of the medical model, but for visualizing a new way to deliver care. Primary care has emerged as such a solution. To successfully meet this challenge, the primary care field itself must be able to navigate the gray areas between the dualities imposed by our overarching dependence on the medical model—health and illness, patient and provider, mental health and physical health, standardized care and individualized care, quantitative measurement and qualitative understanding. The various examples of integrated behavioral health care projects presented throughout this book include creative and well-intentioned attempts to work around, through, over, and under a system ingrained in these dualities, highlighting some of the barriers to, and unintended consequences of, integrating behavioral health and primary care.

Integrated Behavioral Health Care Teams

The infancy stage of formal evaluation around team-based care, team structure, and location leaves many questions. The optimal composition of a primary care team, the proximal location of providers, the role of case management and the professional credentials, and the attributes and core competencies that make for an effective team remain ambiguous. Time demands and space configurations can have an impact on team-based care, but the barriers that impede formation of effective partnerships between medical and behavioral providers extend beyond whether they are housed in separate offices, in primary care, or mental health settings. They are rooted deeply in cultural differences in professional identity and in resulting power and control issues between medical and behavioral health providers.

Hindrances to team-based care begin with traditional training curricula. Medical and behavioral health professionals are exposed to curricula and role models that expose them to different bodies of health research and knowledge, promote disparate ways of conceptualizing health, diagnostic reasoning, and intervention methods, steep them in assumptions, language, and values specific to their professions and, in most cases, perpetuate a bias toward viewing health issues primarily from a biomedical or a psychosocial perspective. Medical and behavioral professions and their respective training programs have done little to bridge the chasm or cross-train their ranks to be more facile with a holistic view of the human condition. Thus, it comes as no surprise that many who work in a integrated behavioral health care team environment describe the experience of disconnectedness between the two fields.

Behavioral health professionals are often quick to project blame on medical personnel, accusing them of being too insensitive or failing to take the time necessary to address and respond to the personal, interpersonal, occupational, or life stress issues that impact their patients' medical presentation. Medical professionals are often not shy about portraying behavioral health providers as inefficient because of their emphasis on "soft" psychosocial issues, their tendency to process clinical information to the point of losing sight of producing observable results, and their resistance to regular, prompt, direct communication with medical providers on shared cases, often citing special ethically based confidentiality constraints. Narrowing such cultural and communication gaps in order to permit formation of effective integrated care teams that can grapple with power, control, and conflict issues takes time; time which currently detracts from billable services.

Identifying Patient Populations

Integrated behavioral health care is often considered applicable only when major psychiatric disorders and/or substance use disorders are present. These inconsistent and often narrow definitions of the term "behavioral" fail to appreciate the role that unhealthy lifestyles and behaviors, normal life stress reactions, and noncompliance with medical directives play in affecting clinical outcomes. To reduce the focus of integrated behavioral health care to only patients with a DSM diagnosis could negate appreciation of the potentially far-reaching benefits of psychosocial interventions for much larger populations of medical patients whose clinical presentations, treatment response, and recovery potential may be largely determined by lifestyle, life stress, and less severe psychosocial issues.

Research clearly suggests that persons with severe, persistent psychiatric disorders are in dire need of primary care services (e.g., integrating primary care into mental health centers). Nevertheless, it is possible that the potential for cost-effectiveness is far greater among more expansive and diverse medical patient populations with far more common yet underrecognized and unaddressed contributory psychosocial issues.

Specifying Clinical Interventions: Inconsistent Definitions of "Behavioral Treatment"

Such narrow operational definitions of "behavioral treatment" are often based heavily upon pharmacologic interventions, as though they, in and of themselves, can be adequate for depression and anxiety in particular. This depiction frequently fails to appreciate, if not disregard, the appropriateness and cost-effectiveness of the full range of nonpharmacologic, evidence-based behavioral interventions. Psychotropic interventions are certainly recognized as a centerpiece in the treatment of psychiatric disorders, such as schizophrenia and bipolar disorder, and play important ancillary roles in the treatment of many forms of depression and, increasingly, addiction disorders. Their applicability in the treatment of anxiety, personality or transitional stress disorders is not always evident and may be outweighed by risks. Most behavioral health professionals and growing numbers of medical professionals also recognize that targeted, focused psychosocial interventions, like certain cognitive behavioral techniques, motivational interviewing, and dialectal behavioral therapy, can be instrumental in not only promoting greater emotional, interpersonal, and occupational well being, but in eliciting healthy behavioral change, in promoting patient engagement, and in improving patient treatment adherence. Unfortunately, research that evaluates the comparative benefits of different combinations of pharmacologic and psychosocial interventions for specific types of clinical presentations by diversely presenting patients in primary care settings is lacking.

Operational Sustainability: Information Sharing and Reimbursement Obstacles

Success of an integrated behavioral health care program depends squarely upon the ability of team members to effectively communicate not only with patients, but among themselves and with relevant external entities integrally involved in patients' care. Such communication is gradually becoming reliant upon sophisticated information technology, like electronic health records (EHRs). Such systems are designed to not only store and share clinical information among involved internal and external providers, but to also perform a wide range of critical support functions (e.g., scheduling, billing, finance management), demonstrate compliance with regulatory requirements, drive continuous quality improvement and, increasingly, provide new ways to promote patient health education and engagement in their own care. CMS and other regulatory and third-party payors for provider organizations have delineated clear expectations for providers to adopt multifunctional information technology systems. Still, many providers resist purchasing and implementing new information technology systems due to the potentially daunting financial investment, the unavoidable modifications to established workflows, and the necessary staff training.

Because payment drives practice, the implementation of integrated behavioral health care models continues to be impeded by fee-for-service reimbursement models that (a) involve separate payors, preauthorization requirements, billing and coding procedures, and reimbursement levels for behavioral and medical services and (b) do not routinely cover consultative and care management functions, hence, providing little incentive for integration. In effect, the behavioral services component of an integrated program are, under traditional reimbursement methodologies, not billed or paid for as medical service components, rendering this service difficult to justify. Moreover, rules vary from state to state in terms of reimbursement eligibility of more than one Medicaid service on the same day (which is common practice in an integrated setting) and in terms of whether Medicaid accepts CMS' HBA billing codes either fully, partially or at all. The net effect of obstacles regarding behavioral services reimbursement is the limited fiscal feasibility of their inclusion into integrated practice. Some integrated programs such as DIAMOND have found some relief from such impediments by negotiating with payors for bundled reimbursement of medical and behavioral services into a single payment, which not only simplifies billing, but allows coverage for the costs of case management and consulting activities not covered under typical reimbursement systems. Within the context of developing ACOs to share the risk for the costs of meeting all the health needs of certain identified populations, support is growing for the concept of bundled payment to cover all services, including primary behavioral care.

Lack of Consistent Measures of Quality, Outcomes, and Value

Long gone are the days when providers could garner support for their services without also offering some type of quantitative evidence of the quality of service or tangible benefit of such expenditures (as in, "Trust us, we're professionals."). Health Care payors, regulators, and increasingly, consumers have grown more sophisticated in their expectations for reliable measures of quality, satisfaction, and effectiveness. Purchasers in particular are increasingly looking for more than process measures of "quality" or satisfaction survey data and are demanding evidence of demonstrable outcomes to evaluate the value of services and justify their health care expenditures. Health Care, and especially behavioral health care, has yet to arrive at a consensual definition of outcomes that are, at once (a) subject to ready, reliable calculation, (b) relevant and meaningful to provider, payer, regulatory, and consumer constituencies, (c) permit reliable comparisons between different providers over time, and (d), perhaps most importantly, can be used to calculate "value" (defined as a product of "cost" vs. "result"). Until data are available to conclusively demonstrate the clinical benefit and cost offset of the integrated behavioral health care model in terms that translate to a "value story," it will remain difficult to make a compelling argument for why it should become industry standard.

Conclusion: Hope for the Future of Integrated Behavioral Health

As the fiscal unsustainability of the current US health care system reaches critical proportions and as calls for health care reform reach unprecedented levels, never before has there been such opportunity for the field of behavioral health to play a key role in reshaping the industry landscape to meet the triple aim of improved individual care, improved population health, and reduced costs. It is truly an exciting era. While there will always be a need for specialized behavioral care systems to meet the needs of those with serious mental illness and addictions and those whose concerns are solely psychosocial in nature, it is time for the behavioral health field to not only advocate for change within the system, but to redefine itself as a central player in health care as a whole, rather than a distinct and separate subspecialty.

A vanguard crusade in this movement to create space for an adapted integrated behavioral health model of care is focused on developing a common lexicon. Through shared dialogue both among advocates of integrated behavioral health care and with external professional, regulatory, funding, and consumer constituencies, it is imperative to (a) consensually define a well-articulated "big picture" of what the ideal integrated behavioral health care system would look like, (b) agree upon what desirable results it will produce, (c) develop a common appreciation of the obstacles in our way and an organized, systematic approach for overcoming them, (d) make compelling business case for integrated behavioral health care (e.g., the "value story"), and (e) get these messages delivered effectively to the right audiences and in a manner that it easily understood by and personally relevant and meaningful to the majority of the US populace.

As we surveyed the landscape of integrated behavioral health care, we have been able to identify the barriers and the opportunities for advancing the field. We have also been able to see parameters and anchor points for behavioral health practices and describe some of these developmental processes and types of approaches for placing behavioral health into the mix of primary care. Table 15.1 depicts these key areas of obstacles and opportunities but more importantly describes the continuum of clinical practices that fall within the lexicon parameters. For example, organizing an integrated team where behavioral health has a role faces obstacles from culturally protective attitudes and disciplines-specific clinical practice silos; however, team-based care offers opportunities for more open communication about patient care and shared responsibilities. Team care also falls on a continuum from parallel practices between mental and medical providers to shared care plans for patients and opening addressing power differentials and control issues between members. Another example of the continuum of integrated care is evident in how teams

Table 15.1 Opportunities and obstacles in the continuum of integrated behavioral health care

Parameters	Barriers	Opportunities	Continuum and anchors
HOW: **Team-based care**	Boundaries Practicing discipline-specific silos Power differentials—status, salaries, practicing at the highest level of training Comfort with confronting differences Passivity Tied to professional identify Lack of integrated behavioral health team care training for all members	Clear roles and responsibilities Accountability Protected team planning time—huddles, weekly/monthly meetings Shared structures (e.g., shared care plans) Patient/family as team members New vehicles for communication—learning lunches, huddles.	Building a culture of shared decision-making, respect, and open communication, addressing issues of power and control
Referral/consultation model Silo practice Separate systems of Control/power	versus		Team-based decision-making
Population	Screening is narrowly defined (e.g., MH diagnoses) No systematic process for screening or identification	Disease registries Systematic screening or identification Stratify complexity level of patient care	Unique patient-specific identification versus population-based screening Screening for mental health and/or behavioral health factors
Clinical	Standard mental health services in primary care setting Traditional clinical time increments Limited training for all providers	Morphing/emerging of mental health and behavioral health interventions Variable clinical time Self-management coaching	Standard, evidence-based, mental health treatment versus behavioral health in routine primary care visits Chronic disease management pathways versus unique, patient-centered needs for BH/MH
SUPPORTED BY: Management: financial and processes	Diverse policies—local, state, and federal Confidentiality protections Separate records or barriers between records. Variable billing practices Many pilot studies, few project/mainstream	Same day billing for MH and PC Shared care plans Shared EHR Health and behavioral codes	Grant-funded, time-limited initiatives versus sustainable funding from federal, state, and local sources Fee-for-service versus population comprehensive care plans

identify a behavioral health patient(s). Provider's process for identifying behavioral health needs may range from ad hoc, patient-specific situations—whoever comes through the door, to systematic screening of all patients—an age group, or patients with a diagnosis. We encourage administrators, providers, and other stakeholders to use this chart to help describe their current level of integration based on the lexicon parameters. This can be one way to unify our language, expand the culture of integrated care, and layout a road map for the group to plot their journey ahead.

If we are to shake off the shackles of the status quo and take health care to a high level of quality, we undoubtedly need to overcome a multitude of far-reaching and well-entrenched system-level barriers. On-going conversation and collaboration among those who are committed to advancing integration of primary medical and behavioral care is a critical element to any successful patient-centered medical home model, ACO-type organization, or overarching health reform plan. Behavioral health advocates need to become actively involved with the professional, advocacy, and legislative entities at the local, state, and national level that are engaged in collective efforts to promote change toward integrated behavioral health care. Examples of these advocacy groups include:

(a) The National Council for Community Behavioral Healthcare's Center for Integrated Health Solutions (http://www.thenationalcouncil.org)
(b) The Patient-Centered Primary Care Collaborative (http://www.pcpcc.net), which also has an active Behavioral Health Task Force (http://www.pcpcc.net/behavioral-health),
(c) The Collaborative Family Healthcare Association (http://www.cfha.net).

Integrated behavioral health care pioneers cannot afford another four decades of narrowly focused research on the establishment of only small numbers of short-lived programs that show minimal impact on health care policy and funding. Despite Thomas Edison's wisdom, "I have not failed. I've just found 10,000 ways that won't work," the additional time and resources required by such a hit-or-miss approach is no longer an option if the integrated behavioral health care model is indeed aiming to fulfill a central role in aiding the overall health care system to achieve its triple aim. Rushing to impose trial-and-error "fixes" at the operational level will result in pouring more money, time, and energy into efforts of limited effectiveness and/or generalizability. Such efforts often result in frustration for the providers due to the lack of ability to measure success in a meaningful way, lack of applicability beyond the localized setting, and lack of fiscal health and sustainability.

Regardless of American political party agendas, health care reform has become a new reality even in the midst of political changes. The goal is for fully integrated behavioral health care and its biopsychosocial underpinnings to become the norm rather than the exception in how health care is delivered and gets paid for. To achieve this, new advocacy strategies are needed and champion leaders need to be supported. We hope that this book adds to the framework and foundation for defining and positioning behavioral health clinicians, administrators, consultants, and thought leaders, and innovative ways to present the case for integrated behavioral health care to the right audiences.

Reference

Peek, C. J. (2011). A collaborative care lexicon for asking practice and research development questions. One of three papers in: a national agenda for research in collaborative care: papers from the collaborative care research network research development conference. Agency for Healthcare Research and Quality, Rockville MD. http://www.ahrq.gov/research/collaborativecare/.

Index

27843486R00212

Made in the USA
Middletown, DE
22 December 2015